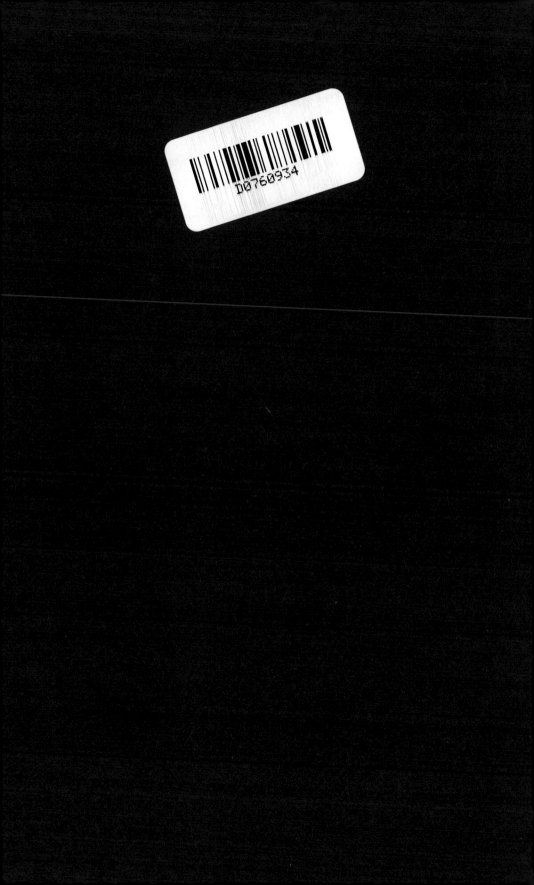

Moonlight, Magnolias, & Madness

INSANITY IN SOUTH CAROLINA

Moonlight,

FROM THE COLONIAL PERIOD

Magnolias, &

TO THE PROGRESSIVE ERA

Madness

PETER MCCANDLESS

THE UNIVERSITY OF NORTH CAROLINA PRESS

Chapel Hill & London

© 1996

The University of North Carolina Press

All rights reserved

Manufactured in the United States of America

The paper in this book meets the guidelines for permanence and durability of the committee

on Production Guidelines for Book Longevity of the Council on Library Resources.

Library of Congress Cataloging-in-Publication Data

McCandless, Peter.

Moonlight, magnolias, and madness: insanity in South Carolina from the colonial period

to the progressive era / Peter McCandless.

p.   cm.

Includes bibliographical references and index.

ISBN 0-8078-2251-5 (cloth: alk. paper). — ISBN 0-8078-4558-2 (pbk.: alk. paper)

1. Mentally ill—South Carolina—History.   2. Social psychiatry—South Carolina—History.

3. South Carolina Lunatic Asylum—History.   4. South Carolina State Hospital for Insane—

History.   5. South Carolina State Hospital—History.   I. Title.

RC445.S58M33   1996

362.2'09757—dc20   95-16641

CIP

00   99   98   97   96   5   4   3   2   1

In memory of my mother

and

in honor of my father

South Carolina is too small

to be a republic,

and too big to be

a lunatic asylum.

attributed to James Louis Petigru, 1860

Contents

Illustrations & Tables

Preface

I owe this book to my wife Amy. It was her decision to enter the M.B.A. program at the University of South Carolina that prompted me to begin research on the topic. We moved to Columbia in the summer of 1981 so she could take the foundation courses for the degree. Once the decision was made, I began casting about for a research project to keep me busy. I had written a dissertation on insanity in nineteenth-century England and was curious about the history of the insane in South Carolina. I knew that little had been written about it, and I soon discovered that enough sources existed to justify a monograph. Most important, I learned that the early records of the South Carolina Lunatic Asylum, the nation's third-oldest state mental hospital, had survived virtually intact. They revealed an institution that was far closer to contemporary northern asylums in inspiration, aims, methods, and clientele than previous historians had indicated.

The existence of these records, along with a wealth of state and local government records, private papers, journals, and newspapers, encouraged me to attempt a state history of the experience of insanity, both within and beyond the asylum walls. It is a history at times inspiring but more often depressing. This is not only because the great hopes of the state's asylum reformers were not realized—that happened everywhere—but also because a combination of severe economic decline, political turmoil, and racial oppression ensured that South Carolina's insane often fared much worse than those in other states. Institutionally speaking, their condition was probably worst around the turn of the present century, when conditions in the state hospital became truly scandalous. At first I had intended to carry the story down to the present. But as my research developed, I decided that the Progressive Era, during which various investigations and reforms brought South Carolina's mental-health policies back into line with those in most of the nation, made a logical ending point.

Some readers may wonder why the book usually identifies patients at the South Carolina State Hospital by name until the 1880s but rarely thereafter. The reason is that the hospital's records are restricted for one hundred years. Special permission is required from the South Carolina Department of Mental Health to access these more recent records, and it is unlawful to identify patients mentioned in them by name. Therefore, I have used initials or commitment numbers to identify state hospital patients after about 1885, unless the information about them was taken from unrestricted sources.

It is a truism that every book has many authors, and this one is no exception. At the outset of my research I was fortunate to receive the first of several summer fellowships at the Institute for Southern Studies at the University of South Carolina. The institute's director, Walter Edgar, and assistant director, Nancy Ashmore Cooper, provided invaluable assistance and direction. Woodrow Harris, Director of Education at the South Carolina State Hospital, told me more about the relevant sources in a day than I could have discovered on my own in weeks. Another hospital employee, the late Inez Nolan Fripp, introduced me to the riches of the institution's manuscript records and regaled me with fascinating stories about its history.

After my first summer of research, the hospital's manuscript records were moved to the South Carolina Department of Archives and History a few blocks away. I have spent untold hours working there and at the nearby South Caroliniana Library. The staffs of both institutions deserve accolades for their kind and patient assistance. I owe numerous debts as well to the staffs of the following libraries and archives: the Waring Historical Library at the Medical University of South Carolina, the South Carolina Historical Society, the Library Society, the City of Charleston Archives, the College of Charleston Library, the Southern Historical Collection at the Wilson Library of the University of North Carolina at Chapel Hill, the Manuscript Department at the Perkins Library at Duke University, and the Pennsylvania Hospital Archives in Philadelphia. Special gratitude is due to Allen Stokes, director of the Caroliniana; to Anne Donato and Elizabeth Newsom of the Waring; to David Moltke-Hansen, director of the Southern Historical Collection and former director of the South Carolina Historical Society; to Susan King of the Charleston City Archives; and to Oliver Smalls of the College of Charleston's Special Collections.

Several grants and fellowships enabled me to undertake the research for this book. Much of the research and initial writing was done with the aid of a year-long fellowship from the National Endowment for the Humanities (Fellowship no. FB-23394-85). The College of Charleston Research and Development Committee provided me with several summer grants. I have already noted the assistance of summer fellowships at the Institute for Southern Studies.

The manuscript has profited from conversations and exchanges with several scholars. Gerald Grob, Ellen Dwyer, and Todd Savitt offered useful suggestions, encouragement, and advice at an early stage in my research. Sam Thielman shared with me his knowledge about therapeutics at the South Carolina Lunatic Asylum and other antebellum asylums. Nancy Tomes provided needed information about the contents of the Pennsylvania Hospital Archives, and Caroline Morris, the hospital archivist, kindly helped me find the documents I sought which related to South Carolinians who were committed to that institution. Whitfield Bell identified letters in the Benjamin Rush Correspondence concerning insane patients from South Carolina. Lee Drago gave me good advice regarding the NEH proposal and helped me gain a basic knowledge of southern history. Attending the Southern Studies Colloquium that Jane and Bill Pease conducted for several years at the College of Charleston helped increase my familiarity with historical scholarship on the region. The Peases also directed me to a number of helpful sources and, along with Bob Stockton, provided needed confirmation concerning some aspects of Charleston architecture.

I have been fortunate indeed to have had the support of the people at the University of North Carolina Press. They have been unfailingly helpful and kind through all the stages of the publishing process. I wish particularly to thank Lewis Bateman for his confidence in me and his good advice; Pamela Upton for nursing me through the preparation of the manuscript for publication; and Karin Kaufman for her thorough copyediting work. I am indebted to JoAnn Diaz for her assistance with the technical aspects of word processing and preparing the manuscript for publication. My thanks also go out to colleagues and friends who have read and commented on part or all of the manuscript, including Bill Pease, Randy Sparks, Woody Harris, and Amy McCandless. Along with the readers selected by the University of North Carolina Press, they have both encouraged me and saved me from some embarrassing errors. For those that remain, I alone am responsible.

Moonlight, Magnolias, & Madness

Introduction

In Columbia, during secession times,
Mr. Petigru was asked by a Northern gentleman,
"where the lunatic asylum was?"
He replied: "The asylum is up on the hill,
but the lunatics are all over the State."
BENJAMIN F. PERRY

When I first began research on insanity in South Carolina, archivists, librarians, and historians jokingly assured me that I should have no difficulty finding material. After all, to quote Mary Chesnut, had not "Mr. Petigru said all South Carolina was an asylum"?[1] Wherever I went, I heard that James Louis Petigru had described his state as an asylum without walls. To Petigru, the state's most prominent antebellum Unionist, secession (like nullification before) was sheer madness. The diagnosis was not, of course, psychiatric; it was political. But whatever one thinks of Petigru's analysis, the history of insanity in South Carolina cannot be understood separately from its political—not to mention its economic, cultural, and social—history.

The state that Petigru diagnosed as politically mad was also one of the first, in the 1820s, to confine the psychiatrically mad in a public mental institution. Yet for reasons that go well beyond the limits of a narrow psychiatric history, most of the state's insane did not experience institutional care before the late nineteenth century. They were "all over the state." Moreover, the events Petigru considered symptomatic of political madness greatly affected the fate of his fellow Carolinians unfortunate enough to be considered psychiatrically mad, both before and after the Civil War. The events themselves were the product of a particular economic, racial, and social milieu that also influenced how South Carolinians perceived and treated the insane. One of the aims of this book is to locate the history of insanity in South Carolina in this broader historical context.

But the story of insanity in South Carolina would have little meaning considered by itself. To give it wider significance, it is necessary to relate it to the rich but perplexing literature on the history of mental illness and psychiatry in the United States and Europe. Until the 1960s historians portrayed the development of mental institutions and modern psychiatry as examples of the humanitarian and progressive nature of modern civilization. The purpose of both was to care for and cure a class of unfortunate beings who had become the victims of mental disease. That the realities of mental institutions and psychiatric practice often fell short of this ideal did not alter their fundamentally benign character. To Albert Deutsch, for example, the nineteenth-century outburst of asylum building in the United States was the proper, indeed inevitable, response of a society growing in wealth, knowledge, and compassion.[2]

This progressive, or Whiggish, view of the history of insanity came under attack from several directions in the 1960s and 1970s. Sociologists such as Erving Goffman and renegade psychiatrists such as Thomas Szasz and R. D. Laing pictured mental hospitals and orthodox psychiatry as repressive and mental illness as a social construct designed to justify the incarceration and control of individuals whose behavior was socially disruptive, economically unproductive, politically deviant, or morally objectionable.[3] The emergence of this antipsychiatry movement coincided with a growing conviction among many mental-health professionals that large numbers of patients in mental hospitals were not benefiting from institutionalization and would be as well or better off in the community. This conclusion was encouraged in large part by the discovery after World War II of psychotropic drugs, which controlled the symptoms of certain psychoses sufficiently to allow many patients to function outside a hospital. Politicians seeking to cut budgets seized upon the idea of community care as a humane and less expensive alternative to custodial care in mammoth mental hospitals. The upshot was the deinstitutionalization movement, which greatly reduced the number of mental hospital inmates in this country and others.[4]

Not surprisingly, these dramatic developments affected historians' attitudes toward mental institutions and psychiatry. The move away from an institutional response to insanity sparked renewed interest in the origins of the response. "Revisionists," led by Michel Foucault, attacked the progressive interpretation of psychiatric history as naïve.[5] The revisionists did not form a monolithic school. They often disagreed sharply with one another and sometimes with Foucault as well.[6] Yet all of them rejected what Andrew Scull calls the "public relations" version of psychiatric history and agreed that asylums in some sense served the cause of social control or hegemony. But they differed over who (or what) was doing the controlling, how, and why.[7]

Revisionist critiques of traditional psychiatric history inform most of the recent work in the field. But much of this work does not fall neatly into any historiographical category. One of the most prolific historians of mental illness in America, Gerald Grob, argues that the history of insanity is more complex than either the progressive or revisionist viewpoints have allowed. Both perspectives, he argues, are marred by a "presentist" outlook, didacticism, and a tendency to generalize on the basis of insufficient evidence. Grob pointedly confesses his inability to explain American policy toward the insane through any "single all-encompassing thesis." The modern response to insanity, he stresses, was shaped by a heterogeneous collection of groups often strongly in disagreement with one another: doctors, philanthropists, politicians, bureaucrats, and the insane themselves. None of these groups could control the way mental institutions developed, yet each helped make them what they became. The results were as much fortuitous as part of any predetermined plan. To Grob, asylums were not simply hospitals, as progressives such as Deutsch claimed, nor were they essentially jails or reformatories as the revisionists argued. They were multipurpose institutions whose nature and function varied according to time, place, and circumstance.[8]

Grob's work, in effect, called upon scholars to transcend the progressive-revisionist divide through in-depth studies of particular institutions, regions, or issues. During the past decade, many historians, whether influenced by the revisionists, Grob, or both, have done exactly that. They have meticulously explored the inner world of individual asylums and their relationships with outside society, the influence of gender on the perception and treatment of insanity, and the perception and treatment of insanity in particular countries and periods. These works have both enriched and complicated psychiatric history. One of the most important results has been a new appreciation of the role of the insane, their families, their communities, and their attendants in creating, manipulating, and altering psychiatric environments.[9]

Although much of the recent literature on the history of insanity deals with the United States, little of it focuses on the South. Books with an ostensible national perspective, such as those by David Rothman, Grob, and Norman Dain, as well as the older work of Albert Deutsch, concentrate primarily on the Northeast and the Midwest. Although these historians do not overlook the South entirely, their comments on the psychiatric history of the region are brief and general. The relative neglect of the South in these "national" works is somewhat surprising, because the first public mental institutions in the United States were in Virginia, Kentucky, South

Carolina, and Maryland. In *The Discovery of the Asylum*, Rothman occasionally refers to southern asylums, but he does not attempt to compare or contrast the South psychiatrically to the rest of the United States. In contrast, Deutsch, Grob, and Dain emphasize to varying degrees distinctions between North and South. Grob and Dain, for example, rightly emphasize how the presence of a large black and (before 1865) slave population complicated the care and treatment of insanity in the South.[10] All of them also portray the South as a psychiatric backwater compared to the North, and in so doing, perhaps justify paying less attention to southern developments. At best, they argue, southerners generally followed belatedly in the American psychiatric mainstream; at worst, southerners were ignorant about innovations in the treatment of the insane or too lacking in civic spirit or resources to implement them. To Grob, Dain, and Deutsch, the founders of the first southern asylums were uninformed about the new psychiatric thinking of the early nineteenth century, with its emphasis on moral therapy and therapeutic optimism. As a result, these historians argue, the early southern asylums were essentially custodial welfare institutions and were neither innovative nor influential.[11]

Comparison of North and South inevitably raises an issue that has long fascinated American historians: the question of southern distinctiveness. Historians since Ulrich B. Phillips have debated the extent of sectional differences and tried to explain how and why the South differs from the rest of the United States. They have variously located the South's alleged uniqueness in its racial, environmental, economic, cultural, or religious patterns. More recently, medical historians have explored the role of disease in contributing to southern distinctiveness. They have investigated the influence of predominately southern diseases, such as malaria, yellow fever, hookworm, and pellagra; the specific disease experience of blacks and poor whites; and the development of the concept of a distinctive southern medicine.[12] The debate over southern distinctiveness raises major questions about treatment of the insane in the region. Was the South psychiatrically distinct as well? In what ways was the southern response to insanity affected by its racial, economic, environmental, and cultural milieu? How did slavery, racialism, and segregation affect the perception, care, and treatment of the insane? To what extent and in what ways did the vicissitudes of southern history, especially the region's economic and political problems after the Civil War, affect the region's insane? To what degree did southern asylums differ from those in other regions of the country, in terms of their internal organization, methods, staff, or patient population? It is difficult to answer these questions, for few historians have analyzed in depth any aspects of the southern psychiatric experience.[13]

This book fills part of this gap in southern psychiatric history by examining the extent to which the experience of one southern state, South Carolina, paralleled or diverged from that of the nation at large. In many respects, South Carolina presents an ideal subject for the study of southern insanity and mental institutions. It is one of the oldest of the southern states, and its impact at the regional and national level has often been out of proportion to its size, population, or wealth. (South Carolina, like the Balkans, has often produced more history than it could consume locally.)

In many respects, the history of South Carolina is representative of the southern experience, although admittedly at its extreme. In the eighteenth and early nineteenth centuries, South Carolina was one of the richest of states, its wealth based on a plantation economy geared to the production of staples such as rice, indigo, and cotton for world markets. By the late nineteenth century, a changing world economy and the ravages of Civil War had transformed it into one of the poorest regions of the United States. In South Carolina, as in all southern states, race has been a powerful historical theme. For most of its history until the early twentieth century, the majority of its population was African American. Looked at from a nationalist perspective, the history of South Carolina, like that of its region, often seems to have been marked by futile, self-destructive tendencies. Wedded to the plantation economy and the peculiar institution that undergirded it, the state was the most consistent defender of slavery and the way of life it produced, the parent of nullification, secession, and Civil War. In the wake of the war, South Carolina spent decades mired in poverty, racialism, and nostalgia for a mythical Old South of moonlight and magnolias.

The unpleasant and idiosyncratic aspects of South Carolina's past have perhaps blinded historians to the ways in which it participated in the American mainstream. The history of insanity is a case in point. During the eighteenth century, South Carolina was one of the first colonies to provide a public institution for the reception of the insane, in the "Mad-House" connected to the Charleston poorhouse. In the 1820s, South Carolina became the first state in the Deep South—and only the third in the nation—to establish a state lunatic asylum. Contrary to most of the literature on insanity in the United States, South Carolina's asylum reformers resembled their northern counterparts in that they were influenced by avant-garde ideas of moral treatment and therapeutic optimism. From the beginning, the South Carolina Lunatic Asylum was intended to be a curative, not simply a custodial, institution. Its officers tried to emulate the practices of the more progressive northern and European asylums. They never succeeded even to their own satisfaction, but the problems they encountered were similar in kind, if not always in degree, to those their northern colleagues faced: insufficient funding, inadequate facilities, a lack of qualified attendants, overcrowding, accumulation of chronic and incurable cases. In many respects the history of the South Carolina Lunatic Asylum, at least during the antebellum period, was not remarkably different from that in many northern states.

Yet the history of insanity in South Carolina does not fit readily into any explanatory thesis, progressive or revisionist. Racial factors alone greatly complicate the attempt. The experience with insanity of the black majority differed fundamentally in some respects from that of whites. The fate of the black insane was marked by an even higher degree of indifference, cruelty, and neglect. These conditions were largely determined by white dominance, both under and after slavery. The care and treatment insane blacks received was primarily dependent upon the attitudes and priorities of whites, who controlled the political, economic, and social institutions of the state. For the most part, white leaders showed little interest in the situation of insane blacks as a group, except when political necessity demanded a show of public concern.

South Carolina's institutional history also defies easy analysis. Many historians have found a common ethos or set of circumstances behind the development of modern social institutions such as asylums, reformatories, penitentiaries, and public schools. The reason for the development may vary: enlightened humanitarianism, a quest for social hegemony, order or efficiency, the impact of market capitalism, the rise of an industrial, urban society, and so on. Whatever the reason, one would expect such institutions to appear in a given area at roughly the same time; that is to say, a society that produces an asylum should also be establishing penitentiaries, reformatories, public schools, and so forth. South Carolina's institutional history does not fit this neat pattern. It was one of the first states to establish a public asylum, but extremely retarded in founding most other types of social institutions. The state did not create a penitentiary until 1866, a juvenile reformatory until 1900, an institution for the feeble-minded until 1918. South Carolina created a system of common schools in 1811, but it was so poorly funded during the antebellum period as to be virtually nonfunctional.

Popular sentiment apparently had little to do with this odd pattern of development. For example, public support for a penitentiary in the first part of the nineteenth century was much greater than that for a public asylum. Why then, did South Carolina build an asylum, but not a penitentiary, during the antebellum period? Michael Hindus's book *Prison and Plantation* may provide part of the answer. Among other things, Hindus examines South Carolina's failure to follow Massachusetts and establish a penitentiary during the antebellum period. He argues that South Carolina's penal-reform movement was inhibited by a political culture dominated by slavery and the planter aristocracy. In the eyes of the ruling elite, he maintains, slaves constituted the largest potential criminal class, and they were already effectively incarcerated by virtue of their bondage. The elite were less alarmed by white crime, which they preferred to handle through traditional modes of punishment: fines, short jail terms, and corporal and capital punishment, leavened by a free use of pardons. Most of South Carolina's leaders were in any case reluctant to follow the lead of abolitionist Massachusetts.[14]

Ironically, Hindus's argument, if correct, would seem to undermine a social-control interpretation of the South Carolina Lunatic Asylum. The asylum was not established to control insane blacks, for most of them were effectively controlled by their masters.[15] With a couple exceptions, it did not even accept black patients for twenty years after it opened and admitted fewer than forty blacks before the Civil War. It can be more forcefully argued that the asylum functioned to control white lunatics. But if so, it was conspicuously unsuccessful. For more than a decade after it opened, the asylum had great difficulty in attracting a sufficient number of white patients to justify its existence to the legislature. Annual admissions averaged only slightly more than twenty during the first decade and did not exceed forty until 1849, the first year the total number of patients in residence surpassed a hundred. Proslavery propaganda to the contrary, the small number of admissions during the antebellum years was not due to the mental benefits of the southern way of life. It resulted from the asylum's exclusion of blacks, minimal support from the state legislature, and the reluctance or inability of whites to patronize the institution. Antebellum censuses no doubt greatly underenumerated the state's insane, but even using those faulty statistics, it is obvious that the asylum was unable to attract hundreds of potential patients. If the founders hoped to create an instrument for controlling a socially disruptive population, they fell far short of achieving their goal. Moreover, the asylum's difficulty in attracting clientele weakened enthusiasm for institutional solutions to social problems.[16]

During the antebellum period, then, there seems to have been little societal pressure in South Carolina to employ the asylum as a means to control the mentally disordered. One of the ironies of the history of insanity in

South Carolina is that in 1821 asylum reformers managed to establish an institution for which there was (at the time) little effective demand. That they succeeded in doing so was almost a historical accident, the result of a temporary conjunction of favorable circumstances. Soon after they achieved the necessary legislation, the circumstances became much less favorable. They had to struggle through seven more years of political and economic adversity to bring the asylum into existence. In the process, they appealed to the same humanitarian, philanthropic, medical, and social-control arguments asylum reformers elsewhere used. But significantly, South Carolina's reformers also repeatedly appealed to civic pride. To found an asylum, they stressed, was an act that would add luster to the state's reputation for humanity and benevolence. It may have been one of the most convincing arguments for creating the asylum. To keep pace with the improvements of an improving age was one way the state's elite could convince the outside world and reassure themselves that slavery, far from inhibiting progress, provided the best foundation for it.

Whatever the reformers intended, most of the state's inhabitants were either satisfied with traditional modes of caring for the insane or for some reason (poverty, racial exclusion) unable to take advantage of the asylum. Indeed, from the colonial period until the late nineteenth century, the great majority of South Carolina's insane were cared for outside the state asylum, by their families, their masters, or the local authorities. The fate of the insane beyond the asylum walls is a major focus of *Moonlight, Magnolias and Madness*. Several chapters examine the situation of the insane in its community context. In contrast, most historical works on insanity have tended to concentrate on asylums and their populations. Historians who have looked outside the walls have mainly assessed how the wider society influenced the creation of asylums, the commitment process, the nature of institutional existence, and so forth.[17] Few historians have thoroughly investigated the situation of the insane in the community on its own terms, rather than as a means to illuminate institutional developments.[18] In the case of South Carolina, an investigation of community care seems particularly imperative, given the virtual exclusion of the black majority and many whites from the asylum until the late nineteenth century. The great obstacle to an inquiry of this type is the relative scarcity and unrepresentativeness of sources, which renders most conclusions tentative at best. But that is no reason for not making the attempt. By drawing on a wide range of sources, including state and local government records, family papers, correspondence, memoirs, newspapers, domestic manuals, and other medical and nonmedical writings, one can gain some insight into the complex situation of the insane in the community and the multitude of social, racial, cultural, and economic influences upon it. The evidence does not support a romantic, Foucaultian conception of liberated lunacy; but neither does it support the view of asylum advocates that community care invariably meant brutality or neglect.

The same influences affected the institutional history of the insane. South Carolina society changed radically in several respects in the late nineteenth century, and in response the state asylum altered its nature and functions. The asylum became increasingly dominated by chronic patients and gradually accepted a largely custodial role, without completely abandoning its therapeutic pretensions. The number of patients increased faster than the staff and facilities, producing severe overcrowding and a general deterioration in the patients' environment. These changes were not unique to South Carolina; many states experienced them. But the changes in South Carolina were perhaps more drastic and sudden than in many contemporary institutions, because its society changed so completely and radically between the antebellum and postbellum eras. Few states have suffered such a precipitous fall from economic grace as did South Carolina during the nineteenth century. One of the wealthiest of states at the beginning of the century, it had become one of the poorest by the end. The antebellum period was a time of relative economic decline. The 1860s and 1870s brought defeat in war, economic dislocation, enormous loss of wealth, the destruction of slavery, military occupation, and federally imposed Reconstruction. Despite the emergence of a textile industry after 1880, the state's inhabitants became more dependent than ever upon the cultivation of cotton in a time of generally falling prices. During the late nineteenth and early twentieth centuries, most South Carolinians suffered severely from agricultural depression and the peonage of the sharecropping and crop-lien systems.

The insane, like others in the state, felt the impact of these developments. The asylum, which received minimal support from the state before 1860, deteriorated badly during and after the Civil War. In the impoverished conditions that followed the war, the asylum authorities found it increasingly difficult to collect payments from patients' families or counties. In 1870, the Reconstruction government tried to aid the institution by shifting the costs of caring for paupers in the asylum from the counties to the state. State care, as elsewhere, brought about a sharp increase in the numbers of asylum admissions and in the proportion of pauper, or "beneficiary," patients, as they now became known. Local officials were more willing than before to commit someone as a pauper lunatic, and many families were more willing to accept state aid than local poor relief.

Racial and political developments also greatly increased the pressures on the state asylum in the late nineteenth and early twentieth centuries. Emancipation, supported by federal troops, fully opened the asylum to blacks for the first time and greatly increased the potential patient population. Large numbers of black patients entered the asylum during and after Reconstruction. They changed the nature of the asylum's population and complicated its administration. For the first time, the asylum became a truly biracial institution, although black patients were not on anything like an equal footing. They were segregated (although sometimes kept in the same buildings as whites), provided with markedly inferior care and accommodations, and worked more and died faster than their white counterparts. Their fate is hardly astonishing, given their former slave status and the racialist assumptions of the state's white rulers. What is perhaps more surprising, given the commitment to racial segregation in the postbellum decades, is how slow the state was to establish a separate asylum for blacks. Several other southern states built asylums for insane blacks soon after the Civil War. The South Carolina legislature resisted proposals for a separate black institution until just before World War I, largely on the grounds of cost. Fiscal conservatism, in this case at least, overrode the segregationist ideal.

The same fiscal imperative ensured niggardly appropriations for the South Carolina Lunatic Asylum during the late nineteenth and early twentieth centuries. The asylum's facilities and staff did not expand commensurately with the rapid influx of patients, with tragic results. The Reconstruction government enacted state care and appointed an able superintendent for the asylum, but it did not provide adequate funding. Under the post-Reconstruction regimes, the asylum fared even worse. From the 1880s to 1914, South Carolina's per capita expenditure on its institutionalized insane was consistently among the lowest of all the states.

Political upheavals exacerbated the asylum's financial problems. The Reconstruction government politicized the asylum to a greater degree than before by making the superintendent and regents political appointees and by enacting state care. The asylum became one of the biggest items in the state budget and a source of political patronage. Those who controlled the state government became more determined than before to control its operation, so that it could serve, or at least not subvert, their political interests. Those who wanted to control the state government often pointed to the management of the asylum as an example of the extravagance or incompetence of the regime in power. The state experienced several political revolutions between 1868 and 1915, each of which brought major changes in the personnel of the asylum.

The greatest losers from these economic and political developments were the asylum's patients. By the beginning of the twentieth century, conditions at the South Carolina State Hospital (as it became known in 1895) had become scandalous. After two major legislative investigations, in 1909 and 1914, Governor Richard I. Manning (1915–18) successfully promoted a series of reforms that remedied some of the worst conditions. The reforms were influenced by progressive ideals of efficiency and the growing mental hygiene movement and improved the situation of the institutionalized insane in many respects. But the improvements aided the white patients more than the blacks, and in any case could do little to change the fundamentally custodial nature of the hospital. By the 1920s, for better or worse, South Carolina was rejoining the nation's psychiatric mainstream.

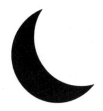

PART ONE

Before the Asylum

1670–1828

One

OUT OF HER SENSES

INSANITY IN EARLY SOUTH CAROLINA

For months, Kate's neighbors along the Santee River had considered her dangerously mad. Thus, they were probably not surprised to hear in June 1745 that this slave woman had murdered a black child. The Craven County authorities lodged her in jail, where her actions convinced the justices of the peace that she was indeed "out of her Senses." Because they deemed her irresponsible, they did not bring her to trial. But they did not know what to do with her. They did not want to release her, because they considered her dangerous. But Kate's owner, Robert Fullwood, was too poor to pay for her confinement, and the colony of South Carolina made no provision for the public maintenance of slaves. The justices remanded Kate to jail and petitioned the colonial assembly in Charleston for relief and advice. The assembly refused their request for remuneration. Instead it passed an act that made each parish in the colony responsible for the maintenance of lunatic slaves whose owners were unable to care for them.[1]

Kate's story may seem a strange place to begin a history of insanity in South Carolina. English settlers had founded the colony seventy-five years earlier, and even discounting native Americans, hers was not South Carolina's first case of insanity. Yet there are several reasons for beginning with Kate. Her predicament (or that of the Craven County justices) prompted the first law in the state's history that dealt specifically with the care of the insane. That the act dealt only with insane slaves was significant and, in a sense, fitting.

By the early eighteenth century, blacks made up a majority of the colony's population. Their numbers and skills went far to shape the nature of South Carolina's culture. Yet the colonial government had never made any provision for their care when attacked by insanity. Until Kate's case, the colony's laws assumed that masters were responsible for the control and care of their slaves; a law of 1717 provided for a fine of twenty pounds for any master who turned out a sick or disabled servant.[2] The act of 1745 remedied, on paper at least, a flaw in that assumption: some masters, like Fullwood, might be unable to control or care for an unproductive slave.

The act was also significant in what it did not do: it did not lead to any general reassessment of public policy toward the mentally disordered. The assembly did not perceive insanity as a widespread problem. The colony's population was low, and its inhabitants were scattered about the countryside on plantations and farms. Charleston was the only town of consequence well into the nineteenth century.[3] Only rarely, as in a case like Kate's, did the insane intrude upon the public consciousness. The insane were few, and the authorities were satisfied with the existing mechanisms for dealing with them.

Governmental interference in the care of the insane before the nineteenth century was minimal. But it does not follow that they were generally abandoned to brutality and neglect, as many historians would have it. In the 1930s Albert Deutsch characterized colonial provision for the mentally disordered as a mixture of "punishment, repression, and indifference."[4] Evidence regarding the insane of early South Carolina is ambiguous and sketchy; but much of it points to a more complex reality, closer to Roy Porter's remark about the fate of the insane in Georgian England: it depended "on who you were, and where you were and who was treating you."[5]

A variety of social, racial, geographical, and medical circumstances influenced the care and treatment lunatics received. Perhaps none was more important than their domestic situation, for nearly everyone viewed the insane as primarily a private, familial responsibility. If a family had the means to do so, they were expected to care for their insane themselves. For such families, the main options were home care or boarding out with another family. Planter families sometimes assigned a slave to care for an insane relative. Ann Richardson awarded her slave Sam his freedom in 1810 as a reward for several years' devoted care of her deranged son Manley.[6] If an insane person had no family, or his family was unable or unwilling to care for him, sympathetic private citizens sometimes accepted the familial role. When a ship's captain named Bernard became "disorder'd in his head" in 1744, Charleston merchant Robert Pringle provided him with a lodging in town and medical care. Reverend Francis Guichard took the deranged shopkeeper Peter Calvett into his own home in 1751.[7]

An insane person for whom no one took responsibility might be left alone as long as he or she did not appear to threaten public safety or tranquility. Documented cases of wandering lunatics, however, are surprisingly few in the early records of South Carolina. Whether this was because they were rare or because they did not arouse much public concern is not clear. Samuel Farrow was allegedly moved to campaign for a lunatic asylum in the early nineteenth century by the sight of a deranged woman who for years had wandered about the upper parts of the state.[8]

The Carolina backcountry probably had its share of characters like Mason Lee, whom some considered insane but who nevertheless lived his life without interference. Lee, who lived in Marlboro County in the late eighteenth and early nineteenth centuries, amassed a considerable fortune in slaves and land. At the age of thirty he was struck by lightning and soon afterward began to exhibit bizarre ideas and behavior. He moved to Georgia, where he murdered one of his slaves. After returning to South Carolina in a successful attempt to avoid prosecution for the crime, he became convinced that his relations, the Wigginses, wanted him dead to get his property. He allegedly accused them of using supernatural powers, including bewitchment, to accomplish their goal. Despite his great wealth, he lived in a shack "worse than any of his negro houses" and possessed no tables, chairs, or dishes. He slept in a hollow log, surrounded by an arsenal of swords, guns, and razors. Convinced that all women were witches, he refused to sleep in a bed made by a woman. He extracted fourteen sound teeth because he was convinced that the Wigginses were inside them. To prevent witches from grabbing his hair during fights, he shaved his head. During the day he slept, so that he could stay awake at night to struggle against witches and the devil.

These oddities and more came out when his relations contested his will, itself decidedly peculiar. Determined to prevent his relatives from gaining by his death, he left his property to the states of South Carolina and Tennessee. After his death in 1820, the Wigginses contested the will on the grounds that Lee was insane when he made it. Witnesses at the trial differed as to Lee's mental condition; some thought him insane, others thought him merely eccentric. But the jury ruled that Lee was mentally competent when he made the will.[9]

The Lee case indicates that early South Carolinians, at least in the backcountry, tolerated a high degree of odd ideas and behavior. Yet Lee's neighbors may have left him alone more out of fear than tolerance. In the early 1820s John Adamson, a man many considered insane, terrorized the area around Camden. Members of the community tried to get Adamson declared a lunatic on several occasions. But he threatened to shoot anyone who claimed he was insane, and potential witnesses refused to testify. Adamson was eventually killed in a fight with a man whose life he had threatened.[10]

The insane who had committed a crime were sometimes sent to jail, as Kate was. Charleston tailor William Linnen was sent to the city's jail twice as a criminal lunatic, the second time after he shot and killed Dr. David Ramsay in 1815. Several patients admitted to the South Carolina Lunatic Asylum shortly after it opened in 1828 had been in local jails for long periods of time, one for fifteen years. But references to incarceration of lunatics are rare in early South Carolina. This may be partly due to gaps in the records, but few jails existed and those that did exist were notoriously insecure.[11]

Early South Carolina had two formal mechanisms, adopted from England, which could be used to deal with the insane whom no one was able or willing to care for: the commission of lunacy and the poor law. The commission of lunacy was a chancery or equity procedure adopted from English law. The ostensible purpose of the commission of lunacy was to protect the property and persons of lunatics, idiots, and other persons of "unsound mind." Family members normally initiated lunacy commissions through a petition to the court. If the court ruled favorably on the petition, it would issue a *writ de lunatico inquirendo* appointing a commission to inquire into the alleged lunacy. If the commission's members found the person to be incompetent, the court would appoint a committee (a guardian or guardians) to handle his or her affairs. In some cases, the judge would also give directions about the care or control of the alleged lunatic. The number of lunacy commissions increased greatly in the early 1800s, when the equity court began to hold sessions in the counties and the power of holding commissions of lunacy and appointing guardians for the insane was given to judges of the court of common pleas.[12]

The court records of early South Carolina include a few lunacy cases. In 1726, for example, a lunacy commission found David Guerard to be "of very unsound Memory and understanding," and the chancery court appointed Rev. Alexander Garden and Benjamin Godin as guardians. Guerard was still under the protection of the court more than twenty years later.[13]

Thomas Drayton's relatives sought to bring him under the protection of the chancery court in 1785, when his behavior began to alarm his neighbors and embarrass his prominent planting family. Drayton was declared a lunatic, but his period under the court's protection was brief. In December 1787, a friend presented a petition from his physician and several other persons stating that Drayton "had recovered his perfect senses." The court superseded the commission and restored Drayton's liberty and control over his property.[14] In 1801, a lunacy commission declared Catherine Wigfall insane for, among other reasons, "speaking of smoking her body until it be as black as a Negroes and living with them."[15]

The commission of lunacy was normally a private procedure, an arrangement between the lunatic's family and the court to safeguard property. But public authorities or concerned citizens might also use the procedure if an alleged lunatic with property had no family or his family failed to control him. In 1749, the vestry of St. Philip's Parish in Charleston petitioned the governor and council to hold a commission of lunacy on shopkeeper Peter Calvett. The vestry had two reasons for wanting to bring Calvett under the guardianship of the court. One was to prevent him from harming others. For some time, the petition alleged, he had been acting in a bizarre, irresponsible, and dangerous manner. Among other things, he had a habit of firing pistols out of his windows at night, terrorizing and endangering the lives of his neighbors. The second reason the vestry wanted to place Calvett under legal control was to prevent him from squandering his property and becoming "burthensome to this Parish."[16]

The vestry's petition succeeded. The lunacy commission declared Calvett a lunatic and appointed two citizens as guardians. But the committee apparently did not perform its duty properly. Two years later, Rev. Francis Guichard petitioned the chancery court, asking that a new committee be appointed to take care of Calvett's property and person. Guichard claimed that the original guardians had failed in their responsibility to Calvett, who was now living at the clergyman's house. Guichard was not anxious to keep him. Caring for Calvett, he stated, "would greatly Embarrass and obstruct him in the Discharge of his ministerial Function." The court appointed a new committee and ordered that Calvett's personal property be inventoried and sold and his home rented out. His subsequent fate is unclear.[17]

The lunacy commission was of little use to those without property to protect. Its use was also probably restricted by ignorance of the law—by the courts as well as by ordinary citizens. In 1793, George Gill petitioned the state assembly on behalf of his insane relative Jacob Castor. According to Gill, Castor owned a large amount of land, but because of his condition, he was unable to support himself. Gill first applied to the Chester County Court to seek some provision for Castor's support. But, Gill claimed, the court did nothing: they knew "of no law authorizing them to lay their hands on the property of persons of his description and have therefore refused to do any thing." Gill then tried to secure poor relief for Castor, but the Chester court ruled that Castor was ineligible for public assistance because of the property he owned. As a result, Gill declared, Castor was "totally unprovided for."[18]

The poor law was the second, and far more common, method by which government became involved in the care of the insane. Along with the other British North American colonies, South Carolina adopted the English poor law, which made each parish responsible for the maintenance of its paupers.[19] Had Kate, the insane slave, been a free white without anyone able to care for her, the justices would not have needed to petition the assembly in her case. They could have charged the costs of her maintenance to the parish poor tax.

South Carolina enacted its first formal poor law in 1695, but the initial unit of administration was the colony as a whole rather than the individual parish. In 1712, the assembly adopted the English system, by which the vestry of each parish was responsible for administering poor relief. The vestry elected overseers of the poor to collect the poor tax and distribute aid to the poor. South Carolina's poor law made no specific provision for the insane, but insanity, like other diseases, inevitably pauperized some of its victims and made them eligible for relief. The colony's poor laws recognized this connection between disease and dependence. The law of 1695, for example, stated that it was designed to relieve "the sick, lame, impotent, old, blind, and such other persons being poore and not able to worke." The statute of 1712 noted that many poor people came from the country to Charleston for the treatment of sickness and stipulated that their home parish should defray the cost of their care and medicine.[20]

Until 1738 aid to the poor in South Carolina took the form of outdoor relief. Outside of Charleston, outdoor relief predominated well into the nineteenth century. Under outdoor relief, poor-law officers relieved paupers in their homes or boarded them out with citizens who agreed to care for them. In addition to money, the parishes often provided medicine and medical care for the sick poor. St. Philip's vestry in Charleston contracted with local physicians to provide medical care for the city's poor. Rural parishes usually paid fees to medical men or others on an individual basis for the care of the sick or disabled.[21] Parish records rarely mention specific diseases, but the recipients of outdoor relief included occasional cases of insanity and idiocy.[22]

Indoor relief of the poor began in 1738, when Charleston opened its first workhouse. The main rationale for the creation of the workhouse in Charleston, as in other urban areas of Europe and America, was a desire to reduce the costs of poor relief. Compared to some northern colonial towns, early Charleston had the reputation of being relatively liberal in its treatment of the poor. The South Carolina low country was perhaps the richest society in the British North American colonies, but most of the wealth was concentrated in the hands of a small class of planters, lawyers, and merchants. Their prosperity and the presence of a slave majority combined to promote an approach to the welfare of poor whites that was allegedly generous by eighteenth-century standards. Charleston was also a major seaport and the only city within hundreds of miles. As such it attracted people from the countryside and other provinces, destitute immigrants, and derelict and unemployed seamen.[23]

By the 1730s, the vestry had become alarmed by the rising poor-tax burden, which they attributed in part to an influx of "Idle, vagrant, and viciously inclined People" who took advantage of the city's charity. The vestry was also concerned about the rising costs of and inadequate facilities for caring for the sick poor. The solution, St. Philip's Parish vestry informed the colonial assembly in 1734, was to build a workhouse and hospital in the city. Two years later, the assembly gave its approval, and the institution opened in 1738.[24]

The Charleston workhouse resembled many similar institutions elsewhere in America and Europe, and it shared their contradictions. Its promoters sought to deter the undeserving and aid the deserving poor within the same walls. After it opened, the vestry ordered that all the city's paupers be removed to it, although before long, some paupers were once again receiving outdoor relief.[25] In the years that followed, the assembly directed the commissioners of the workhouse to receive seamen and disobedient slaves as well. The workhouse became a motley receptacle of the destitute and deviant of all kinds, trying to serve simultaneously as a house of correction, a hospital, and an almshouse. An enumeration of the types of people a local justice could send there indicates the heterogeneity of the workhouse population:

All rogues, vagabonds, lewd and idle persons and beggars, stubborn and obstinate apprentices and servants, (on complaint of their masters and mistresses) and children (on complaint of their parents) common drunkards, common night walkers, pilferers, lewd, wanton and lascivious persons, common scolds and bawlers, tradesmen and laborers neglecting their callings, and leading idle and dissolute lives, and who do not provide for the support of their families, . . . stubborn, obstinate, or incorrigible negroes or slaves.[26]

Such an institution defied the goal of efficient management. In 1750, the vestry complained that conditions within the workhouse were so unpleasant that the poor preferred to beg in the streets.

By this time, insane inmates had become numerous enough within the workhouse to present a management problem, and the vestry sought some means to separate them (as well as slaves, felons, and sailors) from the other inmates. In 1754, the vestry urged the commissioners of the workhouse to consider building an apartment at some distance from the workhouse for the reception of the mad.[27] The following year, the colonial assembly debated the idea of erecting a separate building for confining "Persons disordered in their Senses, Fugitive Slaves and others" so as to make the existing establishment more suitable for the city's poor and sick. The assembly appropriated funds for the construction of an additional building, part of which was allocated to the insane.[28]

A few years later a group of prosperous artisans began a campaign to improve the condition of the colony's insane. They formed the Fellowship Society in 1762 to raise funds for a hospital for the care of "lunaticks, and other distempered and sick poor." A hospital was needed, they argued, because the homes of the city's poor were often unsuitable for treatment and the transient poor had no homes. The solution was to provide a single institution where they could be "under one inspection, and in the hands of skilful Physicians and Surgeons."[29] The society's members were influenced by their knowledge of similar institutions elsewhere in America and England. Experience, they announced, had shown that hospitals greatly benefited society by curing large numbers of persons and restoring them to useful lives. During the eighteenth century, philanthropic groups in several English towns founded hospitals to cope with the problems Charleston was encountering. In America, the Pennsylvania Hospital, opened in 1752, may have served as a model for the Fellowship Society's members, for the Philadelphia institution received the insane as well as the physically ill.[30]

In aiming to bring the insane and sick poor of the city and region together under "one inspection," the members of the Fellowship Society may have been motivated by a paternalistic desire to control the sick and insane poor. But they also felt a sense of kinship with them. Fear of the black majority no doubt contributed to this, but there was another reason. The society's members were artisans, many of whom had only recently become wealthy. They were acutely conscious of the fleeting nature of prosperity, and they envisioned creating an institution that they or their children might someday need: "Our present state, how prosperous soever, hath no stability. . . . [Therefore] how careful should we be freely to distribute a small portion of our stewardship towards the distress of our fellow creatures."[31]

According to David Ramsay, a leading South Carolina physician of the early national period, the Fellowship Society appropriated one-half of its funds toward the care of the insane.[32] Yet it never established an institution for the insane or the sick poor. But its efforts may have convinced the local elite to improve the city's facilities for the insane poor. In 1765, a grand jury investigated conditions at the workhouse and concluded that it was not a proper place for the poor, because it was filled with sailors, criminals, vagrants, and slaves. Charleston, the jury concluded, needed a general hospital or poorhouse to accommodate the large number of deserving poor who congregated there from around the province. The St. Philip's vestry repeated the plea to the assembly the following year and added that it was "an Act of Inhumanity to put the Poor and Sick (who may be, and often are pious and well disposed persons)" in an institution where they had to endure "Correcting of Slaves, [and] a Continual Noise and Disturbance, Cursing and Swearing, from the Seamen and Others Confined there."[33] In 1768 the assembly responded with an act that approved the construction of a separate "Poor House and Hospital" with a building for the insane. The old workhouse became a house of correction (used mainly to discipline unruly slaves).[34] Some political letters and essays of the following year refer to the city madhouse and describe it as a brick structure behind the poorhouse and close to the arsenal.[35]

This location was unfortunate. In 1780, during the War for Independence, an accidental explosion at the arsenal following the British capture of the city leveled the madhouse and some other poorhouse buildings. According to a later account, the blast killed most of the inmates.[36] But the problem of accommodating the insane poor soon confronted the occupying British authorities. In 1782 they directed the churchwardens of St. Philip's Parish to find some place to keep "Persons disordered in their Senses." The churchwardens examined several houses but found none suitable for the care of the insane. They suggested that the top rooms of the poorhouse, if repaired, could provide a temporary home. The British agreed to pay for the repairs and, presumably, the insane returned to the poorhouse.[37]

After the war the care of Charleston's poor was transferred from the St. Philip's vestry to an elected secular board, the commissioners of the poor. Unfortunately, no poorhouse records have survived from the late eighteenth century. In 1796 an ordinance authorizing the commissioners of the poor to confine "Strolling Beggars" noted that the poorhouse had recently been renovated and considerably enlarged.[38] An ordinance of 1801 gave the commissioners of the poor responsibility for caring for "all lunatics or persons disordered in their senses, who may be there confined." In 1800, when the extant poorhouse records resume, the institution included a "Lunatic" or "Maniac" Department, which housed seven insane inmates. The department continued to function until 1856.[39]

The records of early South Carolina tell us something about where the insane were kept and by whom. They are much less informative about how they were treated. The historian is restricted to occasional fleeting (and perhaps misleading) glimpses of the world of the mentally disturbed. The available evidence indicates that the insane in South Carolina were treated much the same as elsewhere in America or Europe, sometimes with neglect and brutality and sometimes with concern and sympathy. The fate of particular individuals depended to a large extent on how they were perceived, and that varied according to community and family attitudes, type of disorder, geographic location, class, race, and gender.[40]

The insane have always elicited varying reactions: fear, disgust, perplexity, embarrassment, ridicule, awe, and compassion. Early America was no exception. Eighteenth-century Anglo-American culture portrayed the insane in varied and sometimes violently contrasting ways: as divinely or intellectually inspired, possessed, animalistic, and sick. The idea that insanity was a physical disease, which physicians since Hippocrates and Galen had advocated, had achieved widespread acceptance by the eighteenth century. The equally ancient view, that the mad were either divinely inspired or possessed by demons, was in decline and was opposed by the hierarchy of the Anglican church. Yet supernatural explanations persisted among people of all ranks and coexisted with natural explanations. This was true of influential theologians such as John Wesley, the English founder of Methodism, and Cotton Mather of Massachusetts. Moreover, people who rejected religio-magical explanations did not necessarily adopt sympathetic attitudes toward the insane. Cartesian rationalism viewed reason as the noblest essence of humanity; man without reason was little more than a beast. Such a perspective could justify brutality and neglect: animal madness was impervious to cold and hunger, and it could only be beaten and starved into submission.

But that was not the only view. Advocates of associationist or sensation-alist psychology (derived from the writings of Locke, Hartley, and Condil-lac) generally viewed the insane more sympathetically. Associationist theory held that insanity was primarily a disorder of the sensory system rather than a total deprivation of reason. The insane were defective human mecha-nisms; they were victims of incorrect thinking, of a false association of ideas. Insanity was often partial and temporary, and the insane often retained the ability to reason correctly on some subjects. They were like children and had to be reeducated. Thus, as some associationists concluded, the insane deserved, appreciated, and benefited from kind treatment. Associa-tionism provided a theoretical basis for the emerging psychological therapy known as moral treatment, discussed below. During the eighteenth century, many physicians accepted associationist theory and sought to physicalize it through various explanations of the working of the nervous system.[41]

Early South Carolinians exhibited this gamut of reactions to the insane. Seemingly contradictory views of the insane sometimes coexisted in the mind of one person. In 1742, planter Eliza Lucas Pinckney visited her friend Mrs. Chardon and was shocked to find her "quite out of her Sences." To Pinckney, Chardon was "as good as woman could be" but in her obsession with goodness had "ceased to be rational." As a result, she had sunk to ani-mality, or worse: "She is now inferior to her own species of which she was lately an ornament. . . . Surely there can not be a more dismal prospect in nature than man, the master piece of this our world, deprived of the noblest principle of his nature and laid on a level with the beasts that perish, and even inferior in some respects to those."

Yet Pinckney's harsh assessment of her friend's state competed with the strongest sympathy for a good friend. Mrs. Chardon, she wrote, was "an object that must greatly move a stranger that had not lost every spark of humanity; what then must it be to an intimate friend! who loves, es-teems and admires her even now that her charming intellects are so much disordered."[42] A similar mixture of alarm, repugnance, and compassion ap-pears in a letter by Joseph Manigault concerning Thomas Drayton: "I saw Tom Drayton this afternoon, whiskered up to the eyebrows, and booted up to the Hips; he looked as fierce as ever. . . . Poor young man, he is really to be pitied, and I think it would be acting a friendly Part, if some Person would have him confined, and not suffer him to expose himself to the Ridicule of all the Blackguards of Charleston."[43]

Perceptions of the insane varied according to the type and severity of the disorder, not to mention the relationship of the insane to those around them. Victims of melancholia (depression) or lesser nervous disorders such as hypochondriasis or hysteria were likely to elicit more sympathy and less fear than those suffering from violent mania. Indeed, the milder nervous and mental complaints became somewhat fashionable among the British upper classes of the eighteenth century. Educated South Carolinians shared similar views. According to Pinckney, her friend Mrs. Chardon's goodness of heart continued to show "through her melancholy veil." Charleston merchant Robert Pringle described his acquaintance Captain Bernard, who suffered from "a fitt of Melancholy," as a "poor man" suffering from "misfortune" who deserved protection and medical care.[44] After Reverend Crallan, an Anglican, became depressed and committed suicide in 1768, his colleague Charles Woodmason described him as "a Saint." Woodmason attributed Crallan's insanity and that of several other Anglican parsons to the local environment, particularly its obstreperous inhabitants: "These flighty, Proud, Ill principled Carolin[i]ans . . . are enough to make any Person run Mad."[45]

The case of Hugh Bryan illustrates another aspect of the thinking of early South Carolinians about insanity: a tendency to associate it with extreme religiosity. The eighteenth century British elite viewed enthusiasm (fanaticism) as a symptom, type, and cause of insanity. Beginning in the later seventeenth century, many English writers argued that the religious enthusiast indulged his "fancies" (imagination, passions, or feelings) to the point where they overpowered his reason and its control over the will. The result was bizarre ideas and behavior, which could lead to disorder and upheaval, as Puritan enthusiasm had produced bloody civil war in the mid-seventeenth century.[46] South Carolina's Anglican elite shared these attitudes, which one can see reflected in Woodmason's comments on a congregation of New Light Baptists in the backcountry. They acted, he wrote, like "a Gang of frantic Lunatics broke out of Bedlam."[47]

South Carolina's elite found confirmation of the connection of enthusiasm with madness through their experience with Bryan. A Beaufort planter, Bryan was an early convert of Rev. George Whitefield, the Methodist preacher who brought the religious revival known as the Great Awakening to South Carolina at the end of the 1730s. The timing of the awakening's arrival was important, for it coincided with the largest slave revolt of the colonial period, the Stono Rebellion of 1739.[48] Not surprisingly, the colony's nervous leaders were greatly alarmed when they learned early in 1742 that Bryan was preaching to large gatherings of slaves. The year before, he had referred to the Stono Rebellion and other recent disasters as examples of God's judgments on the colony's iniquities. In March 1742, the grand jury charged that Bryan was encouraging unlawful assemblies of slaves and making "sundry enthusiastick Prophecies of the Destruction of *Charles-Town* and Deliverance of the Negroes from their Servitude." [49] Eliza Lucas Pinckney claimed that he had also tried to perform biblical miracles: he attempted to divide the waters of a river and to walk upon water. According to Pinckney, his failure to perform these feats brought him to his senses. He apologized to the colonial assembly for his actions, and they dropped the charges against him. He resumed his life as a respectable if somewhat eccentric planter. [50]

Given the widespread acceptance of eighteenth-century ideas about the relation of enthusiasm, madness, and disorder, it is not surprising that some of Bryan's contemporaries attributed his ideas and behavior to insanity. Pinckney's discussion of his case contains a classical rationalist description of eighteenth-century religious madness. Bryan, she claimed, was "very much deluded by his fancys and imagined he was assisted by the divine spirit to prophesy. . . . From thence he went on (as it was natural to expect when he gave himself up intirely to his own whims) from one step to another till he came to working miracles." [51] In his letter of apology to the assembly, Bryan himself admitted that he had been deluded, although he, echoing an older tradition, blamed the wiles of Satan: "I find that I have presumed in my Zeal for God's Glory beyond his Will, and that he has suffered me to fall into a Delusion of Satan. . . . This Delusion I did not discover till three Days past, when after many Days' intimate Converse with an invisible Spirit, whose precepts seemed to be wise, and tending to the Advancement of Religion in general, and of my own spiritual Welfare in particular, I found my Teacher to be a Lier, and the Father of Lies; which brought me into a Sense of my Error." [52]

In typical eighteenth-century fashion, Pinckney's analysis blamed Bryan himself for bringing on his madness by allowing his "fancys" free rein. Yet she showed little animosity toward him, and accepted his sudden enlightenment and confession of error as a piece of "agreeable news." [53] Bryan, after all, was like herself a member of the cohesive planter elite. As he reminded the colonial assembly in his apology, "My whole Life has been spent among you." By acknowledging to his peers that he had been deluded, Bryan saved himself from severe punishment as a fomenter of slave rebellion. But he also reinforced the elite's ideas about the mental and social dangers of religious enthusiasm. [54]

These various perceptions of the mad should caution us against assuming that early South Carolinians treated the insane with indifference or brutality. Yet it would also be a mistake to conclude that eighteenth-century South Carolina was a paradise for the mentally disordered. For one thing, the cases cited above involved people from the upper, or at least educated, ranks of society. For another, the available records contain little information about the care and treatment these individuals received. A few cases from the first two decades of the nineteenth century, all involving planting families, may illustrate the variety of possibilities. None of them explains why the family adopted the methods of care and treatment they did. Their attitudes toward madness were no doubt important, along with the nature and severity of the victim's disorder.

When Hugh O'Neall became furiously insane in 1809, his family kept him "caged like a wild beast" until he suddenly recovered his reason four years later.[55] William Adamson's family confined him in a dark room for about two months in 1810 after extensive medical treatment failed to calm his mind. They subsequently placed him in the Pennsylvania Hospital under the care of Benjamin Rush. The family of Georgina Izard provided much different treatment. When she developed a "disorder in her head" around 1815, they placed her under medical treatment and took her on trips to Niagara Falls and Bordenton, New Jersey, to take the mineral waters.[56]

The husband of Mary Saxon strove to keep her life as normal as possible after she began to exhibit irrational behavior. She continued to see company, although often averse to doing so, and was given to irritability and fits of uncontrollable laughter. Her condition worsened, however, and her husband was advised that traveling might benefit her mind. Around 1811, he took her on a three-month journey through the upper country of the Carolinas, after which "her mind became more tranquil but not restored." She remained in this precarious condition for nine years, during which time she bore four children and continued to manage the household. In 1820, after spending several days and nights at the sick bed of one of her children, her mind became completely deranged. The family called in medical aid, but to no avail, and she remained insane and at home for nine more years before her husband took her to the newly opened state lunatic asylum in 1829. How she was treated during this latter period is unclear.[57]

If we know little about the treatment of the insane from affluent families, we know much less about the insane poor. Poor-law records seldom reveal anything specific about the condition of the insane poor on outdoor relief. A significant exception is the case of Mary Bonnell. Between 1766 and 1770, the parish of Prince Frederick, Winyah, boarded Bonnell out with several residents of the parish. In May 1770, the vestry placed her under the care of Thomas Nowland and his wife Lucretia, who agreed to board her for less money than her previous caretakers. A few months later, Mary suddenly died. The vestry, suspecting that the Nowlands had mistreated

Bonnell, called an inquest to determine the cause of her death. Two neighbors testified that on the morning of Mary's death, they had heard someone at the Nowlands crying out, "O lord, O lord, murder, murder" and heard Mrs. Nowland "Daming and Cursing." Another witness, the coffin maker, claimed that Bonnell appeared healthy and cheerful a few days before her death; when the Nowlands put her in the coffin, however, he had noticed bruises on her arms. The coffin maker's wife testified that she had also seen bruises on Bonnell's body. The Nowlands insisted that Mary had died suddenly after complaining of pains in her stomach and had injured herself falling against a post. The inquest jury learned little from viewing Bonnell's body, which had been buried for more than a month before they saw it. Despite obvious suspicions, they decided that Mary had probably died a natural death. Nevertheless, parish authorities removed two other paupers from the Nowlands' care and placed them with other citizens at a higher rate.[58]

It is impossible to generalize from a case like Mary Bonnell's about the condition of the insane poor under outdoor relief. The evidence even in her case is ambiguous and contradictory. The Nowlands may have mistreated her, but we should also remember that she survived boarding out for four years and that the coffin maker described her as well and hearty only a few days before her death. The reactions of her neighbors and the authorities to her death indicate that they did not take abuse of the insane for granted.

No other case in South Carolina's early poor-law records provides detail similar to Bonnell's. Evidence from the early nineteenth century, although more abundant, is usually vague. In 1822, the poor-law commissioners of Chester District reported that they were supporting six pauper lunatics. Of these, one had "to be confined with a chain"; another was "silly" but able and willing to work. The commissioners said nothing about the condition or care of the rest. South Carolina's poor-law officers, like those elsewhere, were anxious to maintain insane paupers as cheaply as possible. In 1826, Newberry District's commissioners of the poor were letting out their paupers, who included two insane persons, to the lowest bidder. But as the complexities of the Bonnell case indicate, one cannot conclude from this that the care of the insane poor was dictated by economic considerations alone. Moreover, expenditures and methods of caring for the poor varied considerably according to time and place. Robert Mills's survey of the care of the state's poor in 1826 revealed that Fairfield District spent about two hundred dollars a year to maintain about thirty paupers. A third that number cost Marion District about thirteen hundred dollars. Beaufort's commissioners drew a firm distinction between the able-bodied poor, who should be forced to work for their support, and the sick poor, who "should be nourished and comforted." Edgefield's commissioners reported that they had recently begun putting all paupers to work under the direction of a superintendent in an attempt to cut the poor tax.[59]

Few details survive concerning the care and treatment of the insane in Charleston's poorhouse. Antebellum records reveal that the poorhouse insane were given work if they were capable of it, and that may have been true in the eighteenth century as well. One source of the late 1760s states that persons sent to the Charleston madhouse received "straw and other necessaries suited to people in [such] deplorable circumstances" and implies that they amused themselves by making crowns of straw. But the description appears in a political work and seems more metaphorical than realistic.[60]

The poorhouse asylum impressed Abiel Abbot, a Yankee minister who visited Charleston in 1818. He praised its roominess and its garden, paved yards, promenades, and piazzas. He found the wards generally clean and remarked that the "cells" for the "maniacs" were "well contrived for solitude and the admission of sweet air." Some of the inmates were confined to their cells and "too hideous in their appearance to be subjects of investigation." But others were allowed to work or walk about in the paved yard, and Abbot was able to converse with them. One of the inmates he described was a Frenchwoman from St. Domingo "who improved her time, when more regular in mind, in the finest kind of needle work."[61]

Race as well as class influenced the fate of the insane. But the eighteenth-century sources are virtually silent regarding the care and treatment of insane blacks, most of whom were slaves. Economic calculation would suggest that to treat a slave well was to maximize his chances of recovering and returning to work, but slaveholders may not always have reasoned this way. That the law prohibited masters from casting out sick or disabled slaves indicates that economic calculation alone did not guarantee that an unproductive slave would be well cared for. Masters sometimes attributed "crazy" behavior to malingering or an unruly temperament and may have inflicted punishment instead of providing care.

The act of 1745, as we have seen, directed the parishes to assume the costs of maintaining insane slaves when their masters were unable to do so; but the law did not stipulate the nature of the slaves' care. It merely required the justices to confine the slave in a "convenient place," to protect the public and to ensure the slave's subsistence.[62] The number of slaves who came under this law was undoubtedly very small, and the surviving records do not reveal anything about them. Kate, the slave whose insanity prompted the act of 1745, disappeared from history immediately thereafter. In 1768, the St. Philip's vestry sent a slave named "Negroe Harry" to the "Madhouse." It is not clear if the members considered him insane or merely wanted to punish him for misbehavior. A few months later, the vestry ordered the churchwardens to prosecute Peter Johnson for mistreating Harry. Was Johnson Harry's keeper at the madhouse? We do not know. But Harry was not the last black to be sent to the madhouse. During the early nineteenth century many blacks joined whites in the poorhouse lunatic wards.[63]

What medical treatment, if any, did the insane receive for their disorder? Probably not much during the first decades of the colony's existence, at least not from the hands of regular practitioners. The first colonists frequently complained about a lack of medical men. But by the middle of the eighteenth century, the wealth, growing population, and tropical fevers of South Carolina had attracted a large corps of practitioners.[64] Their education and training varied greatly. A minority, clustered primarily in Charleston, were physicians in the European sense; that is, men with university educations. The majority of practitioners were surgeons and apothecaries trained by apprenticeship or people with no formal medical training. Some of them combined medicine with another occupation, such as farmer, minister, or shopkeeper.[65]

South Carolina's elite placed considerable faith in the benefits of regular medicine, for both themselves and their social inferiors. The wealthy regularly consulted physicians. Parish vestries frequently provided medical care for sick paupers. As early as 1733, the St. Philip's vestry began contracting with local physicians to care for the sick poor of Charleston, a practice the city's commissioners of the poor continued during the antebellum period.[66]

Masters also employed physicians to treat sick slaves. Two Charleston physicians were operating a slave hospital as early as 1749; similar institutions existed in the city from then until the Civil War.[67] In 1779, Rev. Alexander Hewett, who lived in South Carolina for many years, asserted that sick slaves received better medical care than the poorest laboring class in Europe.[68] Hardly a ringing endorsement, perhaps, but that many slave owners provided some form of medical care for their slaves admits of no doubt.

The elite's confidence in regular physicians meant that the insane—or some of them at least—received medical treatment for their malady. During the eighteenth century, insanity became increasingly medicalized. Medical men in Europe and America began to assume a dominant role in the care of the insane. Britain, as in so many other respects, was the model for American development. A growing number of medical men began to specialize in the care of the insane, and many of them published treatises on the subject. British philanthropists founded several hospitals for the insane between 1750 and 1800. In 1774, Parliament gave medical men the power to sign medical certificates of insanity and established a commission composed of physicians to inspect the numerous private asylums of the London metropolitan area. These developments coincided with increasing acceptance of the view that insanity was a physical disorder and curable if placed under medical treatment soon after its onset.[69]

The role of medical men in the treatment of insanity expanded in eighteenth-century America, too, although more slowly. The insane ward of the Pennsylvania Hospital (1751) provided a physician, as did the Virginia lunatic asylum at Williamsburg (1773); the founders of both institutions intended them to be curative rather than custodial institutions. Charleston's Fellowship Society's plans for a hospital envisaged placing the insane under the care of a physician.[70]

Given this environment, it is not surprising that many of the planter and merchant elite came to view insanity as a natural disorder within the reach of medicine.[71] In 1744, Charleston merchant Robert Pringle recorded that he had placed the melancholic Captain Bernard under the care of "the Best Physician in the Place and hope that in a Short time he may be Brought to the use of his Reason and Judgement."[72] The vestry of Prince Frederick Parish in the 1760s provided a physician for insane pauper Mary Bonnell in order to restore her "Senses."[73] When a Mrs. Campbell showed symptoms of hysteria in 1777, her family brought her to Dr. Charles Drayton for treatment.[74]

South Carolina's courts also promoted the view that insanity was curable through medical means. In 1813, Judge Thomas Waties rejected the petition of Hugh O'Neall's creditors that too much had been paid for his medical treatment. The judge ruled that the treatments were reasonable in cost, beneficial to the patient, and in the best interest of his creditors. O'Neall's recovery seemed "to be confidently expected," and the judge concluded that the creditors would have no difficulty in collecting their debts once he was able to return to work.[75]

References to medical treatment of the insane in early South Carolina rarely mention specific therapies. But the evidence indicates that South Carolina medical men normally employed the same remedies as their colleagues elsewhere. The standard medical treatment for insanity (as for most diseases) had been the same for centuries: bleeding, purging, and blistering, along with various drugs designed to sedate or stimulate. The rationale for these therapies and the extent of their use might vary considerably according to time, place, patient, and practitioner. For example, physicians might bleed a patient to combat inflammation, calm excitement, relieve congestion, or reduce pain and spasm. They might take a lot of blood or a little; purges might be drastic or mild.[76]

By the late seventeenth century European physicians were abandoning the ancient humoral theories that had originally justified these methods. But the change had only minor effects on eighteenth-century therapy. Whether practitioners accepted humoralism, a new medical system such as that of Edinburgh's William Cullen, or rejected systems in favor of empiricism, they tended to give their patients similar therapies.[77] Most physicians viewed disease as a state of bodily imbalance to be rectified by regulating and balancing the secretions. That does not mean that practice was uniform. Some eighteenth-century physicians relied more heavily than others on opiates and tonics, such as quinine and iron; others experimented with the new force of electricity. Some medical men bled or purged more freely than others. Lionel Chalmers, who practiced medicine in Charleston in the 1760s and 1770s, condemned routine bleeding and claimed that local medical men used the lancet too freely. But in other respects, Chalmers emphasized the typical remedies of the time.[78] Dr. David Ramsay criticized earlier physicians for routinely bleeding, purging, and sweating patients. But the practice of his own time, which he lauded as a great improvement, emphasized drastic bleeding and heavy use of mercury, antimony, and opium.[79]

Ramsay and his South Carolina colleagues probably bled and purged more often and more drastically than their predecessors, thanks to the influence of Dr. Benjamin Rush, physician to the Pennsylvania Hospital. A pupil of William Cullen, Rush developed a medical system of his own that argued that almost all diseases were due to one basic cause — vascular inflammation — and should be combatted with one basic therapy: decreasing inflammation through antiphlogistic (anti-inflammatory) methods. For Rush, this meant removing large quantities of blood and administering powerful cathartics such as calomel (a compound of mercury) and jalap.

Rush, the traditional "Father of American Psychiatry," employed this "heroic" therapeutic regime for a wide variety of disorders, including insanity. In his capacity as physician to the Pennsylvania Hospital, he treated many insane patients. He discussed his ideas about insanity at length in 1812 in his *Medical Inquiries and Observations upon the Diseases of the Mind*, the first American treatise on the subject. Rush, along with most medical men of the time, viewed mental disorders as physical in nature. Insanity, he argued, was essentially a chronic form of fever or inflammation of the blood vessels in the brain, and "the first remedy" in dealing with it was bloodletting. Rush advised the practitioner to remove more blood in cases of mania than in any other disease. At the first attack, the physician should take twenty to forty ounces, which would produce "wonderful" effects in "calming mad people." Repeated heavy bleeding should follow; Rush recalled that he had taken almost two hundred ounces of blood from one insane patient over a two-month period. Rush also recommended many other standard medical therapies for insanity, including blisters, purges, emetics, calomel, a low or spare diet, the cold bath or shower, solitude, and darkness in the early stages of the disease. These therapies had the same purpose as bleeding, to reduce vascular inflammation and calm the patient.[80]

Between the Revolution and the 1820s, Rush probably had more influence in America than any other physician. Many South Carolina physicians of this period trained under Rush at the University of Pennsylvania, and some of them enthusiastically adopted Rush's drastic therapeutics. Rush also secured a corps of devoted followers among the state's wealthy elite, many of whom summered and took their schooling in Philadelphia. An example is Alice Izard, wife of planter Ralph Izard, who became a devotee of Rushian therapies after he successfully treated her son for an ailment in 1809. South Carolina physicians sometimes consulted Rush in cases of insanity. William Adamson's doctors wrote Rush about his case, then followed the Philadelphia physician's therapeutic advice. Adamson was given two courses of calomel and bled copiously. His head was shaved, and he was blistered, given warm baths, and doused with cold water.[81]

Such drastic therapeutics were by no means universally accepted. Lay opposition to bloodletting is indicated by a rhyme in the *South Carolina Gazette* of 1775: "The People alarmed at such Proceeding, Resolve (tho in Fevers) not to be bleeding."[82] Some physicians also opposed heavy bleeding. In 1793, for example, a physician writing in the *Charleston City Gazette* applauded Rush's use of calomel and jalap but claimed that the city's climate "contra-indicated" the use of the lancet in many cases.[83]

Rush's ideas about insanity and its treatment were by no means the only ones available to American physicians of the time. Many European medical men of the eighteenth and early nineteenth centuries wrote treatises on the nature, causes, and treatment of mental disorders. Although most of these works recommended therapies similar to those of Rush, they often cautioned the physician to tailor his therapies to the condition and constitution of the patient as well as the particular form of mental disorder. Writers on melancholia, for example, invariably stressed the need to use gentle purges and to minimize the bleeding of patients in a weakened state.[84]

Regular practitioners, whatever their therapies, were not the only ones who treated the insane of early South Carolina. Many families lived in isolated rural areas, far from the nearest medical man. In contrast to Charleston, the wild backcountry attracted few doctors until after the Revolution. In 1768, Charles Woodmason complained about the lack of facilities for medical care in the backcountry: "How hard the Lot of any Gentleman in this Part of the World! No Physician — No Medicines — No Necessaries — Nurses, or Care in Sickness. If You are taken in any Disorder, there you must lye till Nature gets the better of the Disease, or Death relieves You."[85]

Physicians had become more plentiful in the state's interior by the beginning of the nineteenth century. But to secure regular medical care often remained difficult even for the wealthy. Manley Richardson, a planter who became insane in 1804, lived too far from any physician to obtain the constant attendance his family believed he required. Even in areas where physicians were plentiful, the sick might not be able to afford them. Some people refused, out of skepticism, to patronize the regulars.[86]

People who had no access to or faith in regular practitioners had other options. They could resort to self-medication, using folk remedies and prepared medications. As early as the 1730s, South Carolinians could purchase drugs and patent medicines imported from England such as Godfrey's Cordial, Daffy's Elixir, Hooper's Female Pills, and Lockyer's Pills. By midcentury, Charleston apothecaries sold these English patent remedies, as well as ready-made medicine chests for plantations. At the end of the eighteenth century, Ramsay claimed that the most enterprising planters kept such chests and maintained a sick house or hospital on their plantations. By then, Americans were producing their own patent remedies, some of which they used to treat nervous and mental disorders. In 1815, Alice Izard wrote that Hooper's Female Pills had cured the mental problems of a family friend and recommended that her daughter Georgina take them. Sounding like a twentieth-century advertisement, Izard touted the pills' convenience: "they will be so easily carried, and taken; the directions are sealed up with them."[87]

Families often had access to almanacs and domestic medical manuals containing advice on the treatment of many conditions. The authors of these works included physicians and nonphysicians. The most popular in the eighteenth century were English imports: John Wesley's *Primitive Physick* (1747) and Dr. William Buchan's *Domestic Medicine* (1769). After the Revolution, Americans began to produce manuals of their own. For many early Americans, far from regular medical help and often skeptical of orthodox practitioners, such manuals were a primary medical resource.[88]

Wesley's and Buchan's works provided remedies for mental as well as physical disorders. Wesley believed in witches, devils, and possession, but he recommended natural therapies for insanity. He counseled against both beating and blistering the mad. Most of his suggestions were simple, cheap, and relatively harmless compared to some of the cures advocated by regular physicians. They included the application of vinegar, herbal ointments, and cold water to the head, exercise, moderate diet, temperance, botanical remedies, and electricity. In cases of "Raging Madness," Wesley recommended shaving the patient's head and washing it with vinegar, placing the maniac under a waterfall for as long as he could bear it, or pouring cold water on his head out of a tea kettle. One of Wesley's therapies for mania was decidedly odd: eating nothing but apples for a month.[89]

Buchan, an English physician, discussed the causes, symptoms, and treatment of several "Nervous Diseases," among which he included "Melancholy," "Epilepsy," "Low Spirits," "Hysteric Affections," and "Hypochondriac Affections." Many of his remedies, like those of Wesley, were relatively moderate. For the milder nervous disorders such as hypochondriasis, Buchan stressed a regimen of exercise, fresh air, amusement, and a nourishing and easily digestible diet. He advised abstinence from heavy or fatty foods, spirits, tea, and coffee, and recommended consumption of fruits, vegetables, and grains. The medical therapies he mentioned included old standards such as bleeding, purges, cold baths, and counterirritants. In cases of melancholy, he argued, vomits should be "pretty strong." But most of the purgatives he mentioned were mild, and he cautioned that bleeding should be restricted to the more violent patients of strong constitutions and full pulse. For melancholy and hysteria, he recommended tonics of iron, quinine, and alcohol. Like many contemporary physicians, he recommended various "psychological" remedies for depressed patients, such as music, amusing company, games, travel, and sea voyages.[90]

Early South Carolinians could also turn to an array of irregular healers to cope with mental disorders. In the colonies as in England, a host of folk healers, faith healers, and quacks flourished in the eighteenth century, and their clients were not restricted to the ignorant. Because regular medicine could do little for many diseases, and promised much suffering in the bargain, many people patronized the irregulars as a first or last resort. The irregulars encompassed men and women, Europeans and Africans of a wide range of ability, education, and method. Many of them were illiterate, and few left much trace of their presence.[91]

Many irregulars adopted a form of medical practice only marginally different from that of the regulars. Others relied on herbal concoctions mixed with prayers, astrology, charms, or conjuring. Occasionally, they may also have tossed in a bit of advice about how to cope with life's difficulties. Folk healers of both races sometimes attributed illnesses, including madness, to demons or evil spells, which they tried to exorcise through touch, incantations, relics, and amulets. The religio-magical healing tradition had lost support among the educated elite by the eighteenth century, but it retained a strong attraction for many people into the nineteenth century and beyond.

Germans who settled the central parts of South Carolina in the 1750s brought a form of magical healing called "using," which involved rubbing and blowing upon the affected part of the body while repeating charms or incantations. "Mother" Mary Ingleman of Fairfield, an herbal practitioner of German extraction, was accused of witchcraft in 1792. Joshua Gordon, a reputed witch who lived in York County in the late eighteenth century, left a book of cures for a few common physical ailments, as well as advice on how to combat spells. Black folk healers drew on African traditions for remedies, both natural and supernatural. Planters sometimes employed the services of black healers, who treated whites as well as blacks. In 1754, a free black advertised his services as "Doct. Caesar" in the *South Carolina Gazette*, and the following year the colonial assembly awarded "Negro Sampson" his freedom for revealing his cure for rattlesnake bite. In 1797, a notice in the *Charleston City Gazette* described a runaway slave who practiced medicine in town.[92]

Magic aside, medical treatment was not the only possible therapy for the insane. A number of eighteenth-century medical treatises and manuals recommended psychological therapies for some forms of mental disorder, especially those that might seem to derive from emotional causes such as grief, anxiety, fear, or disappointed love. Buchan is an example, but he was drawing on a tradition that in some respects derived from the ancients: exercise, amusement, music, and so forth might calm the anxious mind.

During the later eighteenth century, a few Europeans specializing in the care of the insane developed a more structured form of psychological therapy: moral treatment (or moral management, as its early advocates often called it). Moral treatment was grounded, in large part, on an acceptance of Locke's definition of madness as a matter of faulty reasoning or false associations. Locke's environmentalist approach encouraged the view that the insane were not submerged in total mental darkness or bestiality. They retained varying degrees of reason, a sense of justice, and a concern with their condition, which careful nurturing could employ as a means of cure. They were like children who needed to be reeducated and encouraged to reestablish their self-control. The key was to break the chain of false associations and reestablish right reasoning. Practitioners of moral treatment aimed to accomplish this through techniques designed to divert the patient's mind from its delusions. These included recreations and amusements, a system of rewards and punishments, and classification and separation of patients by sex, class, and type of disorder.

During the nineteenth century, moral treatment became synonymous in many people's minds with kind and humane treatment, but originally it meant much more than that. The early practitioners of moral treatment generally condemned the idea of beating, chaining, and starving the insane into submission. But they did not abandon all means of coercion, because they believed that a cure depended upon the therapist achieving control over the patient. Control could be accomplished in various ways: by sheer charisma on the part of the practitioner; by appeals to the patient's sense of proper behavior; by granting or revoking privileges; and, failing all else, by intimidation, isolation, or mechanical restraints such as straitjackets or muffs. Above all, practitioners of moral treatment agreed that to succeed, it required the separation of the patient from the environment that had helped precipitate his disorder. To break the chain of false associations, he had to be removed from the familiar surroundings of home and family and confined in an establishment dominated by the father figure of the moral therapist. Moral treatment thus promoted the idea that curing the insane required institutionalization.[93]

Moral treatment was an eighteenth-century development. But before the early nineteenth century its impact on the situation of the insane was limited to the inhabitants of a few European asylums. Shortly after 1800, however, Americans began to discover moral treatment. In 1806, Philippe Pinel's *Treatise on Insanity*, which described the successes of moral treatment in two Parisian hospitals, appeared in English translation. A few years later, Samuel Tuke published *A Description of the Retreat* (1813). Tuke discussed the employment of moral methods at the Quaker institution near York, England, which his grandfather, tea merchant William Tuke, had opened in 1796.[94] These two works soon became accepted as the classical accounts of moral therapy, and contemporaries credited Pinel and the Tukes (somewhat inaccurately) as the inventors of a new approach toward the treatment of the insane.

By the second decade of the nineteenth century, moral treatment had emerged as an important part of a new approach to insanity in the United States and Europe. Benjamin Rush adopted some aspects of moral treatment even before the works of Pinel and Tuke appeared. As early as 1798, Rush asked the managers of the Pennsylvania Hospital to provide a variety of employments for insane patients capable of it. By 1810, he was promoting reforms at the hospital that incorporated much of the ideology and methodology of moral therapy: employment, amusement, classification of patients by sex and type of disorder, comfortable accommodations, and restrictions on visitors. He also discussed moral remedies in his treatise on insanity.[95]

The work of Pinel, the Tukes, Rush, and others helped convince many philanthropic Americans that asylums based on the principles of moral treatment could cure many of the insane. American Quakers influenced by the Tukes opened the Frankford Retreat near Philadelphia in 1817. The Quaker philanthropist Thomas Eddy played a major role in establishing Bloomingdale Asylum as a separate department of the New York Hospital in 1821. Charitable asylums were soon being built in Boston and Hartford.[96]

But knowledge of moral treatment and the new, more optimistic outlook on insanity was not restricted to northern philanthropists. It was quickly absorbed by some members of South Carolina's elite. When Rush died in 1813, one of his many South Carolina pupils, David Ramsay, eulogized him for having "improved the theory and practical treatment of madness."[97] Around 1810, a few wealthy South Carolina families began to send their insane relatives to the Pennsylvania Hospital for treatment. It was a logical choice, as many planting families summered in Philadelphia and knew Rush. But some of the state's citizens desired something more: an asylum, based on the principles of moral treatment, within South Carolina. In 1815, Alice Izard, whose daughter Georgina was suffering from some form of mental disorder, wrote that she had just "read, with great pleasure, the account of the establishment at York, in England, for insane Quakers." Mrs. Izard added that she hoped that an institution similar to the York Retreat could be founded in each of the American states.[98]

By the time Izard wrote, a small but influential band of South Carolinians shared her wish and had begun a movement to bring it about. In 1821 they convinced the state legislature to establish a lunatic asylum based on the principles of moral treatment. To recreate the ambience of the York Retreat in the markedly different environment of antebellum South Carolina, however, would prove a daunting task.

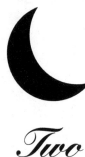

Two

A PROPITIOUS MOMENT

FOUNDING THE ASYLUM

The original building of the South Carolina Lunatic Asylum, constructed between 1822 and 1827, still stands on the grounds of the present state hospital in Columbia. A national historic landmark named for its architect Robert Mills, it was recently converted into a state office building. Until a few years ago, the Mills Building housed a small museum illustrating the history of the state hospital. On the walls of the museum, side by side, hung the portraits of the two men tradition credits as the founders of the asylum — Samuel Farrow and William Crafts. All contemporary and later accounts of the South Carolina Lunatic Asylum's founding agree on the central role of Farrow and Crafts, and there is no reason to doubt them.[1]

But the traditional accounts are somewhat misleading in that they present the asylum's founding as a simple struggle of two enlightened and determined men over ignorance and lethargy. In reality, Farrow and Crafts were only the most visible of a larger group of reformers whose efforts were first aided, then nearly aborted by the state's rollercoaster political and economic fortunes between 1815 and the 1830s. This is not to imply that the campaign for a state lunatic asylum in South Carolina was in any sense a popular crusade. It attracted little attention in the press or in other public forums outside the state legislature. Public demand for a state prison was far greater than for an asylum; yet South Carolina did not build a penitentiary until the late 1860s. But neither was the asylum the outcome of a two-man movement.

As in many other states and in Europe, asylum reform in South Carolina was the work of an elite but diverse coalition of physicians, educators, lawyers, legislators, and social activists. Many of them were active in other philanthropic and reformist endeavors. They shared the general enthusiasm for improvement that characterized much of the antebellum period, and their reforming activity was motivated in part by a desire to enhance the state's reputation for public benevolence. They were aware of the new ideas of moral treatment, and they wanted to put South Carolina in the forefront of efforts to ameliorate the condition of the insane. The South Carolina Lunatic Asylum was as much an expression of civic pride as of humanitarian, medical, or social-control arguments.[2]

Farrow and Crafts were typical of this reforming group. The story of their collaboration provides one of those inspiring tales that public-spirited citizens love to relate. They presented, moreover, an intriguing study in contrast. Except for the fact that both were lawyers and legislators, they had little in common. Colonel Samuel Farrow of Spartanburg was a crusty veteran of the Revolutionary War who had come to South Carolina from Virginia in the 1760s. His face still bore a prominent scar inflicted by a British sword.[3] In the postrevolutionary years he became a Republican and a strong supporter of the War of 1812. After serving as lieutenant governor (1810–12) he was elected to the U.S. Congress. According to tradition, he gave up his seat in 1815 to enter the South Carolina House of Representatives and work for the establishment of a state asylum.

Like most early settlers of the upcountry, Farrow was a rough-hewn character with little formal education; but his contemporaries respected him for his energy and determination. John Belton O'Neall, who served with Farrow at the bar and in the legislature, remembered him as the most "zealous and indefatigable" member he had ever seen. Farrow's lack of education often showed in his speech, O'Neall recalled, but "when one looked upon his face, and saw the scar, inflicted by the wound of the enemy, his incorrectness of speech was quickly forgotten, and his auditors were irresistibly borne to his conclusion."[4] In the case of the asylum, however, it seemed that Farrow's persuasiveness and persistence would not be enough. For more than a decade his pleas for such an institution merely earned him a reputation as a monomaniac "who ought to be the first inmate."[5]

Farrow's cofounder, William Crafts Jr., was a younger and more polished man. Born in 1787, he was the son of a Boston merchant who had settled in

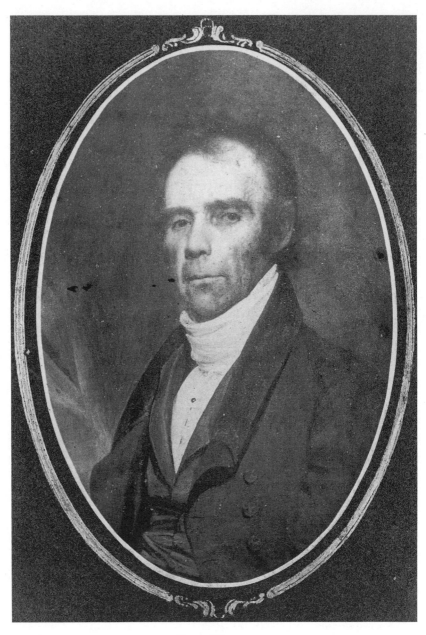

Samuel Farrow.
(Courtesy South Caroliniana Library, University of South Carolina)

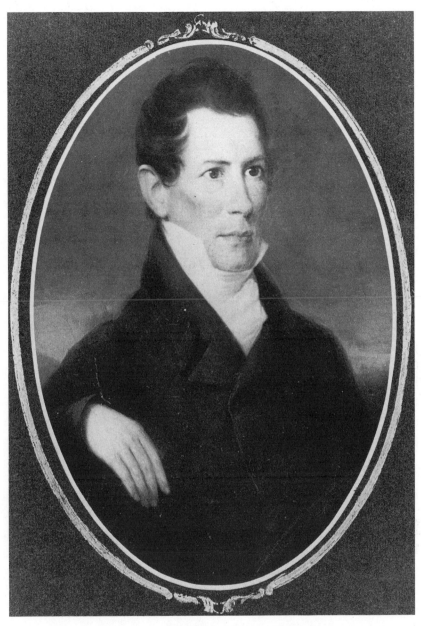

William Crafts Jr.
(Courtesy South Caroliniana Library, University of South Carolina)

Charleston at the end of the Revolutionary War and amassed a considerable fortune. Crafts received a good classical education and went on to Harvard, where he graduated with distinction. Returning to Charleston, he quickly achieved local prominence as a writer and orator. He was elected to the state legislature several times, but his attempt to get elected to Congress in 1816 was rebuffed. Some contemporaries attributed his lack of major political success to indolence bred by early and easy triumphs. Others complained that he wasted too much energy on unattainable political and literary goals. Crafts's ambitions were probably also hindered by being the son of a Boston merchant and a Federalist who opposed the War of 1812. His politics put him in opposition to the dominant Republican and prowar sentiment in South Carolina, and his mercantile origins may have reduced his influence among the low-country aristocracy. Despite the fact that their fathers had often been merchants, the great planters of the early nineteenth century tended to look down on the men of the countinghouses.[6]

Yet Crafts played a significant role in the history of several reform movements in South Carolina. He helped Catholics and Jews to expand their rights, and he supported the successful campaign to establish the Medical College of South Carolina. In 1813 he delivered what many contemporaries considered his greatest speech in a successful effort to prevent the abolition of the new system of free schools. He was also a strong advocate of education for the deaf and dumb. Indeed, it was apparently his desire to establish a state school for the deaf and dumb that brought him into alliance with supporters of a state lunatic asylum sometime around 1821.[7]

That the asylum movement succeeded in South Carolina when it did was due in large part to a momentarily favorable political and economic environment. Politically, it benefited from the decline of sectional antagonism within the state. Since late colonial times, the men of Farrow's upcountry had accused the low-country elite of trying to monopolize the power and wealth of the state. The men of Craft's low country, meanwhile, tended to view the inhabitants of the upcountry as a pack of ignorant and uncouth backwoodsmen unfit to govern. By the early nineteenth century, however, this antagonism was moderating as the result of political compromise and the spread of a plantation economy to the upcountry.[8]

Broader political and economic conditions influenced the timing of the asylum's creation. Farrow began his movement at a time when the state and nation were divided and preoccupied by the conflict with Great Britain that culminated in the War of 1812. One contemporary account notes that Farrow's attempts to gain support for an asylum during this period failed because the "country required all its monied resources in resisting a powerful enemy." [9] The war and the embargo that preceded it also produced economic distress for many of South Carolina's planters and increased their reluctance to embark on costly public projects.

After the war, however, the political and economic climate was much more favorable to public spending. The animosities and party divisions of the previous decade gave way to a short period of relative political calm marked by the absence of distinct party divisions. Economically, the state enjoyed the effects of an equally brief boom in the prices of cotton and rice. Momentarily at least, the general outlook of the state's leaders was expansionist and optimistic. With surpluses piling up in the state treasury, many legislators became infected with enthusiasm for projects and reforms they believed would enhance South Carolina's economic fortunes and her reputation for progress and benevolence. In 1817 the legislature embarked on an ambitious scheme of internal improvements and public works, including roads, canals, and buildings. A year later, legislators appropriated one million dollars for these purposes to be spent over a four-year period. [10]

This short era of euphoria and freewheeling spending gave birth to the South Carolina Lunatic Asylum. Legislators who a few years earlier or later would have balked at the expense were willing to fund a novel experiment in state benevolence. In the session of 1818 the state house of representatives yielded to Farrow's persistence and appointed a special committee to investigate the situation of the insane. The committee, chaired by Farrow, reported that the state contained many lunatics who needed the protection and care of an asylum and recommended that the legislature fund one. With little dissent, the general assembly passed a series of resolutions calling for the construction of a state asylum to be located in Columbia. Legislators chose the state capital because its central location would help draw patients from all over the state, and because they could inspect it during their annual sessions. The resolutions directed the state engineer, John Lyde Wilson, to prepare an economical plan for such an establishment and present it to the next session of the assembly. [11]

In 1819, Wilson submitted two sets of plans based on works and reports about European and American asylums. But when Farrow brought in a bill to establish an asylum, the state house of representatives rejected it by a large majority. The reason for the sudden change in legislative sentiment was almost certainly economic. The financial panic of 1819 had led to a sudden drop in cotton prices, severe deflation, numerous bankruptcies and foreclosures, and a deficit in the state treasury. One result was a loss of enthusiasm for public projects, particularly in the upcountry, where the depression was most severe. [12] More than two-thirds of the upcountry legislators voted against the bill, as opposed to just over half of those from the low country. Following the failure of Farrow's bill, the Charleston-dominated Medical Society of South Carolina established a committee to study the feasibility of establishing a lunatic asylum in or near their city. But nothing came of this idea.[13]

The asylum proposal was not revived in the legislature until 1821. Farrow lost his South Carolina house seat in 1820. Crafts failed in attempts to get elected to the state senate in 1819 and 1820.[14] Farrow was still absent from the legislature when it assembled in 1821, but Crafts gained a seat in the senate in a by-election. He quickly succeeded in convincing the legislature to pass a bill to establish a lunatic asylum and a school for the deaf and dumb. In a few days he achieved the goal that had eluded Farrow for years. A contemporary ascribed Crafts's triumph to sheer oratorical ability: "In a propitious moment, William Crafts . . . carried captive to his eloquence the hearts and minds of the legislators. With zeal and earnestness they addressed themselves to the work of love and mercy, and our Asylum arose."[15]

It was indeed "a propitious moment." For a brief time, antipathy to public projects had eased, as it seemed that the state was recovering from the effects of the Panic of 1819. But the South Carolina economy soon turned down again and remained depressed into the early 1830s. During these years, opposition to spending for public works became increasingly intense. Had Crafts failed in 1821, South Carolina might not have constructed an asylum until many years later.[16]

Yet the efforts of Farrow and Crafts might have been in vain had their cause not attracted the energetic support of a small but influential group of like-minded reformers. Even before the act establishing the asylum passed, the political and economic climate in South Carolina was turning against the project. Building the asylum and bringing it into operation proved a drawn-out and troublesome process; seven years elapsed between the act of 1821 and the admission of the first patient to the state asylum. Because Farrow died in 1824 and Crafts, who had been ill for some time, died in 1826, others bore the burden of accomplishing this work.

Perhaps no one did more to see the asylum to completion than Dr. James Davis, a prominent Columbia physician. Davis, who came to upper South Carolina from Maryland in 1774 while still a boy, had trained as a physician under the apprenticeship method. After serving as a state senator from Union District between 1804 and 1808, he moved to Columbia and achieved local eminence as a doctor and a public-spirited citizen. Like Farrow, Davis had a reputation for sternness, energy, and persistence, qualities he needed to prevent the asylum project from being abandoned during the troubled economic and political climate of the 1820s. He supported Farrow's campaign for an asylum prior to the act of 1821, served on the commission that oversaw the construction of the asylum and the board of trustees that brought it into operation, and became the first visiting physician in 1828. Daniel Trezevant, who succeeded him as physician, asserted that Davis ought to share equal honors with Farrow and Crafts as a founder of the asylum. Davis's obituary claimed that the institution "owed its origin, its completion, and its final organization, to his benevolent, untiring efforts."[17]

Davis was one of several Columbians who supported the establishment of a state asylum. Another was the man who Mrs. Anne Royall claimed was "at the head of everything in South Carolina," Thomas Cooper. A native of England, Cooper came to South Carolina from Pennsylvania in 1819, only two years before the asylum was founded. But he quickly achieved a dominant if controversial position in the state's intellectual and political arena. He came to Columbia to serve as professor of chemistry at South Carolina College. Within a few months he was the college's acting and then permanent president. Soon after he arrived, he initiated a successful campaign to establish a medical college in the state and became involved in the movement to establish an asylum.

Cooper came to South Carolina as an advocate of public asylums. In 1819 he published *Tracts on Medical Jurisprudence*, a volume of English works to which he added his own notes and a digest on the law of insanity. In this work, he castigated the private madhouses of his native England as a danger to individual liberty, noted that America had the good fortune not to have any, and expressed the hope that the states would build enough public asylums to render private ones unnecessary. He served on the asylum's board of trustees from 1822 to 1828 and briefly as a member of its governing board of regents. Several members of Cooper's circle supported the asylum movement, including D. J. McCord and E. W. Johnstone, who served as editors of the influential *Columbia Telescope*; Robert Henry, a professor and future president of South Carolina College; and William C. Preston, a prominent lawyer and politician who was a trustee of the college.[18] Other Columbians involved in the early history of the asylum included Abram Blanding, the state superintendent of Public Works, and several physicians, lawyers, and planters.[19]

Outside this "Columbia connection," the supporters of the asylum are more difficult to identify. The official positions that indicate involvement in the movement, seats on the various asylum commissions and boards, were dominated by Columbians, because of their proximity to the institution. John Blake White, a Charleston artist and writer, served on the 1818 committee that recommended the erection of an asylum and the following year was among the minority who voted for Farrow's bill. White was typical of many early-nineteenth-century asylum promoters in that he supported many reform movements. He opposed capital punishment, advocated a state penitentiary, and promoted the temperance movement.[20] Two governors during the 1820s also strongly supported the asylum: John L. Wilson and Richard I. Manning. Wilson, a Georgetown planter, submitted the first plans for an asylum in 1819, when he was state engineer. The legislature named him to the asylum commission in 1821, and he remained on it until the end of his governorship in December 1824. During the next few years, he continued to plead the cause of the institution in the state senate. Richard Manning of Clarendon staunchly defended the project during his governorship (1824–26), at a time when the legislature seemed ready to abandon it.[21]

The asylum reformers in South Carolina resembled those elsewhere in that they tended to be involved in other social-reform movements, especially education. Nearly all of them were connected as teachers or trustees with an educational establishment or were proponents of some educational movement. So many of them were professors or trustees of South Carolina College that the asylum must have seemed just another branch of that institution. Several were active in the campaign to establish a state medical college or were strong defenders of the free schools. Crafts supported both these movements and a school for the deaf and dumb.

There was a natural connection between the promotion of schools and the promotion of asylums. Much of the impetus for founding an asylum derived from an enthusiasm for moral treatment, which was in essence a method of reeducation. Crafts expressed this connection in his speech at the laying of the cornerstone of the asylum: "The beauty of reason is to propagate itself. The honour of States is to disseminate knowledge. [If education be important] to the Philanthropist, does not as strong an inducement exist to aid by public care and exertion, the *recovery* of reason, as to cultivate it where it exists?"[22]

Most South Carolina asylum promoters shared these beliefs. But many of their fellow citizens did not. Not only were the reformers more "progressive" than most citizens of the state in their ideas about insanity and its treatment, they were also more enthusiastic about the role of the state in dealing with social problems. South Carolina's asylum reformers, like those elsewhere, envisaged government as a paternalistic, positive force that elites could use to both aid and mold the citizenry. The preamble to the report of 1818 recommending a state asylum, plagiarized from the British physician James Currie, would probably satisfy the most zealous advocate of the interventionist state: "Man demands our constant attention. To inform [men's] minds, to repress their vices, to assist their labours, to invigorate their activity, and to improve their comforts—those are the noblest offices of enlightened minds in superior stations."[23]

In common with many northern antebellum reformers, Crafts viewed the state in an almost millennial, perfectionist light. The establishment of a state asylum, he proclaimed, was an act that assured "every individual among us of the guardian sympathy of the State" and showed that "South Carolina tenders to the children of misfortune." The present age was marked by "a growing sense of the necessity of adapting the administration of government to the public good." Through this means, "the amelioration of Society" would progress until the evils that afflicted it gradually disappeared and the earth returned to "the period of its early and original innocence."[24]

The majority of South Carolina's leaders and citizens may not have fully accepted this expansive view of the state's role. But the heady prosperity of the post–War of 1812 era encouraged assent to appeals to public benevolence. So did the current vogue of republican virtue, with its emphasis on civic responsibility, and the evangelical revival, which underlay so many antebellum reform movements. The asylum reformers skillfully blended their arguments to appeal to these sentiments. Farrow's committee proclaimed that it was their duty "as politicians and Christians" to ameliorate the condition of the helpless insane. According to Crafts, God placed man on earth to be happy. But man could achieve happiness only through virtue, and the test of virtue lay in benevolence, "the basis of God's throne." Of all our fellow creatures, Crafts argued, none were more deserving of benevolence than those who had lost their reason. Without reason, which he defined as "the consciousness of the spirit of God," virtuous action— and therefore happiness—was impossible. To assist a lunatic to recover his reason was to "revive in him the knowledge of the blessings of God." Crafts also appealed to the civic patriotism of the people of South Carolina, and to their concern for the reputation of the state abroad: "And may not one State, in the wisdom of its laws, and the purity of its institutions, the liberality of its endowments, its sense of honor and its dread of shame, generously strive to outshine its neighbors?"[25]

The reformers made many such appeals to civic pride during the period of the asylum's construction. Yet they failed to achieve a consensus of public support for their goals. Looking back from 1842, Daniel Trezevant, the asylum's second visiting physician, lamented that the institution had never been popular. He traced the asylum's low public image to the period when the establishment was under construction. Those responsible for the planning and building of the asylum, he alleged, had "grossly deceived" the legislature about its costs and wasted state appropriations. By the time it was completed, legislators had become so "thoroughly disgusted" that it had become "a reproach, and its friends hardly dared advocate it." Growing legislative antipathy toward the project prevented the institution's officials from securing sufficient money to outfit it properly for the care and treatment of its patients. The rhetoric and actions of the legislature in turn influenced public opinion, which for long thereafter viewed the asylum with distrust.[26]

Trezevant's analysis was generally accurate. The construction of the asylum involved mistakes, waste, and perhaps even deception; certainly many legislators believed so, and their views influenced public perception of the institution and contributed to its later problems. But the problems were due to more than the blunders of its founders. The state's leaders held markedly different views about the nature and functions (and in some cases, the necessity) of a lunatic asylum. Similar difficulties affected all the pioneering public asylums of the period. But they were exacerbated in the case of South Carolina by the severe economic and political crisis through which the state passed in the 1820s.

In 1821 no one foresaw how troublesome, costly, or drawn out the construction of an asylum would turn out to be. The commissioners appointed to superintend the asylum's construction moved quickly to purchase a four-acre site just outside the Columbia city limits, procure plans, and begin building.[27] Already they had altered their aims in one respect. The act of 1821 authorized the building of two institutions: an asylum and a school for the deaf and dumb. But they decided to build only an asylum. Probably they realized that the thirty thousand dollars appropriated by the general assembly was insufficient to build one, let alone both, structures.[28]

The commissioners sought to incorporate recent ideas about the care of the insane into the design of the asylum. They appointed a committee to gather information on lunatic asylums in Europe and the United States. They also sent the superintendent of construction, Benjamin Williams, to visit the new asylums in New York, Connecticut, and Philadelphia. The commissioners considered several asylum plans and selected that presented by the new state engineer, Robert Mills (who later became one of antebellum America's most renowned architects). The Mills design, they claimed, was preferable to the others because it could easily be extended "without detriment to the proportions and symmetry" and because it appeared "to embrace the principal improvements of the experience of modern times in Europe and in this Country." Moreover, because Mills was on the spot it would be easy to confer with him when problems arose. The other plans presented, the commissioners added, were more extensive and would cost more than the general assembly had appropriated.[29]

Ironically, by the time the commissioners reported this decision to the legislature in December 1822, they had already decided to make several changes in the original design that, together with other factors, were to send the cost of the asylum far beyond the original estimate. The changes, recommended by Mills, involved erecting a ten-foot wall around the structure, constructing some outbuildings, and rendering the asylum fireproof. Mills had already introduced the principle of fireproof construction in another building he had designed, the Records Office in Charleston, and it was a perfectly sensible alteration for an institution such as an asylum. By adding such changes after his design had been selected, however, Mills laid himself and the commissioners open to charges of deception and incompetence.[30]

Mills designed a handsome neoclassical structure with wings receding at an oblique angle from a central block. He intended the wings, when extended, to eventually enclose a semicircular garden in the rear of the building. The design also envisaged courtyards with gardens on the roof and an extensive garden in front of the structure. Mills's plan was influenced by British architectural innovations in the treatment of the insane, particularly those advocated by Samuel Tuke of the York Retreat. The asylum incorporated many of Tuke's suggestions concerning window frames, heating, corridors, bedrooms, and day rooms.[31]

Initially, construction of the asylum progressed quickly. The cornerstone was laid in July 1822, and several months later a legislative committee predicted that the asylum would be opened for patients within a year. At the same time, however, they noted that changes in the original design would require an additional appropriation of $16,500. They recommended granting the money on the grounds that the changes would make the building safer and more convenient than the original design. The legislature assented, believing that the structure was nearly complete and no more state funds would be required. When the general assembly reassembled in 1823, however, the asylum was not finished. The commissioners explained that the work had been slowed by "unavoidable interruptions" and promised that it would be completed within six months. They asked for and received another $5,000.[32]

Each year, until 1827, the legislature heard the same refrain: explanations

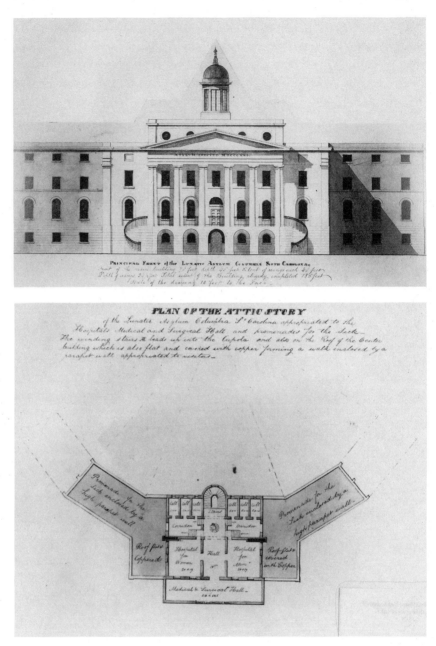

Two views from Robert Mills's plans for the South Carolina Lunatic Asylum, 1822.
(Courtesy South Carolina Department of Archives and History)

as to why the asylum was not quite finished, promises that it soon would be, and requests for additional appropriations. Many legislators concluded that the asylum's promoters had first deceived them by low estimates and then mismanaged the building's construction.[33] Their frustration and disenchantment with the project is evident in the report of a legislative committee that the institution was finally completed:

> [We] waive all discussion upon the wisdom and propriety of the act establishing this institution, as well as all remarks upon the frequent and mortifying disappointments of successive legislatures, when instead of finding the buildings finished as they had so often been assured they would have been, they saw little more than a beginning had been made, and that they were literally in the awkward dilemma of having stepped in so far that to recede was as bad as to go on.[34]

The commissioners were undoubtedly guilty of poor judgment and some mismanagement. Whether they engaged in deliberate deception is less clear. Like many reformers, they may have been oversanguine about the difficulties they faced and the ultimate prospects of the institution they were championing. They often underestimated costs, but, they claimed, they were relying on estimates provided by Mills and the contractors. In one of their reports the commissioners claimed that they had to ask for an additional appropriation because "Mr. Mills . . . again erred in his calculations."[35] The erroneous estimates were probably due less to incompetence than to circumstances beyond anyone's control. The sheer number of public projects the state and federal governments had embarked on in the 1820s created scarcities of labor and materials, which led to numerous delays and unanticipated increases in costs. On one occasion the work was stopped because of difficulty in procuring copper for the roof; on another by an epidemic among the workers. More generally, the commissioners found it difficult to keep skilled workers on the job simply because so many others were competing for their services. The legislature itself increased the commissioners' problems through its own attempts to retrench. They had engaged Mills as architect partly because as state engineer his services would be free. But in December 1823 the legislature abolished the position of state engineer as an economy measure, and from then on the commissioners had to pay Mills a fee of five hundred dollars a year to complete the project.[36]

Faced with such difficulties and desiring to keep the work going, the commissioners sometimes acted in legally and fiscally questionable ways. When their appropriation for 1824 was expended, they borrowed money from a local bank and convinced the workers to keep working without pay by promising them that the state would reimburse them when the legislature met. Because the commissioners had no legal authority to contract such debts, their actions annoyed many legislators.[37] Responsibility for the commissioners' questionable financial practices probably lay with Governor John L. Wilson. A staunch advocate of an asylum since 1818, Wilson had an unfortunate reputation for carelessness with public money which probably increased legislative suspicions of the asylum project. His disinclination to attend to the drudgery of fiscal details led to charges of corruption after he left the governorship in 1824. Two years later, he was nearly impeached as a judge for refusing to account for his use of the contingency fund while governor. Wilson was also an intimidating man who was involved in a number of duels; his formidable personality may have made enemies for the asylum.[38]

By the mid-1820s many legislators were running out of patience with the slow pace and mounting costs of construction. At the same time, wider political and economic concerns distracted legislators and contributed to the growing frustration. Politically, the state's leaders were becoming increasingly distracted by the issues of slavery and states rights. The Missouri Debates over slavery in Congress, the Denmark Vesey conspiracy in Charleston, and the beginnings of an abolitionist movement raised anxieties over the "peculiar institution" to levels never before reached. Simultaneously, the Tariff of 1824 and the growing federal program of internal improvements aroused fears of a powerful central government that might be used to advance northern interests at the expense of the South, even to the extent of abolishing slavery. From the mid-1820s to the mid-1830s the South Carolina legislature was often preoccupied with such issues to the detriment of domestic concerns such as the asylum.[39]

The political crisis was exacerbated if not largely created by a severe economic crisis. Despite a general drop in the cost of living during the decade, the price of the state's agricultural products, especially short-staple cotton, was dropping faster. Many upcountry planters, who specialized in the short staple, became impoverished. The surpluses in the state treasury, which had produced enthusiasm for public projects, gave way to deficits and a movement for retrenchment. This movement, dominated by upcountry legislators, succeeded in reducing state expenditures for public projects such as roads, canals, and public buildings.[40]

These political and economic conditions made it increasingly difficult for the asylum's advocates to secure the funds they believed they needed to complete the structure properly. By the end of 1824, opposition to the mounting costs of the asylum had increased to the point that the general assembly voted only nineteen thousand of the forth thousand dollars the commissioners had requested. The following year the legislature refused to appropriate anything for the asylum, and by the beginning of 1826, if not before, the work had come to a halt. The *Charleston Courier*, a staunch supporter of the project, blasted the "miserable parsimony" of legislators who had stopped the progress of the building when it was nearly completed and turned it into a "monument of prodigal penury, and a scandal to the State."[41]

By the end of 1826 the prospect of securing sufficient state funds to complete the asylum seemed so unlikely that one legislator proposed that the structure should be sold or leased to private individuals who would agree to finish it and apply it to its original purpose. The Committee on Public Buildings rejected such a proposal as dishonorable to the state but declared that the design of the asylum was unnecessarily extravagant. They recommended that new commissioners be appointed to complete the building according to a more economical plan.[42]

The supporters of the asylum countered legislative opposition with a variety of arguments. The most obvious by the mid-1820s was that the state had already invested so much in the institution that it would be foolish to leave it unfinished. The reformers also appealed to the sense of honor and local patriotism of the state's leaders. To fail to complete the institution properly would tarnish the state's reputation for benevolence and liberality. Governor Wilson pleaded that he wished to "see the land of my nativity unsurpassed in all these acts which are calculated to shed a lustre upon our history. . . . [T]he pages will not be full, unless we are recognized as the friends of human misery."[43]

Advocates of the asylum also claimed that it was a masterpiece perfectly adapted to its purposes; elegant, yet inexpensive compared to others of its kind. Governor Manning declared that those who had examined it, including many visitors from other states and nations, had proclaimed it to be one of the finest such buildings in the United States. Indeed, several travel accounts of the period praised the architecture and conveniences of the structure and called it "magnificent," "splendid," "handsome," and "superior to anything of the kind."[44]

The asylum reformers' arguments prevailed, up to a point. At the end of 1827, the legislature heeded their plea to finish this "experiment in the cause of humanity" and provided funds to prepare the asylum for the reception of patients.[45] But the reformers' triumph was far from complete. The institution that opened the following year lacked facilities its backers considered necessary to proper treatment of the insane, particularly those designed for the occupation and amusement of the patients. Many legislators, who did not understand or accept the principles of moral treatment, considered such things frills rather than necessities.

The disagreement over the issue of facilities reflected a wider divergence of opinion among the state's leaders over the nature and functions of an asylum for the insane. From the beginning of the asylum campaign there was controversy and uncertainty over the number of patients who needed to be provided for, what type of patients should be served, and what kind of care the asylum should offer.

When Samuel Farrow's special committee reported in 1818, it claimed that "according to the best information," there were "a great many lunatics" in South Carolina who needed the care and protection of an asylum. The committee did not provide any statistics or sources for their statements, however, and some legislators were not convinced that the number of insane in the state justified the expense of erecting a lunatic asylum. The act authorizing the asylum required the local commissioners of the poor to report the number of lunatics in their districts. The results of this survey seemed to support the skeptics. The commissioners' returns reported only fifty-five lunatics and idiots. This number was embarrassingly small, as the asylum commissioners had by that time already commenced a building designed for eighty to one hundred inmates. A legislative committee favorable to the asylum noted, however, that several districts had not sent in returns, and predicted that when the others reported, the number of the insane would probably exceed one hundred. But the small number of insane reported undoubtedly confirmed legislators' fears that the asylum might have difficulty finding tenants.[46]

The reformers' conflicts with the legislature were exacerbated by disagreements over the functions of the asylum. From the first, the reformers desired to create a multiclass institution that would admit anyone who needed its services. (Any white person at least; the care of the black insane did not become an issue until after the asylum opened.) As Farrow's committee put it in 1818, an asylum should "provide accommodation for the poor suitable to their circumstances, and . . . make provision for those of a superior station who are able to remunerate the expense."[47] In his oration on the laying of the asylum's cornerstone, William Crafts addressed his well-to-do audience in terms that made it clear that he expected the institution to benefit people of their station. The establishment of a lunatic asylum, he emphasized, "tells you, that if your relative be unhappily bereaved of reason you shall not be doomed to hear his piercing cries without knowing how or being able to relieve him."[48]

The reformers also intended the asylum to be a therapeutic institution. Crafts spoke repeatedly of the recovery of reason as one of the primary objects of an institution for the insane. Farrow's committee intimated that the curability of insanity was what made the creation of an asylum so desirable: "If the victims of this fearful malady were incapable of relief, we should have to tremble at their fate, and to mourn over the degradation of our nature. But the science of medicine and experience teaches us that their situation is by no means hopeless."[49]

The reformers' goals were admirable. But many of their fellow citizens were dubious. Many people in the early nineteenth century viewed hospitals and asylums as disreputable institutions for individuals whose families were too poor to provide care at home. The number of such institutions was small, and they served a predominately lower class clientele. Significantly, the only hospital in South Carolina prior to the establishment of the state lunatic asylum was connected with the Charleston poorhouse. Most respectable folk would have agreed with the brothers of a low-country lunatic, who in 1822 told Christ Church Parish commissioners of the poor that they had enough property to support their brother in comfort and scorned "the idea of his becoming a burden to the community."[50] Thus, sending a relative to an asylum was an act that might seem to reflect negatively on the family's reputation, for a public asylum was likely to be no more than a poorhouse for lunatics. The widespread perception that insanity itself was dishonorable discouraged resort to asylums for fear of exposing the family "shame."

The reformers knew that to succeed they would have to overcome the antipathy of the public toward asylums. Farrow's legislative committee of 1818 repeated an argument that asylum advocates often used elsewhere: although the rich might be able to command "every assistance at their houses" in other diseases, insanity was a malady that generally could be treated successfully only in an institution specially designed for its cure.[51]

But the reformers' campaign to convince the public of the advantages of asylum care was complicated by disagreements with the legislature. Many legislators did not understand or could not accept the reformers' goals and assumed that the South Carolina Lunatic Asylum was supposed to be a custodial pauper institution. Legislators used this assumption as a rationale for paring down expenditures on the institution: a state suffering from economic woes such as those afflicting South Carolina, they argued, could not afford to build a palace for paupers. In 1826 a legislative committee erroneously claimed that the asylum was originally intended for pauper lunatics. The committee went on to state that the asylum commissioners had added many extravagances to the design not contemplated by the founders, and that many of these were not necessary for paupers. Among the things the committee deemed unnecessary luxuries were gardens and pleasure grounds, indoor plumbing, cattle, horses, and carriages—items many asylum reformers considered essential to effective moral therapy.[52] By cutting funds for these purposes, the legislature greatly increased the asylum's difficulties in attracting pay patients and implementing the therapeutic ideals of its promoters.[53]

The reformers also clashed with the legislature over the question of the asylum's financial support. From the beginning, they had assured legislators that the institution would support itself from patient fees. In 1827 the board of trustees predicted that the asylum would be financially independent of state appropriations after its first year.[54] At the same time, they asked the general assembly for seven thousand dollars to fit out the asylum for the reception of patients. The legislature complied, in the hope that the trustees' prediction would prove correct.[55] But some legislators were not optimistic about the institution's chances of becoming self-sufficient. The state house committee on the asylum reminded their colleagues that the reformers had often been wrong in their financial calculations. The committee predicted that the proportion of pauper patients would be so great that the asylum would be unable to survive without regular state appropriations. The general assembly should therefore anticipate having to allocate about five to ten thousand dollars a year for its maintenance.[56]

Had these cautions been heeded, some of the problems the asylum faced in its early years might have been avoided. But the majority of the legislators insisted that the institution support itself. They made this explicit in 1827, when they passed an act to bring the asylum into operation. The act required the asylum's governing body, the board of regents, to set patient fees at levels high enough to obviate any need for state aid. To prevent people of means from imposing on the state, the act made each district responsible for the expenses of pauper lunatics its officials sent to the asylum. The committee that drew up the act explained this policy by stating that "when a tax is to be levied upon a small community, it is guarded with the same selfish vigilance of pecuniary interest, as when the charity is private and voluntary."[57]

The legislature thus served notice that the fledgling asylum would have to survive without state aid for either operating or extraordinary expenses. Just how unrealistic this position was would quickly become clear to those charged with operating the asylum, but it would take decades to convince a disgusted and increasingly tight-fisted legislature that the institution could not adequately support itself. The reformers themselves contributed to this outcome by minimizing potential problems and mismanaging the institution's construction. They were hindered, too, by deep-seated antipathies toward asylums and public hospitals. Perhaps most important, the political and economic crisis that struck the state in the 1820s deprived the institution of attention and resources that might have made its early history less turbulent and uncertain.

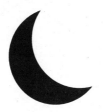

PART TWO

The Antebellum Asylum

1828–1860

Three

GIVE THE EXPERIMENT A FAIR TRIAL

SUSTAINING THE ANTEBELLUM ASYLUM

In the spring of 1828, the South Carolina Lunatic Asylum opened its doors to receive patients. Much to its officers' surprise and consternation, none appeared. More than six months passed before the first patient arrived. Admissions remained low for several years, and in 1831 the asylum nearly closed down for lack of funds. Its financial condition continued to be extremely precarious until the late 1830s. Insufficient revenues, in turn, increased the difficulties of attracting and retaining competent staff and supplying the needs of the patients. All of these problems contributed to a low public image of the asylum, already damaged by the delays and cost overruns of the period of its construction. Critics who had doubted the demand for such an institution found confirmation in its inability to attract enough patients to sustain itself financially. Before the late 1840s, annual admissions averaged in the twenties. The number of patients did not surpass one hundred until 1849. In the late 1830s, writer William Gilmore Simms declared that the asylum was unpopular in South Carolina because it was "known to be unprofitable, and was believed to be unnecessary."[1]

To some extent, the problems of the early South Carolina Lunatic Asylum derived from its experimental nature. The asylum's officers could draw upon an existing body of knowledge about the management of asylums. But none of them possessed practical experience; that could come only through trial and error. The problems of launching such an experiment were complicated by traditional images of lunatics and madhouses. To many people, the whole subject of insanity was distasteful. The insane were frightening, alien beings; asylums were places of torture at worst, little better than poorhouses or jails at best. A visit to the new asylum by Governor Stephen Miller in 1829 illustrated the problem. James Davis recorded disdainfully that Miller's "manner [was] unnaturally precipitate. He ran from room to room with a singular haste—and when he came to the patients he became nervous. He saw nothing and would hear but little. His fastidiousness and squeamishness at the thoughts of an insane person (either natural or affected) was so great as to lead me to doubt who discovered the most insanity, the Governor or the [patients]."[2] The attitudes and feelings Miller exemplified proved more difficult to overcome than the asylum's founders expected.

South Carolina's political and economic climate during the early years also hurt the asylum. Some lawmakers long remained angry about what they viewed as mismanagement and waste during its construction. With the state's economy depressed, many of them viewed the asylum as a luxury the state could ill afford. Even legislators well disposed toward the institution found their energies absorbed by the nullification crisis and their scope for action circumscribed by a persistent economic depression. Under these circumstances, the problems of a fledgling institution of doubtful utility were not a high priority.

Sustaining the asylum required considerable resourcefulness from its officers. By the later 1830s they had succeeded sufficiently to assure the institution's survival. It took longer to achieve widespread public acceptance, but even during its first decade it managed to attract patients from some prominent families. The admission of pauper patients gradually increased, despite the reluctance of cost-conscious local authorities to send them. Sporadic efforts to increase the patient population by opening the asylum to the black majority did not succeed until the late 1840s. Few black patients were admitted until after the Civil War.

In 1827 the legislature passed an act to bring the asylum into operation. The act placed the organization and general superintendency of the institution into the hands of nine regents, whom the legislature elected. All of the regents lived in or near the Columbia area; several had served on the Board of Asylum Commissioners or the board of trustees during the asylum's construction. The legislators chose Columbians because their proximity to the asylum would facilitate regular meetings and inspections. Columbians continued to dominate the regency throughout the antebellum period.[3] Despite considerable turnover in its membership during the early years, the antebellum regency attracted the services of a number of able and prominent men determined, as they put it, "to give the experiment a fair trial."[4]

One of the first and most problematic tasks the regents faced was recruiting staff. The rules they drew up for the asylum called for the appointment of a visiting physician or chief medical officer, a resident assistant physician or apothecary, a superintendent to manage the internal affairs of the house, a matron to oversee the care of women patients, keepers or attendants, and servants. The regents initially left some positions unfilled because of lack of funds. They found it difficult to fill others, in part because few people had the requisite skills for asylum work.

The regents unanimously elected James Davis, one of the asylum's founders, as its first visiting physician. But Davis was plagued by recurring illness, and for several months during 1833 and 1834 he was unable to perform his duties. He resigned in January 1835, and the regents replaced him with their president, Daniel H. Trezevant.[5] Trezevant was born in 1796 into a Charleston family of Huguenot ancestry. Like many contemporary physicians, he began the study of medicine through the apprenticeship method, then pursued a formal medical degree at the College of Physicians and Surgeons in New York. After several years' practice in rural South Carolina, he moved to Columbia sometime in the 1820s. He became involved with the asylum movement, joined the board of regents in 1828, and became the board's president in 1830. As regent and as visiting physician, a job he held until 1856, Trezevant played a dominant role in the history of the antebellum asylum.[6]

In order to save money—and against the wishes of Davis—the regents initially decided to leave the post of resident or assistant physician temporarily vacant. They did not fill it until nearly two years after the asylum opened. The first two appointees, again against the wishes of Davis, received no salary, only room and board. Neither stayed long.[7] The asylum did not have a salaried resident medical officer until December 1836, when the regents appointed Dr. John W. Parker to the positions of assistant physician and superintendent. Parker was born in South Carolina's Edgefield District in 1803. He studied medicine at the Medical College of South Carolina and the University of Pennsylvania, where he took his medical degree. He practiced in Spartanburg and Abbeville Districts for several years before accepting the asylum appointment.[8]

Parker was the asylum's fourth superintendent in eight years but the first who was a physician. Lay asylum superintendents were not unusual in eighteenth and early-nineteenth-century asylums. By the 1830s, however,

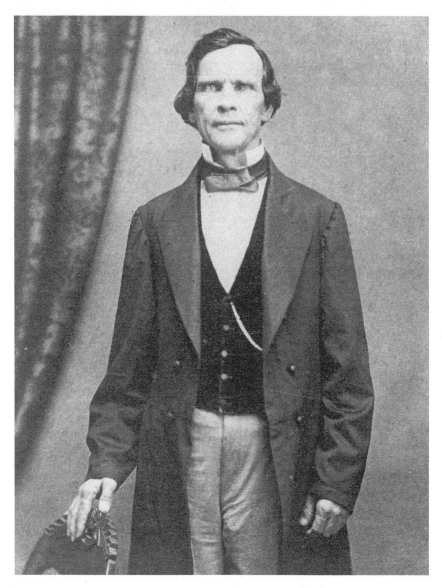

John W. Parker.
(Courtesy South Caroliniana Library, University of South Carolina)

the trend was toward the appointment of medical superintendents. None of the early superintendents at the South Carolina Lunatic Asylum, including Parker, seem to have had any asylum experience, but that was not unusual either. Because there were only a handful of lunatic asylums in the United States before the 1830s, few people possessed what we would call psychiatric expertise.

William Hilliard was technically the asylum's first superintendent, but his abilities were never put to the test. He resigned soon after the asylum officially opened after being arrested for an unspecified crime. His replacement, Archibald Beaty, was not appointed until the first patient arrived in December 1828. Beaty had some experience caring for the insane at his home in nearby Fairfield District. His performance initially pleased the regents, but they soon began to accuse him of negligence and poor record keeping. In 1832, several regents charged him with incompetence and forced his resignation. E. W. Harrison, who replaced Beaty, was more successful. When he left at the end of 1836, the regents praised his ability and kindness.[9]

When they elected Parker to replace Harrison, the regents seemed to be joining the accelerating trend among mental institutions toward appointing medical superintendents. But Parker's appointment was in some respects an anomaly. Unlike most of the medical superintendents then taking over American and European asylums, Parker was not the supreme medical officer. He was subordinate to the visiting physician, Trezevant. Parker's job was to carry out the day-to-day administration of the asylum and to implement the orders of the visiting physician relating to patient care and treatment. At first, Parker does not appear to have resented this division of responsibility, but in the 1850s, the two men came into bitter conflict over their respective spheres of authority. The anomalous situation ended in 1856 when the regents forced Trezevant's resignation and appointed Parker as superintendent and chief medical officer. He administered the asylum until the Reconstruction government removed him in 1869.

The asylum's staffing problems did not end with the physicians and superintendents. In March 1828 the regents elected a matron, but they discharged her a few months later. They had not appointed a replacement by the time the first patient was admitted in December 1828. As an interim measure, they persuaded the patient's mother to serve as temporary matron until one could be found. She left with her daughter a couple of months later, however, and the regents did not appoint anyone else until June 1830. None of the early matrons remained long; there were at least four during the first decade. Attendants, or keepers, as they were called during the early years, also had a rapid turnover rate. Many of the early keepers remained only a short time before leaving for other employment or being dismissed for cruelty, negligence or insubordination. Few stayed more than several months; some left after only a week or two. Their sudden departure sometimes left the asylum badly understaffed. Occasionally a convalescing patient was hired to act as a temporary keeper during the early years.[10]

Initially, state laws exacerbated the asylum's personnel problems. The staff were liable to be suddenly called away to perform jury, road, militia, or patrol duty. Periodic service in the patrol, which was designed to facilitate control of the state's large slave population, was incumbent upon all of South Carolina's adult white males. In 1829 the regents protested to the legislature that the performance of such duties placed an undue hardship on the asylum because of the difficulty of finding adequate substitutes for employees called away at short notice. The regents' concern was highlighted by an incident that occurred when superintendent Beaty had been required to go to Winnsborough to serve as a witness in court. While he was gone, Davis reported, the patients "took advantage of his absence and raised a riot in the court . . . which required almost more than all the physical force that we could command to subdue." In order to prevent such scenes in the future, Davis asked the legislature to free the asylum's staff from public duties requiring prolonged absence from the institution. He added that such an exemption would make it easier for the asylum to attract qualified personnel.[11] The legislature passed the necessary legislation, and the male staff of the asylum became the only group of white men in the state exempt from the sacred obligation of patrol duty.[12]

The new asylum had as much trouble securing patients as staff. During the spring of 1828, the regents advertised the asylum's opening in the Charleston and Columbia newspapers. The announcement contained information about the rules and charges and attempted to counter popular prejudices by assuring the public that no punishment would be inflicted upon the patients beyond solitary confinement.[13] By advertising only in the Charleston and Columbia press the regents may have lost some potential support for the asylum elsewhere. The *Camden Journal* protested that the asylum's advertising policy seemed to indicate that only the readers of those papers needed to know about its rules and regulations and expressed the hope that "they will have the monopoly of the institution."[14]

For several months after the asylum opened in May 1828, it seemed that the regents themselves would have the monopoly. By July no patients had been admitted, and the regents decided to publish their advertisement in handbill form and circulate it throughout the state. In December, the regents admitted the first patient; about twenty-two more had arrived by the end of 1829. For several more years, however, admissions remained well below that needed to support the institution. By the end of 1831, only fifty-eight patients had been admitted to the asylum, and only thirty-five patients were in residence in an institution designed for about one hundred.[15]

The officers attributed the difficulty in attracting patients to the unenlightened attitudes of both the public and local officials. Too many families retained the old negative stereotypes of asylums. Too many poor law officers were more interested in saving a few dollars or a little trouble than in restoring an insane pauper to sanity. The commitment law also inhibited admissions. The act of 1827 restricted the classes of persons who could initiate commitment proceedings to the husband, wife, or closest relative of the patient; judges of the equity and common law courts; and commissioners of the poor. Moreover, no one could be committed unless he or she was examined by a justice of the peace and two licensed practicing physicians. The only exception was the insane from other states, who could be admitted on the basis "of such evidence . . . as the Regents regard sufficient." The law gave local officials considerable discretion in deciding whether to commit the pauper and criminal insane. It also implied that only insane paupers deemed curable, or dangerous or annoying to the community, had to be sent to the asylum.[16]

In order to increase the patient population, the asylum's promoters adopted several strategies. First, they tried to combat public prejudice against the asylum by means of a campaign in the press. They wrote articles and letters that praised the design, facilities, and officers of the institution and pointed out its advantages to the insane and their friends. The public, they argued, did not yet understand the advantages such an institution could confer on the insane, their families, and their community. Once properly informed about the nature of the asylum, people would come to appreciate and patronize it. In a letter to the *Charleston Mercury*, Davis complained that "everything pertaining to [the asylum's] nature, character, and prospects, seems to be but little understood." The *Mercury*'s editor, Henry Laurens Pinckney, predicted that the asylum would have no trouble attracting patients once its advantages had become generally known. In an appeal to nascent sectional patriotism, Pinckney argued that just as it was time for southerners to stop sending their children to the North for education, it was also time to stop sending their lunatics there for care and treatment. The South Carolina Lunatic Asylum was no more expensive than any similar institution in the North, and it transcended them all in point of "comfort and accommodation."[17]

A correspondent of the *Columbia Telescope* combatted what he called a "mistaken fastidiousness on the subject of sending a friend to an asylum, as if something like disgrace attached to it." The real disgrace, he implied, lay in withholding the benefits of an asylum from those who needed them. People naturally scorned the idea of accepting public charity and feared that public exposure of the disorder would bring dishonor on the family.

But to send a relative to the South Carolina Lunatic Asylum should not wound the pride of any family, because the institution required them to pay according to their ability and the type of accommodations and care desired. If the family's great concern was to shield the patient from the public gaze, this could be better accomplished by sending him to the asylum than by keeping him at home. In short, the new asylum was an unqualified boon to families: "They will no longer be reduced to the necessity of either sending [insane relatives] far abroad to distant asylums, at a great expense, or else (to the perpetual annoyance of their own domestic happiness) of keeping them in a state of imprisonment at home, necessarily destitute of very many of the comforts and advantages an asylum affords."[18]

The asylum cause gained important supporters in the legal profession, such as Judge Henry W. DeSaussure. Chancellor of the Court of Appeals in Equity, DeSaussure was a popular and respected jurist who supported many reforms and benevolent causes. His son William and his son-in-law Abram Blanding, also lawyers, were both members of the asylum's original board of regents. Judge Desaussure was better informed than most people about the condition of the insane, because the equity court handled cases involving the property and custody of lunatics. Many of them, he claimed, suffered severely from a lack of proper treatment, which the asylum was prepared to provide: "A skilful physician has the charge of the patients and performs his duties faithfully and kindly. He proceeds on the plan of moral discipline, the effects of which have been very visible, in a short time, on several patients who had been long and severely afflicted."[19] Another judge whose experiences led him to support the asylum was John Belton O'Neall. As a youth, he had seen his insane father consigned to a cage for several years. O'Neall sent his sister to the asylum in 1833 when she became insane and wrote a laudatory portrait of asylum founder Samuel Farrow some years later.[20]

Some physicians also promoted the asylum. Dr. Thomas Y. Simons of Charleston wrote a brief treatise on insanity the same year the South Carolina Lunatic Asylum opened. Although he did not mention the institution by name, he stressed the great improvements that had recently occurred in lunatic asylums: "Kindness and humanity," he wrote, "[have been] substituted in all properly regulated institutions, for brutal violence, or solitary seclusion in dreary dungeons."[21] In the 1840s, Simons sent his son to the South Carolina Lunatic Asylum and urged other families to patronize the institution.[22] A student at the recently established Medical College of South Carolina, where Simons was a professor, advertised the new asylum in his 1829 medical thesis on mania. He noted that the state had recently opened "an institution intended for Maniacs in our own State, which . . . might be infinitely beneficial . . . in . . . alleviating the sufferings of this unfortunate class of our fellow men. The regulations . . . are similar to those of the most approved institutions of the kind both in Europe, and this country." The asylum, he concluded, was "worthy the consideration of our citizens."[23] By the 1840s, Simons's colleague at the Medical College, Samuel Henry Dickson, was writing that everyone now acknowledged asylums to be essential to the treatment of the insane. Few cases, he claimed, could be safely or properly treated at home. Only in an asylum could one achieve and maintain the "salutary influence over the insane" required to prevent harm to the patient or others and to maximize the chances of cure or improvement.[24]

Yet old attitudes about asylums persisted. In 1842, William Gilmore Simms lamented that "a foolish prejudice, the equal result of pride and ignorance, prevails with most persons and makes them regard the transfer to an asylum of a near and dear relative as something like inhumanity, or at least, humiliation."[25] The views Simms spoke of were not confined to the poor and uneducated. Some physicians shared them, to judge from several theses on insanity written by medical students during the 1840s and 1850s at the Medical College of South Carolina. The students questioned the advisability of asylum care and repeated traditional negative stereotypes about asylums. One thesis warned medical men not to be too quick to diagnose a patient insane, lest they consign him to the "dreadful walls" and "horrors" of a lunatic asylum. Another student condemned the tendency of families to place a relative too quickly in an asylum, where he was "surrounded by a choir of moaning, gibbering beings, from all of whose eyes, 'the light of madness glares.'"[26] On the eve of the Civil War, the asylum's officers were still complaining that such prejudices prevented prompt commitment of the insane.[27]

By the late 1830s and 1840s, however, increasing numbers of prominent families showed a willingness to patronize the asylum. Positive comments about the asylum from its promoters and prominent physicians helped remove doubts about the propriety of asylum care. The experiences of a few pioneering families also aided the asylum cause. It is important to realize that for a wealthy family of the early nineteenth century to send a loved one to an asylum was a difficult choice, often arrived at after considerable agony and subject to continual second-guessing and recrimination.

One can see this dynamic in the correspondence of the Townes family, upcountry planters who sent John Townes to the South Carolina Lunatic Asylum in 1835. John's brother Henry repeatedly sought to assure his family (and one suspects, himself) that they had pursued the proper course. After taking John to the asylum, Henry wrote to his mother, praised the asylum and its officers, and declared himself "confident [John] will be restored to you as well as he ever was."[28] Mrs. Townes's concern about her son continued, however, and she visited John at the asylum in July 1835 to see for herself. Following the visit, Henry seemed assured that her anxieties about the propriety of John's commitment must now have vanished: "I hope, Mother, you returned home safe and much better satisfied than you were previous to your visit to Columbia. Have you any doubt now that John will not be well and kindly and skillfully attended to, and allowed every genteel accommodation and comfort warranted by his peculiar situation? I am sure you will say you have no longer a doubt."[29] In the event, Henry Townes's confidence seemed justified. After a few months, Dr. Trezevant pronounced John cured and sent him home to his relieved and happy family.

The successful termination of cases such as that of John Townes helped increase public confidence in the asylum. Henry Townes himself had been encouraged to learn that one of the patients at the asylum was a woman from his neighborhood who was about to be discharged as cured. Extremely grateful to the asylum for John's restoration, the Townes family undoubtedly related their experience to their friends. The Townes may have influenced their relations, the Calhoun family, to send John C. Calhoun's brother Patrick to the asylum in 1838.

After Patrick Calhoun became seriously depressed in May 1838, his relatives discussed the possibility of sending him to an asylum. Initially, they viewed such a course as a last resort. John C. Calhoun argued that Patrick should not be sent to the asylum unless his mind was completely alienated: "Short of that, I cannot but think, it would be fatal to him. It would at least be felt to be a great cruelty."[30] A few days later, however, Patrick tried to cut his throat with a razor, and John C. agreed that if he did not quickly recover through treatment at home, he should be sent to the asylum, "as painful as it would be."[31] The Calhoun family committed Patrick to the asylum a few days later. To their great relief, he was discharged much improved in April 1839.[32]

The patronage of wealthy families like the Calhouns and the Towneses helped make the asylum a respectable alternative to home care, boarding out, or a private asylum in the North. Physicians who were convinced of the advantages of asylum care could also play a key role in a family's decision to commit a relative. In 1848, Mary P. Allston's relatives decided that her insanity had become too severe to be controlled at home. They hesitated between boarding her out and sending her to the asylum. They consulted Dr. Thomas Simons, who recommended the state asylum, and they sent her there. Her grandson, who took the lead in securing her commitment, explained that "with Dr. Simons' opinion so clearly expressed I cannot assume the responsibility of adopting the measure of private restraints. I regard the asylum as the most humane and efficient remedy and as better calculated to lead . . . to a partial restoration of her reason."[33] Another relation, R. F. W. Allston, also agreed with Simons that the asylum was best; there, he argued, "she would be surrounded by as much care and attention to her well being and considerate kindness . . . as in any place of the kind."[34]

Because of the regents' initial difficulties in attracting private patients, they resorted to getting them from wherever they could, including nearby states. The act of 1827 designed to bring the lunatic asylum into operation allowed the regents to admit lunatics and idiots from other states, as long as citizens of South Carolina had first preference. At the time South Carolina's asylum was the only one south of Virginia. Georgia did not have an asylum until 1844; North Carolina, Alabama, and Florida did not open theirs until 1856, 1860, and 1877, respectively. The regents decided to seek patients from other states as soon as it became clear that the asylum was not going to be filled quickly by South Carolinians. In March 1829 the board resolved to advertise the asylum in the capitals of Georgia and North Carolina and to admit out of state patients on the same terms as citizens of South Carolina. This tactic brought rapid success; two months later the first of many Georgia patients was admitted to the asylum. Others soon came from North Carolina, Alabama, and Florida. Throughout the antebellum period the asylum continued to receive patients from these and other southern states.[35]

The regents also sought ways to increase pauper admissions. They knew that the asylum needed to attract a significant number of paying patients to insure its financial integrity, but they became convinced that until the institution had developed a reputation for excellence in the treatment of the insane, the wealthy would prefer to keep their insane at home or send them to out-of-state institutions such as the Pennsylvania Hospital. The best way to earn the confidence of the rich, the regents concluded, was to succeed in the care of the poor. But attracting pauper patients was initially as difficult as attracting pay patients. During the first year of operation, the asylum received only about a dozen pauper lunatics.[36] The regents attributed the low number of pauper admissions to the reluctance of commissioners of the poor to increase local taxes. The cost of caring for an insane pauper in the asylum was two to three times higher than the cost of community care. To remedy the problem, the regents proposed that the law require local authorities to transfer their indigent insane to the asylum or that the state pay part of the cost for pauper patients.[37]

Most legislators initially resisted both of these options. An act of 1829 required sheriffs to send pauper lunatics in the jails to the asylum and stipulated that the state would pay the expenses of transient (nonresident) paupers. But this did not produce a significant increase in admissions. The regents continued to press for a law compelling the transfer of all pauper lunatics to the asylum.[38] The legislature finally complied at the end of 1831, when the regents threatened to close the asylum due to a lack of patients and revenue.[39] The act of 1831 initiated a modest but steady stream of pauper admissions. But it did not end the reluctance of local officials to send pauper lunatics to the asylum. It also required the counties to pay the entire costs of their maintenance and did not include any penalty for noncompliance. The commissioners in some districts at first ignored it or complied at their discretion.[40]

The most important holdout was Charleston, for the twenty-odd lunatics the city maintained in its poorhouse could have filled most of the vacant rooms in the asylum. Paradoxically, while the asylum was being constructed, the Charleston authorities showed every intention of transferring their pauper lunatics to it when it opened. In 1824, the city council recommended that the poorhouse commissioners establish a maternity ward as soon as the insane were removed to the new state asylum. In 1829, however, the commissioners and the city council decided that it would be more expedient to expand accommodation for the insane in the poorhouse than to send them to Columbia.[41]

Charleston's change of policy regarding its lunatic poor was related to the depressed economy of the state. Hard times produced a strong movement for retrenchment in the legislature, which resulted in a sharp reduction in state grants for the maintenance of transient paupers. As a seaport and the state's largest city, Charleston supported a large number of transient paupers, and the cutback was a severe financial blow. To send the pauper insane to the asylum in Columbia would have increased expenditures on the poor at a time when the city's revenues were declining.[42]

Charleston sent only one pauper lunatic to the asylum before 1833, despite sharp criticism from upstate. The *Columbia Southern Times* charged in 1830 that it did not reflect "credit on . . . Charleston that while the State possesses an institution so excellent as [the South Carolina Lunatic Asylum] is growing to be, and one in which the rate of pay for pauper patients is so low, they should still continue to immure in their *poor house* about twenty-five lunatics, whom the utter want of arrangements fitted for a system of discipline or cure, or comfort, condemns . . . to perpetual insanity and wretchedness."[43]

In May 1832, the regents informed the Charleston City Council that the law required them to send their pauper insane to the asylum.[44] Now the Charleston authorities agreed to comply, for the lunatic department had become badly overcrowded and was in need of extensive repairs.[45] Yet Charleston did not send any pauper lunatics to the asylum until February 1833, when it sent nine.[46] From then on, the city sent pauper patients to the state asylum at intervals, as part of what English writer Harriet Martineau referred to as the "periodical clearance" of the Charleston poorhouse. Yet until the mid-1850s, Charleston continued to maintain between twenty-five and forty insane paupers in its lunatic department.[47]

One quick way to increase the number of admissions at the asylum would have been to admit blacks. The institution began to receive applications for their admission soon after it opened. The regents considered the option but rejected it. They concluded that the institution's charter did not expressly forbid it but decided not to admit blacks for two reasons. First, because the acts concerning the operation of the asylum did not expressly permit their admission; and second, because their presence would require additional expense and complicate the running of the institution. They could not "be mingled with the whites, and a separate keeper and a separate [exercise] yard would be necessary." If the legislature intended the asylum to receive blacks, the regents agreed, it should amend the law to state so explicitly.[48]

The regents reported these views to the general assembly in 1828 and 1829, but did not press the matter. By 1832, they seemed more eager to receive blacks, possibly because they were having so much difficulty in securing white patients, or because they had decided that a real need existed that only the asylum could fill. "We have been repeatedly solicited to receive colored persons into the Asylum," they reported. The regents declared that they could provide inexpensive accommodation for blacks at a short distance from the main building, if the legislature would approve it.[49]

The legislature did not act on this proposal, but the issue persisted. Harriet Martineau, who visited the asylum in the mid-1830s, reported that the physician was determined to obtain an asylum for blacks. On several more occasions during the 1830s and 1840s, the regents advocated the reception of black patients. In 1839, a committee of the regents argued that the state should erect a separate building or fix up one of the existing outbuildings for the reception of insane slaves. Five years later, another committee deplored "that no provision is made for the insane Blacks among us. . . . How far this is compatible with our enlightened philanthropy, [we] will not decide."[50]

Ironically, one of the first patients the asylum received, in May 1829, was a fourteen-year-old black slave named Jefferson. He was received as a favor to his owner, a planter who had sent his brother to the asylum. Jefferson was not housed in the main building with the white patients, but in the yard. His name was not recorded in the asylum's admission book. But Davis kept a history of the case, in which he stated that Jefferson was admitted as "an exception to a general rule not to receive blacks." Jefferson remained for several months but did not improve, and his owner removed him.[51] The asylum received one other nonwhite patient before 1850, a mulatto man named David Duncan, who spent several months there in 1839. Why he was admitted is not clear.[52]

When the legislature finally voted in 1848 to legalize the admission of blacks, the move was in large part a public-relations effort designed to counter abolitionist propaganda. To be sure, the act's advocates stressed the standard humanitarian, medical, and social control arguments for asylum care. They argued that the state had a moral responsibility to care for faithful servants and to protect slaveholders families from the dangers of living in proximity to lunatic slaves. But proponents of the act also stressed the political dangers of refusing to admit blacks to the asylum. Charleston writer William Gilmore Simms had warned as early as 1842 that antislavery propaganda might be given credence by "discrimination between the sufferings of [insane] blacks and whites."[53] A legislative committee used the same argument in 1848: admitting blacks would enhance South Carolina's reputation for humanity and serve as a rebuke to the "idle and vicious fanaticism" of the abolitionists.[54]

That the act admitting blacks to the state asylum was largely a political exercise is supported by the minor impact it had on their situation. Between 1850 and 1859, only 30 blacks were admitted to the South Carolina Lunatic Asylum, as opposed to more than 600 whites. At the end of 1858, 7 of the 180 patients in the asylum were black. The state legislature was willing to make a gesture aimed at northern opinion, but not to commit substantial funds to the care of the black insane. Indeed, it is likely that the act admitting blacks passed only because Parker assured legislators that the asylum could provide facilities for black patients without a large special appropriation.[55]

The accommodations the asylum provided for blacks were much inferior to those of the white patients, consisting of a couple of small brick outbuildings placed near the main asylum structure. Moreover, soon after the first black patients arrived, the physicians protested that the provisions for them were unacceptable, from both a medical and racial standpoint. It was impossible to give the black patients the exercise their condition demanded, because their building was located in the white patients' exercise court. The proximity of the blacks, the physicians insisted, distressed the white patients and inhibited their recovery. The asylum also had to provide a special attendant for the few black patients, because the regular attendants refused to care for them. The officers tried using slave attendants for the black patients, but did not find the results acceptable. Parker announced in 1858 that white attendants were caring for the black patients because the asylum was unable to "get negroes sufficiently trustworthy and kind." [56]

Because of these problems, the regents decided in 1858 to release the black male patients and admit no more until the state agreed to fund a proper building and grounds for them. The asylum continued to admit a few black women, but it turned down numerous applications for the admission of male slaves. In 1860 Parker reported that many masters had requested that the regents petition the legislature "for some provision to be made, which will relieve them from the responsibility and danger of keeping such patients at home, without the proper means of comfort and cure." [57] The outbreak of the Civil War a few months later prevented action. In 1865, the asylum contained only five black patients. [58]

South Carolina's refusal to provide sufficient accommodations for insane blacks was not unusual, although the state's large black population made its consequences significant. Prior to the Civil War, most asylums in the United States either did not accept black patients or provided them with separate and inferior facilities. Psychiatric consensus held that the natural antagonism between the races was such that the insane blacks and whites should not be mixed together. As Thomas Kirkbride of the Pennsylvania Hospital put it, "The idea of mixing up all colors and classes . . . is not what is wanted in our hospitals for the insane." [59] The Eastern Virginia Lunatic Asylum was exceptional among antebellum asylums in that it accepted large numbers of black patients and cared for them in the same facilities as the white patients. But until 1846, it accepted only free blacks. [60]

The admission of black patients could in any case have done little to solve the South Carolina Lunatic Asylum's financial problems. The fees for black patients, like those for white paupers, were below the cost of their maintenance. The difference had to be made up from fees paid by white paying patients. But the revenue derived from paying patients was seldom sufficient to offset the costs of the paupers, who normally made up a majority of the asylum's residents. Because of this situation, the officers were often hard pressed to meet expenses. During the early years of the asylum's operation, the regents were forced to appeal to the legislature for aid nearly every year.[61]

It was not an auspicious time to be making such requests. The asylum had the misfortune to be born at a time when the ailing economy of the state and the fever of the nullification crisis left political leaders with little money or time to devote to domestic needs. Convinced that the state's economic problems had been caused or aggravated by the high tariffs of 1824 and 1828, many South Carolinians proclaimed that Congress had no constitutional authority to enact the tariffs and that each state had the right to "nullify" or prevent the enforcement of the tariff within its own boundaries. During the late 1820s and early 1830s, many of the state's leaders were preoccupied by the nullification issue and the need to prepare for a possible conflict with the federal government. Simultaneously, the state's economic woes produced a strong movement for retrenchment within the general assembly. In 1828, upcountry legislators succeeded in cutting the state budget by 20 percent, and for years thereafter the legislature showed little enthusiasm for spending on public projects.[62] Adding insult to injury, some legislators used the asylum's financial difficulties as an argument against further forays into public philanthropy. An attempt to resurrect the project for a school for the deaf and dumb in 1831 got nowhere. A state senate committee that opposed the project noted that the problems of the lunatic asylum showed that "Public institutions for the most benevolent purposes do not always succeed."[63]

The regents, on the other hand, blamed a parsimonious legislature for the asylum's plight. They argued that economizing during the period of construction had created many of its difficulties by making it impossible to fit up the asylum for the reception of wealthy patients. In spite of inadequate facilities and society's prejudices, the asylum had managed to attract some patients from "the first families of the State." But in order to keep them and attract others, it was imperative to extend and improve accommodations for paying patients.[64]

The asylum's financial condition remained extremely precarious throughout its first decade. At several points in the early 1830s it was in danger of closing for lack of funds. In 1829 the regents reported that they did not have sufficient revenue on hand to continue operating the asylum during the coming year. They could not support the institution without attracting more paying patients, yet they did not have the funds to fit up rooms for new paying admissions.[65] At the end of 1830, they declared that they could not support the asylum from patient fees as the law required and that additional state support would be needed to provide the proper level of comfort and care for the patients.[66] When angry legislators rejected the argument, the regents threatened to resign unless Governor James Hamilton provided emergency aid from the state contingency fund. They were forced to this extremity, they explained, by the law, which made them personally liable if they spent more money than the asylum took in.[67] When the legislature convened again at the end of 1831, the asylum had a cash balance of $9.11, and the regents warned that they would have to release the patients unless they received an appropriation from the state.[68] Faced with the imminent closure of the asylum, legislators provided $3,000 for furnishings, clothing, and repairs. Most legislators saw this as an emergency measure. They continued to insist that the asylum support itself and refused to establish a system of annual appropriations.[69]

At times during the first years, the institution was hard pressed to supply the patients with the basic necessities. Davis blamed the death of Daniel McHenry in January 1832 on "careless exposure barefooted in the court in the long continued intense cold of this winter." The physician added that a number of patients had been going barefoot for some time.[70]

The problem was not simply negligence. The patients destroyed or wore out clothing, shoes, and bedding faster than the asylum could afford to replace them. After McHenry's death, the regents ordered Superintendent Harrison to be especially careful to ensure that the patients were provided with sufficient clothing and shoes. But he reported in the fall of 1832 that many of the patients desperately needed blankets, clothing, hats, and shoes. Such conditions may have contributed to the high mortality of the early years of the asylum. More than half of the patients admitted in 1832 and 1833 died (thirty-two of fifty-nine). Between 1835 and 1842, mortality averaged 26 percent of the patients under treatment. Other circumstances undoubtedly added to the death rate. The drastic therapies physicians employed during the early years, discussed in the next chapter, surely hastened the demise of some patients. The physicians themselves often blamed the moribund condition of many patients when they arrived at the asylum. But inadequate funding probably contributed to increased mortality.[71]

In 1833, the regents requested another appropriation of three thousand dollars, but in spite of the dire conditions at the asylum, the legislature refused. By this time, however, admissions had increased to the point that revenues for the year slightly exceeded expenditures. As a legislative committee reported in 1833, the financial situation of the institution was more favorable than at any other time since it opened. The committee added, however, that the asylum would probably remain dependent on the state unless it were enlarged so as to receive a larger number of patients. The male wing was already overcrowded, and there were many more insane outside than inside the asylum. Were these to seek admission, they would have to be refused, and the asylum would lose an opportunity to be fully self-supporting. As proof, the committee noted that as the number of patients had increased, the receipts and expenditures had become more closely balanced. To take advantage of the improving situation, the committee recommended an extension of the men's wing. The legislature did not appropriate the money.

By 1835 the men's wing had become so badly overcrowded that the regents reported that they could receive no more patients and would probably have to discharge some. According to law, the first to go would be the out-of-state patients who paid high fees. Their departure would make it impossible for the asylum to support itself. This time the regents' arguments — aided no doubt by a recent upswing in the state's economy — succeeded, and the legislature appropriated eight thousand dollars for an extension to the west wing.[72]

The approval of the new extension, along with the appointments of Trezevant and Parker about the same time, marked a turning point in the history of the asylum. If it had not entirely overcome legislative hostility and public prejudice, it had achieved a modicum of administrative stability and acceptance. Many legislators remained reluctant to give the asylum money, but few were willing to let it close. It had also won the confidence of some of the state's leading inhabitants. During the 1840s and 1850s, it was able to attract enough paying patients to support itself without state aid except for further extensions. The experiment had survived its trial, but barely.[73]

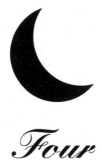

Four

A HOUSE OF CURE

THERAPY AT THE ANTEBELLUM ASYLUM

History has not been kind to the early southern lunatic asylums. Historians have generally dismissed them as custodial welfare institutions largely uninfluenced by the therapeutic optimism that motivated asylum founders in the antebellum North. In his seminal work on the history of mental illness in the United States, Albert Deutsch claimed that the "dominating motive" behind the establishment of the South Carolina and Kentucky asylums in the 1820s was "custody rather than cure." Following Deutsch, Norman Dain argued that with the exception of Virginia, southern asylums were "particularly bad," and that until the 1840s, they were "pauper institutions" designed to control rather than cure the mad. No state asylum, Dain concluded, was founded as a therapeutic institution before 1833—the year Massachusetts opened its asylum at Worcester. Similarly, in his study of nineteenth-century American mental institutions, Gerald Grob called the Kentucky and South Carolina asylums "little more than" custodial poorhouses before 1840.[1]

For South Carolina at least, this argument needs to be revised.[2] The founders of the South Carolina asylum intended to create a curative institution that would admit patients of all classes. Like the reformers who established several other early state asylums, including that at Worcester, those in South Carolina modeled their institution to a large extent on the corporate asylums of the northern states.[3] These asylums were designed to be multiclass institutions, and they were based on a therapeutic optimism derived from the adoption of the new system of moral treatment. The results the South Carolina reformers achieved, in terms of both the social makeup of the asylum's clientele and the proportion of patients cured, did not match their expectations. Yet their aims, methods, and results were not markedly different from those of many other contemporary asylums in the United States and Europe.

In common with most antebellum state asylums, the South Carolina Lunatic Asylum never attracted as many paying patients as its supporters wished. But its clientele was not that of a poorhouse. Its first decade (1828–38) produced a slight excess of pay over pauper admissions. Paying admissions continued to outnumber pauper admissions in most of the antebellum years for which information is available.[4] Moreover, as in other public institutions, some pauper admissions were not true paupers in the usual sense. They were persons whose families would have been pauperized by the costs of their treatment. In 1831, for example, several citizens of Anderson District successfully petitioned the legislature to admit John King to the asylum as a pauper even though he possessed property valued at about seven hundred dollars. The petitioners pointed out that forcing King to pay for his care would reduce his family to "poverty and beggary." Because King was the father of nine children, this was no small consideration: "Instead of one pauper on their hands [they] are likely to have many."[5] The paying patients were often people of modest means, but some belonged to elite families such as the Calhouns, Allstons, Middletons, and O'Nealls.[6]

The asylum's authorities were dissatisfied with this achievement. Despite the preponderance of pay admissions, paupers normally constituted a majority of the resident patients because they tended to remain longer than paying patients. The officers ascribed this outcome to a lack of facilities attractive to the paying class. A committee of the regents lamented in 1842 that the asylum was "becoming a Pauper Institution" because of "the want of proper accommodations for the higher classes."[7] The regents' concern was understandable. They needed to attract a large proportion of paying patients to make the asylum self-sufficient. But their rhetoric was exaggerated. At no point during the antebellum period did the numbers of publicly supported patients in the asylum justify labeling it as a pauper institution.

In addition to serving all classes, the antebellum South Carolina Lunatic Asylum resembled the corporate asylums in another respect. Supporters of both viewed the cure of the insane as one of the most important functions of an asylum. They ascribed to what Albert Deutsch called the "cult of curability": the belief that insanity was highly curable if placed under

TABLE 1. *Paying and Pauper Admissions to South Carolina Lunatic Asylum, for Selected Periods, 1828–1852*

Period	Paying	Pauper
1828–38	117	110
1837–41	68	59
1848–52*	118	65

Sources: South Carolina State Hospital, Admission Book, 1828–38; *Annual Report*, 1842, 1848–52.
*Statistics for 1842–47 and 1851 are unavailable.

TABLE 2. *Average Number of Paying and Pauper Patients Resident in South Carolina Lunatic Asylum, for Selected Periods, 1830–1859*

Period	Paying	Pauper
1830–34*	15	18
1840–44	26	39
1845–49	34	49
1850–54	68	78
1855–59	88	97

Sources: South Carolina State Hospital, *Annual Report*, 1831, 1833, 1842–59; Minutes of the Board of Regents, 1 May 1830; Journal of the South Carolina House of Representatives, 1834, pp. 164–65.
Note: Averages are rounded to the nearest number.
*Statistics for 1832 and 1835–39 are unavailable.

proper treatment in an asylum in the early stages of the disease. As we have seen, the founders of the South Carolina Lunatic Asylum emphasized the therapeutic advantages of such institutions.[8] To James Davis, the asylum's first physician, insanity was "a curable disease in a great majority of cases, especially under the facilities of a well regulated Asylum." The South Carolina Lunatic Asylum, he argued, should be not merely "a place of comfort" but also "a house of cure."[9] In his first annual report (1829), Davis echoed the claims of a number of asylum physicians that recent cases placed under proper treatment in an asylum were "curable in a ratio of something like 90 per cent."[10] Daniel H. Trezevant, who succeeded Davis as physician in 1835, accepted the same position. "In ordinary Insanity," Trezevant wrote, "five out of six would recover if attended to early, and even a larger proportion."[11]

Therapeutic optimism in South Carolina, as in the North and Europe, was largely based on a faith in the ideology of moral treatment. Several months before the asylum opened, the regents established general guidelines for carrying out moral therapy, including the provision of regular employment and amusement and the necessity for kind and gentle treatment. In common with early asylum reformers elsewhere in this country, those in South Carolina lacked practical experience of how moral treatment ought to be implemented. To remedy this deficiency, the regents sent Dr. Davis to visit several northern asylums that had gained "the universal approbation of the public."[12] Soon after the South Carolina Lunatic Asylum opened, they advertised that it was conducted "on the plan of moral discipline" he had observed in the northern institutions.[13]

Descriptions of moral therapy at the asylum are remarkably similar to the classical account contained in Samuel Tuke's *Description of the Retreat*.[14] South Carolina's asylum, according to its officers, was governed on a "system of kindness," in which the "barbarous practice of torture" associated with the old madhouses was completely excluded. Mechanical restraints and other forms of coercion were to be employed only when necessary for medical or safety reasons and applied "with the utmost lenity and kindness." The keepers were instructed to speak as well as act toward the patients in "the most kind, soothing, and conciliatory manner" and to eschew the sort of "trifling, ridicule, and satire which are particularly wounding to the sensibilities of the insane."[15]

Moral treatment was predicated on the notion that the insane were often capable of a large degree of self-control. Its major goal was to encourage that ability to help the patient to internalize proper habits of behavior. Once this process began, it became possible to abstract his mind from his delusion or hallucination and either cure or alleviate his insanity. To achieve these goals, Davis noted that he employed psychological remedies designed to divert the patient's mind from the "painful associations" that he, like many antebellum alienists, saw as a primary cause of insanity. The asylum's patients were encouraged to engage in various employments and amusements and to develop habits of cleanliness, order, and propriety.[16]

The officers' descriptions of moral treatment represented an ideal. The implementation of moral therapy, discussed more fully in the following chapter, was less thorough and satisfactory than the discussion of its principles might imply. Inadequate finances and personnel problems severely hampered efforts to supply the facilities and personal attention to patients that moral treatment demanded. As we have already seen, the asylum's officers during its first few years were sometimes hard pressed just to keep the patients clothed and fed. The case records of these years indicate that the visiting physicians left the details of moral therapy to the lay superintendents, Beaty and Harrison. The superintendents did not elaborate their aims and methods in their reports. To judge by their writing, they were not particularly well educated, and their conception of moral therapy was probably not too sophisticated. For example, Beaty recorded in July 1832 that "the patients were quiet and done any work we asked them to do, so far as they could do."[17] Nevertheless, references to employment and amusement in the asylum records indicate that the officers tried to employ moral methods within the limits of their resources and understanding. During the 1840s and 1850s, Trezevant and Parker employed moral treatment in a more thoroughgoing and sophisticated manner, although inadequate facilities and personnel problems hindered their therapeutic efforts as well.

Moral treatment at the South Carolina Lunatic Asylum, as elsewhere, was not synonymous with an unproblematical "kindness." Coercion in the form of mechanical restraint, seclusion, and cold showers played a major therapeutic role. Their object, as the regents put it in 1830, was to encourage efforts at self-control by convincing the patient that he or she was still "considered a responsible being . . . for whose welfare and prosperity we are deeply interested."[18] Davis claimed that restraint was therapeutically beneficial if used discreetly. During the first decade, the asylum staff used restraint frequently, but not always discreetly. Refractory, highly excited, or suicidal patients were routinely strapped down in a tranquilizing chair or placed in strong rooms, often for long periods of time. Other restraints in common use included straitjackets and various straps, muffs, and stays to restrict the movement of the limbs, hands, and feet.[19]

Under Trezevant and Parker, the use of mechanical restraint declined. They gradually rejected Davis's view that restraint was therapeutically beneficial and tried to minimize its use. Soon after Davis retired in 1835, Robert Gardiner Hill pioneered the "non-restraint" system at England's Lincoln County Asylum. Hill's successful experiments with nonrestraint soon led other British asylum superintendents, including John Conolly of London's Hanwell Asylum, to imitate him. Conolly's conversion to nonrestraint, and his effective propaganda on its behalf, soon led to its widespread adoption in Britain.[20]

American asylum superintendents were generally much less enthusiastic than their British counterparts about the viability of total nonrestraint.

Some were actively hostile and echoed the arguments of British skeptics that nonrestraint was a misnomer, because it did not actually involve the total abolition of restraint. Not only were the patients restrained by the institution itself, but often mechanical restraints were merely replaced by seclusion or manual restraint by attendants. Most American superintendents argued that mechanical restraints were less harmful and more humane than these alternatives, especially given the low quality of most asylum attendants. Nevertheless, many American alienists came close to adopting nonrestraint without accepting the term.[21] Trezevant and Parker fell into this latter category. Neither openly advocated the total abandonment of mechanical restraint, but they did not share the antipathy of some American superintendents toward the nonrestraint movement. Although neither of them took part in the heated discussions of nonrestraint at the meetings of the Association of Medical Superintendents, both expressed their views on the subject in the asylum's annual reports.[22]

Trezevant was the more unequivocal in his support for nonrestraint; he frequently praised John Conolly, whom he called a greater British hero than Wellington. Parker was perhaps less convinced; on one occasion he quoted with approval the argument of Dr. Isaac Ray of Butler Hospital for the Insane that the use of a light article of restraint was preferable to the manual force of the attendants' hands. Nevertheless, Parker joined Trezevant in rejecting Davis's view that mechanical restraint could play a positive therapeutic role in the treatment of the insane. During the 1840s and 1850s, both men condemned its use in all but the most violent and suicidal cases. In 1844 Trezevant claimed that despite having admitted "some of the most noisy violent patients this year, that we have ever had in the Asylum," they had used little coercion.[23] A few years later Parker reported that they had concluded that "a kind word, followed by the warm bath, will generally effect more in subduing the furious maniac than either solitary confinement or any restraining apparatus that has yet been invented." In the place of mechanical restraint they had come to rely on "kind and mild treatment . . . combined with firmness and forbearance." The only mechanical means of restraint they employed were the leather belt and wristbands and the light bed straps. Even these were used only in extraordinary circumstances: "During the past twelve months we have had one hundred and three patients under treatment; in but two or three instances have we resorted to any kind of restraining apparatus, and then using a very light and simple article for a short time."[24] After visiting several other institutions to the north in 1858, Parker claimed that in none had he seen as much freedom of movement among the patients as in his own.[25]

Moral treatment was only part of the therapeutic arsenal at the asylum. The physicians also employed traditional medical remedies for insanity. Like most early-nineteenth-century physicians, Davis viewed insanity as a somatic illness and was careful not to minimize the claims of medicine in treating it. The rise of moral treatment presented a potential threat to the medical profession's newly won control over the care of the insane. The experience of the York Retreat and other institutions seemed to show that a layman could successfully administer moral therapy — it did not require formal medical training. The regents of the South Carolina Asylum initially agreed with this view, because they left the day-to-day management of the patients in the hands of lay superintendents until 1837. Moreover, a total reliance on moral remedies might imply that insanity was a psychological rather than a somatic disorder.[26]

Davis reconciled this apparent contradiction much as did many early-nineteenth-century physicians. Without enquiring too closely into the exact nature of the relationship, he argued that mind and body interacted in such a way that the condition of the one influenced the condition of the other. Mental anxiety might lead to bodily disease, and physical illness could disturb the function of the mind. Insanity might originate from physical causes or psychological causes, but in either case it ultimately produced both bodily and mental dysfunction and required both medical and moral remedies:

> We know that the intellectual and corporeal systems are so intimately connected that "like two friends in harmonious cooperation they mutually support one another, *in health*; but in disease, and especially in *mania* like enemies they act and react upon one another with the most destructive malignity"; and whether it be the mind, or whether it be one of the physical organs . . . that constitutes the primary link in the chain of this morbid affection, the physician will have very little success to boast of, who does not administer his moral remedies with a reference to the condition of the mind, as well as his physical agents with a reference to the state of the corporeal structures.[27]

Davis's approach to the relationship of moral to medical treatment, like that of many antebellum asylum physicians, was thus pragmatic. Although uncertain how it worked, he was convinced that moral treatment was effective, and he viewed moral and medical treatment as complementary rather than antithetical.[28]

Davis exhibited the same pragmatic bent in his approach to medical therapeutics. He did not openly espouse any particular medical system,

which may indicate that he shared the growing skepticism of many antebellum physicians toward systems. This does not mean that he was not influenced in some ways by the ideas of the systematizers. His description of
the post mortem of a patient in 1832, for example, indicates that he adopted
to some extent the view of the French physiologist F. J. V. Broussais that
insanity resulted from irritation of the tissues: "The cerebral irritation in
this case I should think was primary in the brain and did not depend upon
a sympathy with any other morbid tissue—and I should conclude the irritation originally was purely mental."[29] Davis was undoubtedly familiar with
Broussais's ideas, because his friend and fellow asylum reformer, Thomas
Cooper, translated the first American edition of Broussais's *On Irritation
and Insanity* (1828) in 1831. The extent to which Davis was influenced by
Broussais's therapeutic ideas, however, is not clear.[30]

Davis's detailed case records show that he was willing to experiment
in a rather eclectic fashion with a large variety of remedies. He emphasized depleting and anti-inflammatory (antiphlogistic) measures. Like most
early-nineteenth-century physicians, he purged, puked, bled, and blistered
his patients. But he did not prescribe routinely. He tailored his treatments
according to his perception of the patients' condition. Sometimes he employed drastic medical measures; at other times, he desisted from active
medical therapy altogether or employed more moderate techniques. Davis
was not shy about using the lancet, but he did not bleed automatically or
drastically. He seldom took more than fifteen to twenty ounces of blood,
mainly by cupping, and usually the amount was less than ten ounces. Only
on rare occasions did he bleed a patient as a first resort or more than once
or twice. Like many contemporary asylum physicians, he seems to have
limited bleeding to patients whose conditions indicated "inflammation"—
those suffering from fits, fever, or a racing pulse.[31]

His aversion to massive bleeding was not the result of squeamishness,
for it was balanced by a reliance on the administration of drastic purging.
Among the medicines he used most frequently were powerful cathartics and
emetics such as calomel, jalap, croton oil, aloes, iodine, and tartar emetic.[32]
Like many antebellum physicians, Davis favored calomel and tartar emetic
because of their multiple uses. In addition to their ability to cleanse the
system, they often operated as sedatives, alteratives, and antiphlogistics,
leaving the patients in a calmer and less excited state. He also made occasional use of laudanum, morphine, and hyoscyamus (henbane) to produce
calm or reduce pain.[33]

Davis supplemented these drugs with other traditional antiphlogistic
treatments such as blistering, low diet, and cold water. When a patient was

flushed or unnaturally hot around the head, Davis would often order that his hair be cut off and a cold shower or bath be given. Sometimes this was done in an emergency and ad hoc manner. The day after James Flournoy, an epileptic, arrived at the asylum, he suffered a series of fits of "terrible strength." Davis was summoned, and when he arrived "dashed [the patient's] head with Pitchers of cold water. [The fits] instantly ceased." The next day the physician directed the superintendent to cut off Flournoy's hair and give him a shower bath.[34] Davis sometimes prescribed a low (mainly vegetable) diet to calm excited patients. In one case he put a patient on a diet of turnips.[35]

In his use of medical therapy, Davis, like many antebellum physicians, was influenced by what John Harley Warner calls the "principle of specificity": that treatment should be tailored not so much to the disease as to the specific constitutional and environmental characteristics of the patient. Warner argues that this principle produced regional variation in therapeutic principle and practice, and that in the South it led to calls for a distinctively southern medicine. Davis's reliance on calomel and limited use of bleeding follows a pattern Warner found to be prevalent among antebellum southern physicians. Although there is no evidence that Davis advocated a distinctive southern therapeutics, one of his pupils, Josiah Nott, did.[36]

When a patient was first admitted to the asylum, Davis recorded all the information he could get about the history and nature of the case (which was seldom much). He added his own observations (including a physical description of the patient and sometimes a guess at his "temperament" "habit," or "complexion") and then decided whether or not to pursue a course of active medical treatment. For example, Davis recorded the following in the record of John Stokes: "As I have not a syllable of the history of this case, I am without any clue to the necessary treatment. He is a fair haired, and dark eyed man under the middle stature. Appears to be in good bodily health; but obstinately taciturn. He has not the countenance of an idiot, nor is he a melancholic."[37]

If the patient's disorder was recent or acute—if he was excited, dangerous, violent, severely depressed, or suffering from fits of some kind—Davis generally ordered medical treatment immediately and continued it until the patient recovered, was removed, died, or sank into a quiescent and stationary condition. When Elizabeth Caldwell was admitted, Davis recorded that her case, which was recent and acute, provided "ground to hope for a cure," and the next day he began her on a course of purgatives that continued until her family removed her several months later.[38]

If a patient was quiet and docile upon admission and showed no obvious symptoms of physical disorder, Davis tended to forego active medical treatment. This was particularly true if the patient's disorder was of long standing and was marked by a loss of mental power rather than some form of delusion or hallucination. When Steven Parkman was admitted in December 1832, Davis diagnosed him as "extremely stultitious and doubtless incurable." Parkman received no medical treatment except for various physical ailments before dying about a year later.[39] After Archibald Baynard had been in the asylum for several months, Davis noted that his disease showed "so little signs of acuteness that it seems hopeless to put him under treatment." A few months later the physician reported that Baynard had shown no change and was best left "to the discipline of the House and its moral influence."[40]

Patients like Baynard were not always left without medical treatment for their mental disorder. If the malady suddenly became "active," changed in some way, or if Davis concluded that it was functional rather than organic, he viewed this as a hopeful sign and commenced vigorous medical therapy. When Mary Saxon entered the asylum in 1829 after having been insane for many years, Davis judged her to be probably incurable. But after she had been in the institution for about two months, he became more optimistic: "From the lively state of her mental operations I begin slightly to hope [her insanity] may partake enough of the acute character to be relievable. I shall therefore try a course of the tincture of iodine."[41] Nathaniel Snow arrived at the asylum in 1829 in "good health" and behaving in a "polite and affable" manner. After remaining in this state for several months without active medical treatment, he suddenly began to show signs of "Hysteria," excitement of the brain, and costive bowels. During the next few weeks Davis dosed him with a series of drastic purgatives. When his disorder refused to show any significant improvement, the physician stopped active treatment until Snow had an "apoplectic fit" in January 1832. Davis bled and purged to no avail and the patient died the same day.[42]

In keeping with his concern for the individual patient's constitutional idiosyncracies, Davis varied his prescriptions and dosages considerably from one patient to another. The more depleting medications and the higher dosages he gave to patients whose disorder he considered to be in a "high" or active state, that is, suffering from delirium, mania, fits, or extreme despondency. Patients whose condition he viewed as being in a "low" state—suffering from extreme debility, weak pulse, or mental torpor—he commonly treated with stimulants or tonics such as iron, alcohol, or quinine. If he considered a patient to be "robust and strong," like Allen

Griffin, he might prescribe truly heroic doses of some drugs. Davis gave Griffin 60 grains of calomel on two occasions and a total of 240 grains in a thirty-day period. On top of this, Davis subjected Griffin to an almost constant course of various purgatives and blisters. Griffin's wife removed him in June 1830, ostensibly to save him from the effects of Columbia's summer heat. She may well have saved him from a premature dissolution at the hands of his physician.[43]

Some patients tolerated such drastic medication even over a considerable period of time. Griffin was remarkably little affected by the large doses of calomel he received. Other patients quickly became debilitated or experienced unpleasant or dangerous side effects. Mere debility was, of course, no cause for alarm from the physician's point of view. As he was often trying to calm the patient and make him more manageable, a state of exhaustion might well be seen as the first step to recovery. If nothing else, the drastic evacuation produced by a purge or emetic often had a composing effect on a refractory patient. After administering a purge to Saxon, Davis recorded that it had "operated profusely," and that, "obviously debilitated," Saxon was "much more quiet and good tempered—slept at night."[44]

Such strong drugs sometimes reduced patients to a state of extreme and dangerous exhaustion. Davis countered these conditions with stimulants and tonics, and sometimes by stopping the more drastic medicines. For patients who showed signs of being unable to tolerate the more powerful drugs, he often used more gentle purgatives, such as epsom salts, cream of tartar, or castor oil. When James McMillan reacted too drastically to a purge of croton oil and aloes, Davis concluded that "hypochondriasis will not bear intestinal irritation" and ordered that McMillan be put on a course of minute doses of mercury with the object of producing a "gentle but permanent mercurial stimulus upon the extreme nerves and vessels for a long time."[45]

In some cases, the effect of the medicine was opposite to what Davis intended. He gave laudanum to calm one patient and help her sleep, only to find that the drug had "distracted her sadly." She was unable to sleep and became much worse the next day.[46] Many of Davis's patients also developed griping (colic) or severe diarrhea, perhaps brought on by the heavy use of purgatives. Davis fought these conditions by administering chalk, ginger, laudanum, and hyoscyamus.[47] Patients he treated with calomel sometimes showed signs of mercury poisoning: excessive salivation, sore mouths, spongy gums, and loose teeth. He often wished to produce salivation, but when he noted the other symptoms he generally stopped the calomel and turned to some other medication. To this extent his practice was more moderate than that of some contemporary physicians, who persisted with calomel until the patient's teeth fell out or his jaw rotted.[48]

Davis's antebellum successors, Trezevant and Parker, initially followed a similar pattern of medical therapy. But they gradually came to place less emphasis on active medical treatment for insanity. In this they were following trends evident in other American and European asylums in the 1840s and 1850s. Unfortunately, the case records of the Trezevant and Parker years are not as complete or generally as detailed as those of Davis. There are no extant patient records for the mid-1840s or for most of the 1850s. The records that do exist vary greatly in the amount of information they contain; some reveal little more than the patient's name, date of admission, and sometimes the outcome of the case. The less detailed records of Davis's successors may be explained in part by the larger number of patients with whom they had to deal. Trezevant sometimes complained about his inability to keep up with his work at the asylum, combined as it was with private practice. The lack of detail about medical treatment may also reflect Davis's successors' heavier reliance on moral therapy.[49]

At first, Trezevant's approach to medical therapy was similar to that of Davis, except that he seems to have blistered less and bled more often.[50] The case of John Townes is typical of the active medical treatment Trezevant's patients often received in his first few years. When Townes arrived at the asylum in May 1835 in a highly excited state, Trezevant put him on a course of tartar emetic, then followed with jalap, cream of tartar, calomel, croton oil, nitre, and several other purgatives. Townes's head was shaved, he was cupped (bled) several times, treated with cold water, and put on digitalis.[51]

After several years, Trezevant became more skeptical of the advantages of active medical treatment for insanity. He noticed that some patients recovered or improved with little or no medical therapy, whereas others failed to improve or got worse despite receiving every treatment he could devise.[52] In the case of James Nauher, Trezevant tried medicine in vain, and the patient disliked it so much and became so irritable that he decided it was "better to desist and try what mild means will effect in the absence of all exciting causes."[53] After one woman had been in the asylum more than two years, he concluded that a return to her children and the affectionate care of her sister would do more to restore her "than all the medicine in the country."[54] By 1842, he was reporting that experience had convinced him that "lunatics do not require and will not bear very active treatment."[55] A few years later he asserted that the longer he had remained at the asylum the more convinced he had become of "the necessity for close attention to the moral government of our patients, and the less necessity for the medical." [56]

Trezevant did not suddenly or completely abandon active medical treatment for insanity. He continued to bleed and purge occasionally in the case of highly excited patients. From the later 1830s, however, depleting measures increasingly gave way to restorative, sedative, and stimulating ones. Like many other antebellum alienists, he began to use medicine in a less drastic and more supportive fashion. The object, as he said of one patient, was to "restore her general health and see what effect it will have on her mind." [57] If he believed that the patient's bowels, liver, or uterine system were "deranged," he medicated to restore their "normal" function. He tried to build up the strength of debilitated patients through a regimen of rest, tonics, stimulants, and generous diet. Excited patients he tried to calm and keep quiet through the use of sedatives and seclusion. Once a patient's bodily health was restored and excitement subdued, Trezevant generally left it to the moral discipline of the asylum to effect a cure.

Mary Couterier had received medical treatment at home for two years before she arrived at the asylum in 1844 and was "much reduced in flesh and feeble." Trezevant reported that he "abandoned medicine, put her on a generous diet, and attended to the bowels and catamenia." [58] Densby Dorn, who had been treated "very actively" and bled "rather too freely" before admission, was kept quiet and provided a more generous diet than he had been receiving at home. Others were treated for constipation or liver ailments and then induced to work. [59]

Parker agreed with Trezevant's trend away from active medical treatment. In 1847 he reported that they relied mainly on moral treatment and used little medicine, "never having found a necessity for physicking patients because they were insane." [60] Ten years later, after he had become the asylum's chief medical officer, Parker stated that he never medicated a patient "as a specific for insanity, but according to his or her physical condition." [61] In 1859 he noted with satisfaction that the heroic measures long employed routinely and indiscriminately in asylums had "passed into merited disrepute, and are religiously ignored by every scientific and conscientious man." In the place of massive and repeated bleeding and purging, Parker advocated the "masterly inactivity" of Pinel and the other great practitioners of moral treatment. This did not mean that medicine should be ignored entirely. Rather, it should be used to assist the "recuperative power of Nature" and "combat the forces which embarrass its operations." [62]

Few of Parker's surviving case records mention specific medicines. But those that do indicate that he used medicine sparingly and primarily to combat physical disorders as they arose. When he noted medical treatment, it was usually in the case of patients suffering from extreme debility or some form of bowel disorder, particularly chronic diarrhea. John Cline, who was suffering from severe diarrhea, was treated with "minute doses of blue mass, opium, and camphor, with restricted diet and confinement to room." When his condition worsened, he was given various astringents, opiate enemas, and burnt brandy, until he died.[63] John Smith, suffering from anemia and severe debility, with symptoms of dropsy, bronchitis, and other problems, was given a course of tonics, stimulants, diuretics, and expectorants before he, too, died.[64]

Like his predecessors, Parker used drugs to calm highly excited patients. When Robison Marsh became severely agitated after a visit from his father, destroying his furniture and crockery, he was calmed by the warm bath, cicuta, and ipecac. John Mayo, who arrived "handcuffed and furious," was given the same treatment, along with oil for constipation. After a few days he became quiet, the medicine was stopped, and he was allowed to "exercise freely in the yard." [65]

The changes in medical therapeutics under Trezevant and Parker reflected wider trends in both asylum and general medicine. Samuel Thielman has shown that antebellum alienists gradually moved away from a reliance on drastic, depleting therapies toward a more supportive and calmative therapeutics that emphasized tonics, sedatives, and stimulants. John Harley Warner has chronicled the same trend for the antebellum medical profession as a whole. Both Thielman and Warner stress the complex nature of this process, in particular the persistence of older therapies along with the new. This reflects what was occurring at the South Carolina Lunatic Asylum during the antebellum period.[66]

Therapy at the antebellum South Carolina Lunatic Asylum failed to achieve the expectations of the institution's founders and officers. The promised cure ratio of 80 to 90 percent of admissions did not materialize. In the early years the number of cures claimed was disappointingly small. During Davis's tenure (1829–1834), the avowed cure ratio was about 19 percent.[67] But many of these patients had been insane for years before coming to the asylum. Trezevant and Parker reported greater success. They claimed to have cured almost 45 percent of the patients admitted from 1835 to 1860. These results, as Trezevant declared, compared favorably to those being reported at many other asylums in both Europe and America.[68]

Assessment of such claims is problematic, given the lack of any fixed standard of what constituted a cure. The South Carolina Lunatic Asylum's physicians never clearly explained what they meant by a cure. Like many alienists elsewhere, they seem to have considered patients recovered when they were "rational" and able to function adequately according to contemporary normative standards. The goal of the asylum was to repair damaged human mechanisms so they could return to society mentally and physically able to cope with its demands. It was no easy matter for the physicians to judge when that aim had been achieved, because they had nothing but outward manifestations of behavior on which to base their decision. Moreover, their judgments concerning cures were sometimes influenced by their sociocultural preconceptions and values, which were those of a slaveholding patriarchal society.[69]

This was most obvious in the case of women patients. The asylum's physicians shared much of the patriarchal outlook that dominated thinking about gender relationships in contemporary society (which slavery reinforced in the South). The success of the plantation and the maintenance of slavery demanded the subordination of women as well as slaves. As one South Carolinian put it: "The Slave Institution of the South increases the tendency to dignify the family. Each planter is in fact a Patriarch— his position compels him to be a ruler in his household. From his early youth, his children and servants look up to him as the head, and obedience and subordination become important elements of education. . . . Domestic relations become those which are most prized."[70] The southern lady was worshipped as the embodiment of innocence, selflessness, piety, modesty, and graciousness. Yet at the same time, she was expected to be totally submissive to her husband or father.

The nineteenth-century asylum replicated in many respects the patriarchal values of the surrounding society. Moral treatment involved the domestication of the asylum; its internal order was modeled after that of the family, with the physician the dominant father figure. At its best, the asylum demonstrated that the insane could be managed without overt cruelty. Some scholars have argued that its very success in this regard made it attractive as a means of enforcing sociocultural norms. Elaine Showalter asserts that the Victorian asylum was particularly repressive toward women because it was dominated by males imbued with the values and assumptions of patriarchal society. One of the main goals of asylum therapy, she claims, was to restore in deviant women a proper regard for domestic virtues and ladylike behavior. Showalter's thesis has not gone unchallenged, however; several historians have argued that it exaggerates the repressiveness of nineteenth-century asylums toward women.[71]

It would be simplistic to argue that the physicians of the antebellum South Carolina Lunatic Asylum functioned as guardians of patriarchy. As we shall see in the next chapter, Trezevant was capable of challenging contemporary notions about proper feminine behavior. But the case records of women patients indicate that the physicians sometimes judged their mental state with reference to such notions. They seem to have considered a woman well on the road to recovery when she showed interest in the domestic duties and affections and began to behave and speak in a ladylike fashion. When Martha Smith entered the asylum in April 1839, Trezevant recorded that she was "noisy and uses exceedingly coarse language." A few months later, he reported that she seemed to have recovered, citing the fact that her mind was "clear, she has fattened much, does not swear, makes no noise, and is mild and ladylike in her deportment."[72] Davis decided that Rachel Seybert was recovering when she became quiet, bashful, and seemed to be developing "a sense of shame and self-respect."[73]

The physicians viewed a woman patient's interest in the domestic duties and virtues as both therapeutic and as signs of recovery. For example, when Josephine Catonet began to improve, Trezevant suggested that her relatives remove her and "try whether the occupations of the Household . . . would not completely restore her."[74] A show of maternal instincts could also be seen as a sign of recovery. When other efforts failed to restore one of his patients, Trezevant had her children brought to her in the hope that it might spark her recovery:

> Mrs. Inhan's sister came to see her by my advice and brought her children with her. She took no notice of them at first but upon putting the youngest on her lap and making her throw her arms around her neck and kiss her mother, the feelings of the mother became aroused and she gradually pressed the child to her bosom then kissed it and cried. Day after day she has improved and I have hopes that she will eventually under the kind and affectionate treatment of her sister recover her health.[75]

As in other contemporary institutions, some of the patients the physicians listed as cured were suffering from a disorder other than insanity, or simply from someone's bad judgment. Some were victims of alcoholism, who frequently improved rapidly after a period of "drying out" in the asylum. In May 1829, Thomas Martin, suffering from *mania a potu*, was admitted as a case of temporary insanity. The following week, the regents dismissed him as cured. Patrick Flanagan, who came from Lancaster Jail in 1830, was said to have been insane frequently for short periods of time, "especially after fits of intemperance." Davis dosed him with croton oil and discharged him as cured two months later.[76] The officers occasionally claimed cures in the cases of patients whose insanity they questioned. A few days after G. F. Williams arrived, Davis recorded that he could "discover no real insanity upon him. He is an ignorant, weak man, but does not show real derangement." After several months, Williams still did not exhibit any signs of insanity, yet he was discharged as cured.[77] Cases of this sort, although apparently not frequent, increased the number of alleged cures. Moreover, just as in other asylums, patients discharged cured were sometimes readmitted and "cured" a second or even a third time.[78]

The asylum's officers were never satisfied with their therapeutic achievement. They explained their failure to cure a larger percentage of patients much as did asylum authorities elsewhere: the admission of too many chronic or incurable cases, the lack of proper facilities for occupation and amusement, inadequate and overcrowded buildings, and an inability to get and keep a sufficient number of adequate attendants. In a more general sense, the officers blamed the unenlightened attitudes of the wider society for the asylum's failure to cure more patients. In common with their peers at other asylums, they constantly decried the tendency to delay sending patients to the asylum, thus squandering the best chances of obtaining a speedy and lasting cure. Because of the public's ignorance, parsimony, and prejudice against asylums, too many patients arrived at the asylum after their disease had become chronic and incurable.

At the end of the asylum's first full year of operation, Davis noted that only two of eighteen patients admitted were recent cases. The rest had been insane from one to fifteen years. The regents predicted, correctly, that few cures were likely to result from such unpromising cases. In 1842, the regents reported that more than 80 percent of recent cases (of less than one year's standing) admitted in the previous five years had been cured. Of the chronic cases, who made up two-thirds of the admissions during that period, less than 3 percent had been discharged as cured. In 1857 Parker lamented that of 182 patients in the asylum, only 6 had been insane for less than a year, so that 176 "had passed the most favorable period for recovery."[79]

By the end of the antebellum period, hopes for improving the cure ratio still hung partially on an anticipated change of community attitudes. A legislative committee reported in 1859 that the "extreme reluctance on the part of friends, to place patients in the asylum early after the appearance of insanity . . . is the reason why the percentage of cures is not much larger." The committee predicted, as had others before, that when "more enlightened views prevail this reluctance will be gradually overcome, and more of these unfortunate creatures restored to reason."[80]

Like the officers of public asylums everywhere, those in South Carolina accused local officials of sacrificing the insane poor to the demand for lower taxes. As Trezevant put it, "Though the law has made it an imperative duty on the Commissioners of the Poor to send their Lunatics here, yet it is constantly evaded, and they will, to save a few dollars, often detain a patient for months."[81] The commissioners could not seem to understand that by keeping pauper lunatics out of the asylum, they were practicing a false economy. True economy—and justice to the insane—lay in securing them prompt treatment and thus increasing their chances of cure and financial independence.[82]

The asylum's officers often accused families of similar shortsightedness. Relatives had a tendency to jeopardize the chances of cure by meddling with a patient's care or removing him prematurely. The problem was encountered with the asylum's first patient, Eliza Fanning. Davis blamed the unenlightened behavior of her parents (along with the disorganized state of the new asylum) for his failure to cure her. When Fanning arrived, the asylum had not yet hired a matron, and her mother agreed to remain and serve temporarily in that capacity. Much to Davis's dismay, her father stayed as well. The parents opposed many of the physician's therapeutic measures, until her father, "a drinking man and extremely ignorant," decided to take her home. Davis recorded angrily that he would

> have succeeded in the cure of this case under a proper organization of the House. But her parents who were extremely ignorant . . . were so overwhelmed with false tenderness . . . as to make the most improper keepers in the world. They were in the way every step of the treatment. They embarrassed me perpetually—they repressed my measures—and thwarted my plans, and moreover by their unintelligent manner towards her . . . they greatly aggravated her mental irritations and utterly prevented the formation of any new mental associations. . . . She twice manifested . . . the most encouraging signs of restoration—but relapsed in consequence of the foolish indulgence of her mother in diet—and of moral improprieties of treatment.[83]

The physicians firmly believed that they were the best judges of when a patient was so far recovered to be removed. When their judgment was questioned, ignored, or overridden, their anger—as in the Fanning case— sometimes overflowed into their reports. When one man removed his wife against Davis's wishes, the physician recorded peevishly that "her husband who is a great Jack Ass this day removed her."[84] Trezevant cited a similar case to illustrate how the poor judgment of families sometimes destroyed a patient's chances of cure: "To the foolish intercession of her friends and a want of firmness in her husband, she, who was nearly well, has been returned to us an incurable maniac, and must now spend the balance of her life as an inmate of the Asylum." Parker was less outspoken than Davis or Trezevant in criticizing premature removals, but he too was irritated by them.[85]

The patients' families were not the only ones the physicians blamed for premature removals. During the asylum's early years, the regents sometimes discharged patients against the recommendation of the doctors or even without their knowledge. When one patient appeared to recover quickly, the regents discharged him as cured despite Davis's contention that the man's brain was still in an excited state and required a longer period of confinement for complete recovery. In 1837 Trezevant threatened to resign after the regents, without consulting him, released a patient he considered not yet recovered. A few years later, a similar case led the regents to pass a rule that no pauper patient would be released except with the advice of the physician.[86]

It is evident that the antebellum asylum did not achieve all its founders' aims, in terms of the clientele it attracted, the facilities and staff it could provide, and the number of patients it cured. But it is equally evident from the records of the asylum's founding and early years that it was not intended to be—nor did it function as—a custodial welfare institution. It may not have been the "house of cure" its founders envisaged, but in terms of its clientele, goals, therapeutics, successes, and failures, it was closer to the mainstream of antebellum asylum reform than historians have hitherto allowed.

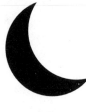

Five

A WELL-REGULATED COMMUNITY

LIFE IN THE ANTEBELLUM ASYLUM

Soon after the South Carolina Lunatic Asylum opened, Dr. Davis described its inhabitants as a happy and contented family. Moral treatment, he claimed, had transformed the patients, many of whom had languished in jails or in close confinement for years. Most had arrived in a "ragged, filthy, and haggard" state, and all were "turbulent, irascible, violent and . . . dangerous." Once they had been cleaned up, given decent clothing, and exposed to the "decencies, order, comforts, and discipline of the house," they quickly became "tranquil, submissive, contented, and comparatively cheerful and happy." Images of chaos, filth, and misery gave way to their opposites to produce an improved replica of the wider society: "They are already a well regulated and subordinate little community, and actually exhibit a considerable share of self-government. . . . They take their meals decently and in good order — play at nine pins, and other sports, and really seem to enjoy themselves remarkably well."[1] More than a decade later, Dr. Trezevant painted a similar picture of contentment: "The term happiness may appear strange, when the subject is that of an inmate of a Lunatic Asylum, but can any one pass through our Court yard, and see the cheerful manner and content countenance of our people, and refuse to acknowledge that they are happy?"[2]

Such descriptions abound in the reports of early-nineteenth-century asylums. They were part of the language of moral treatment. The advocates of moral therapy sought to restore patients to reason by placing them in a community that would replicate the best aspects of "normal" society, a community in which they could gradually learn, or relearn, the principles of correct behavior or self-government. The officers of these establishments frequently compared the inhabitants to a happy family, in which the physician or superintendent played the role of the wise and benevolent father and the patients were allotted the part of children. As children, they needed to be educated and disciplined, but in a kind and restrained manner. When asylum officers described their institutions in terms of the ideals of the patriarchal family, they were both defining their mission and attempting to allay the public's fears and suspicions of madhouses. Were they also describing reality? Did the asylum regime in fact produce such an orderly and contented community?

The evidence is ambiguous, and most of it comes by necessity from the records of the institution itself. Visitors to the antebellum asylum sometimes recorded their impressions of the institution, but these usually tell us little about the context of life within its walls. A woman who visited the asylum in 1854 to "see the maniacs" was disappointed that, because it was not a visiting day, she was not admitted to the building. While viewing the greenhouse, however, she came upon a patient she knew taking a walk in the garden: "He was making a wreath of flowers, and appeared quite contented and happy. . . . [H]e shook hands with us all. . . . He looked quite crazy, although he spoke rationally." [3] In 1855, a student from nearby South Carolina College wrote that he had spent part of the Washington's birthday holiday visiting the asylum. He found the patients, at least the women, somewhat less content and orderly: "The women were much worse than the men; some dancing, some walking about, and others just raving. The men were all very calm, most of them sitting and lying down upon the ground and benches in the yard." [4]

Relatives of patients occasionally commented on the asylum and its staff. After one patient committed suicide, her brother wrote Parker to assure him of the family's appreciation for "the kindness which our deceased relative received from you . . . and also from the kind lady who nursed her." [5] Families were not always so pleased. Trezevant angrily recorded his reaction to the ingratitude one patient's relatives showed for her recovery: "Though cured in less than four months time and contrary to their expectations, they were so kind and candid as to say that it ought to have been done in less time." [6] Trezevant had a much more pleasant relationship with the Townes family. When Abbeville planter Henry Townes took his brother John to the asylum in 1835, he was impressed by "the order, mildness, and gentility of the institution, and . . . the politeness and kindheartedness of the physician and superintendent." After being admitted to the asylum, Henry reported, John had "remained cheerfully and contentedly." Henry assured his concerned family that Dr. Trezevant was a kind gentleman and skilled physician who would give John "every comfort and attention that his situation requires." A few months later, Henry wrote John and urged him to obey the instructions of the asylum's officers:

> You must do everything you can to facilitate your cure, and nothing you can do will contribute so much towards it as paying the strictest attention to the advice and directions of your physician. Dr. Trezevant has a very great regard for you, John, and is exerting all his skill to cure you. . . . You ought to be well satisfied that any restriction the Doctor and the superintendent Mr. Harrison impose on your liberty or your diet, etc., proceeds from the kindest motives, and it ought to be a pleasure to you to cheerfully submit to any thing they desire you to do. No man when he is sick is allowed to do anything he pleases, if he is under the charge of a physician and nurse, but if he wishes to get well he must be governed *entirely* by them.

It is obvious from Henry Townes's letters that he wanted to believe the best of the asylum and to assure his family that they had done the right thing in sending John there. But his praise of the institution and its officers was genuine enough. After John recovered and returned home, Henry insisted that he and other family members should write letters of thanks to Dr. Trezevant and his wife for the kindness they had shown him.[7]

Unfortunately, John Townes did not leave us his impressions of the South Carolina Lunatic Asylum. One antebellum patient who did was Mary P. Allston. Allston's grandsons committed her in 1848, when she was sixty-five. A member of a prominent low-country planting family, she was boarded at the asylum's highest rate and had every indulgence and convenience the institution could offer. She had a private nurse and apartment and could send out for whatever special foods she wanted. (For a time, she ate nothing but pound cake!) When she expressed dissatisfaction, the physicians moved her to a larger apartment so her nurse could sleep in the same room and she could enjoy a fireplace. Parker assured her grandson that the asylum staff did everything they could to make her comfortable, and this seems to have been true. Allston herself praised the kind attention of Trezevant and Parker and claimed that they had relieved a vaginal problem from which she was suffering. Yet she was unhappy with her situation; like many an asylum patient, she frequently pleaded with her relatives to remove her. Remaining in the asylum, she claimed, was making her worse:

"My poor weak shattered Nerves are truly harassed and tortured by being confined in a Madhouse or perfect Bedlam! [I] would now rather suffer the most excruciating death than be confined here." The worst part of being in the asylum, she insisted, was being deprived of the "refreshing sea air" and being subjected to "the incessant noises and cursing and swearing and Dialogues passing continually between the violently deranged." The constant tumult, she wrote, "has tormented and agonised [me] to such a degree that I should have gone mad also, if my blessed Savior had not prevented it, for I can scarcely understand what I am writing or reading or thinking of." She declared, "Nothing on Earth would induce me to confine any human being in [a Madhouse]."[8]

If one reads through the daily records of the South Carolina Lunatic Asylum, especially during its first decade, the impression that emerges often seems closer to Allston's Bedlam or to anarchy than to a contented and well-ordered community. At times, the staff were hard pressed just to protect themselves and keep the inmates from destroying the asylum's property or escaping. The early admissions included some patients who were particularly difficult to handle, perhaps because of previous mistreatment or because the asylum staff was inexperienced. After arriving from Richland Jail in 1830, John Hollingsworth became, in the words of Superintendent Archibald Beaty, "as outrageous as possible." Beaty ordered him restrained with straps and the muff, but he became worse, and Beaty restrained him in the tranquilizing chair. The result was anything but tranquil: "From this with the strength of a giant he broke out—got hold of a common chair, broke it in pieces and with it broke down the door and escaped out the gate of the court." Hollingsworth then found some bricks and other missiles with which he kept the staff at bay. He tried to escape into nearby woods but was soon recaptured. The attendants put him back in the repaired chair, where he continued to rage and try to get out for more than twelve hours.[9]

During the early years the officers frequently reported that they had punished patients for striking or cursing the staff or fellow patients; for attempting to escape; for destroying clothing, bedding, chamber pots, windows, and shrubbery; for uncleanliness; for being "outrageous," "crazy," or "making a great noise."[10] Escapes and attempted escapes were common; sometimes as many as three or four patients escaped in one week. On at least one occasion the patients staged a riot, and on others they were on the verge of rebellion over the quality of the food and the treatment they received. Beaty reported the patients' complaints about the food with a mixture of sympathy and anxiety: "There has been some dissatisfaction . . .

as respects our Victuals—that they are . . . not fit to eat. The victuals . . . are good enough for me but perhaps not as they ought to be. This dissatisfaction has . . . made some of [the patients] express themselves that they will leave us at all risques and that if any of us attempts to stop [them, they] will give us a mark."[11]

One of the most rebellious patients during the early years was Patrick Hayes, whose rule breaking and frequent attempts to escape were not inhibited by any punishment he received. Like Randle Patrick McMurphy, the hero of *One Flew over the Cuckoo's Nest*, Hayes seems to have been a born rebel against what he saw as oppression and mistreatment. Hayes had come to the asylum from Camden Jail, to which he had been consigned for "preaching sedition amongst the negroes." In August 1832, he was confined to his cell for several hours for complaining about the treatment of another patient, who had received a bloody mouth and a black eye in a scuffle with his keeper. Later, Hayes spent time in seclusion and in the chair for giving bread to a fellow patient, an epileptic whom Davis had put on a light diet, after being ordered not to. Hayes was frequently punished with seclusion or restraint for attempting to escape, but with little effect on his subsequent behavior.[12]

The South Carolina Lunatic Asylum, like most early-nineteenth-century asylums, used mechanical restraint and solitary confinement for a variety of reasons. Physicians referred to restraint as therapy, punishment, coercion, and prophylactic. It was a means of controlling and altering patient behavior, of preventing patients from injuring themselves or others, or of getting them to take their medicine. From the patients' point of view, however, restraint must often have been indistinguishable from punishment. Moreover, whatever the ostensible rationale for restraint, there was always a danger that the staff might use it to free themselves from the annoyance of a troublesome patient or to gratify a desire for retribution. This seems to have happened in the case of a patient who refused to take his medicine. Beaty recorded that when they had tried to force him to swallow the medicine, he began to kick wildly at everyone around him. The superintendent ordered that the patient be put in the tranquilizing chair, "poured the medicine in him and let him remain in the chair till the next morning, about eight hours. On the next morning he remained on the bench in the Privy for upwards of half an hour. His keeper tried to bring him away [but] he made considerable resistance for which his keeper put him in the chair again. He remained in the chair the second time about seventeen hours."[13]

The shower bath or cold plunge bath, which the physicians used to calm and soothe excited patients, was another therapeutic tool whose use could be hard to distinguish from punishment. When one patient persisted in uncleanliness, Davis ordered that he be submersed in the cold bath "immediately after each offense" and noted that he intended this "partly as a moral and partly as a physical remedy."[14] For another unclean patient, Davis prescribed several duckings or showers a week. Two weeks of this treatment produced no improvement, but Beaty noted that he and Davis remained hopeful that they could "break him of his uncleanliness." The cold showers and baths continued for about two more weeks, after which, Beaty reported, the patient "departed this life."[15]

The physicians also tried to influence patient behavior through the denial of privilege. The system of moral treatment encouraged the giving of privileges to patients, such as a greater degree of liberty or some amenity, in order to promote a sense of personal responsibility. After Rachel Seybert had spent days in the dark room, Davis released her and permitted her the privilege of associating with the other women patients in the common room. A few days later, he reported that this indulgence seemed to improve her behavior.[16] But these privileges could also be taken away if the patient reverted to unacceptable behavior. As Davis put it, "Privations judiciously imposed are remedies in all cases."[17] Superintendent Harrison reported to the regents that he had barred a patient from the building's portico area for disobedience "and also as a punishment for his filth . . . since he was allowed the privilege of occupying the portico [he has been] a great annoyance to visitors—and also to my family."[18]

Patients normally remained in restraint or seclusion only a few hours at a time, but in a few cases such confinement lasted weeks. Harriet Gray spent nearly a month in a dark room in 1830, and Rachel Seybert suffered three months of solitary confinement between December 1831 and April 1832. It is not clear if they were kept in the dark room constantly or only part of each day. In June 1832 Beaty reported that two patients had their feet constantly confined, although one was occasionally freed to do work or go out for walks with an attendant. One particularly refractory patient appears to have been under some form of restraint during most of the year he spent in the asylum.[19]

John and Anthony, two slaves admitted in 1851, seem to have been kept locked up continuously. They were, Trezevant reported, "two of the worst cases of raving madness ever in this Institution. Their raving was incessant; and with Anthony it was impossible to give him any liberty. It would be dangerous to leave him loose for a moment."[20] The physicians justified close confinement of the blacks on the grounds that they were violent and dangerous. But there was another reason for keeping them in seclusion: to keep the white patients from being disturbed by their presence.[21]

The officers often used restraint, or the threat of it, in order to persuade patients to conform to the rules of the asylum. Harrison recorded in June 1836 that Zachariah Goodson did "not seem disposed to come under proper government. . . . Dr. Trezevant thinks it best to keep him confined until he is convinced that he can be made to obey us."[22] If a patient expressed contrition for misbehavior, he might escape with mild or no punishment. When Jonas Robinson was returned to the asylum after trying to escape, he was not punished, because, as superintendent Harrison reported, "he seems sorry for the offence and promises not to do the like again."[23] Two other patients who tried to escape were put in the chair but released after a few hours when they "promised to behave better for the future."[24] Longer punishments awaited those who refused to make such an acknowledgment. One patient spent two weeks in the dark room before he promised to behave himself. Restraint sometimes produced the desired effect of calming a patient, if only because he exhausted himself attempting to break free. After spending a day frantically trying to get out of the restraining chair, Davis reported, John Hollingsworth became "thoroughly subdued in mind and body . . . [and] promised if we would release him he would behave himself." Davis ordered his release and recorded that the patient was "much benumbed by his long continuance in the one posture and complained of being very sleepy. As far as I can learn he has not slept a wink in the last fortnight."[25] Although such punishments often succeeded in securing promises of improved behavior, patients sometimes remained defiant. After Christian Rumph had been in the chair for eleven days for refusal to take his medicine, Davis reported that he was still as "obstinate" as he had been before his confinement. The physician decided that Rumph seemed "too much exhausted to venture to persist any longer" and ordered his release.[26]

Beginning in the late 1830s, the physicians gradually reduced the use of mechanical restraint and dark rooms. They increasingly relied on seclusion in the patients' own rooms, and they abandoned some forms of restraint, such as the tranquilizing chair and the straitjacket, altogether. Trezevant reported in 1842 that the only punishment the asylum inflicted was "to seclude the violent [patient] from the others, and to keep his hands so confined as to prevent him injuring himself or his companions."[27] The patients so punished, he claimed, were "exceedingly destructive" or "annoying to the other patients."[28] In 1859 Parker claimed that the asylum had long ago abandoned punishment. To some extent, no doubt, this was just a matter of semantics. The physicians still employed shower baths and seclusion, but they never referred to them as punishments. As Parker explained, "The effects of the shower bath, it is true, have not been abandoned, but its uses are restricted to the cases where its sedative and soothing influences are clearly demanded, and is never used as an instrument of torture. Confinement, too, for a few hours among our most dangerous and destructive patients, is often found indispensable; but it is always done with assurances, on our part, tending to disabuse the patient of all idea of punishment."[29]

The adoption of milder methods of controlling patient behavior produced beneficial results. By the 1840s, the South Carolina Lunatic Asylum was a more orderly community than during its first decade. As in many other asylums and hospitals, this achievement was secured in part through an increasing reliance on rules, regulation, and routine.[30] Before the asylum opened, the regents established a set of rules for its governance that stressed the need for order, regularity, and cleanliness. But the early rules were vague; they did not prescribe a set routine for the patients, and they were often laxly enforced. For example, the rules stated that the keepers should as far as possible always be in a position to exercise direct control over the patients. But patients were sometimes able to move about the grounds and house without the direct supervision of an attendant. Gradually, the officers concluded that the laxity of the regime was a source of disorder, escapes, and suicides. From the 1830s to the 1850s, the regents revised and elaborated the rules in an attempt to produce a more orderly and secure environment. Changes in rules did not always have the desired effect; attendants sometimes ignored them or, perhaps, did not understand them. But on paper at least, the rules introduced a more rigid routine in which patients were to come and go, rise and retire in a body.[31]

By the 1840s the ideal routine had become well established. At five o'clock in summer and six in winter, Superintendent Parker began the day by ringing his bell. The patients rose, washed, and dressed under the eye of the attendants and proceeded to breakfast. After their meal most of the patients were taken to the courtyards for exercise while the staff and some patients cleaned the house. During the rest of the morning the attendants tried to engage the patients in occupations and amusements. At midday the patients returned to the building while the attendants prepared the dinner. In the afternoons the patients could walk, read, or rest. After supper, they were supposed to retire at ten o'clock in summer and nine in winter, but this was not always adhered to. Trezevant complained that the attendants sometimes sent the patients to bed as soon as it was dark so as to free up their evenings.[32] Moreover, the attendants sometimes left patients unsupervised in the yards while they busied themselves with tasks elsewhere. In November 1850 the regents forbade this practice after a patient left alone in the yard had burned herself to death. A committee of the regents that investigated the suicide exonerated the attendants from blame but concluded that had one of them remained in the yard the patient would not have died. Emphasizing the necessity for a "perpetual vigilance and an incessant supervision . . . over the afflicted beings committed to our care," the committee recommended and the regents approved a rule that one keeper should always be present in the yards while any patients were there.[33]

Patients and attendants were not the only ones who could disrupt the orderly routine of the asylum. Visitors presented another potential source of disorder. Soon after the asylum opened, it became a popular attraction for Columbia residents and travelers alike. The top of the building's cupola provided an excellent view of the town and surrounding countryside, not to mention the patients below in the airing courts. The asylum's gardens, laid out in the 1840s, also enticed visitors.

The officers claimed that they wanted people to visit the asylum. A committee of regents explained in 1844 that visitors helped the patients by providing assurance that the outside world was concerned about them and saw them "not as idiots or brutes, but as members of the great family of intelligent creatures." A steady stream of visitors also undermined prejudices against the asylum, revealed its true character, and encouraged public benevolence. The visitor would see that the institution was "conducted on the most humane and enlightened principles" and presented "none of those revolting pictures which . . . fancy may sketch." The interests of the asylum and its patients demanded that it open its door "to the knock of the intelligent and benevolent stranger—let him penetrate its most secret recesses: he will hear no clanking chains, but his tender heart will be moved to new and nobler impulses."[34]

But regulating visitors to the asylum was a complex problem, one which aroused much disagreement among its officers. Visitors might be welcome in the abstract, but particular visitors caused problems. They came at inconvenient times, disturbed the patients' routines, and distracted the staff. Moreover, not all visitors were intelligent and benevolent. Some of them came not to be enlightened but merely to be entertained.

Physicians and patients alike complained about gawking or insensitive visitors. Parker reported in 1849 that he was trying to end the tradition of visitors viewing the patients from the top of the building. The practice, he claimed, was a nuisance and offensive to many of the patients, who objected to "being looked down upon from the top of the house, from which place they are occasionally mortified by impertinent questions."[35] A few years later, Trezevant complained that visitors sometimes taunted the patients with cruel remarks or flung tobacco at them for the sport of watching them fight for it. As a result, some of the patients refused to go out into the courtyards. In 1855, several women patients asked Parker to approach the regents about placing some restrictions on visitors to the gardens: "Mrs. Comstock and Mrs. Wray informed me that they seldom walked in the Garden without being . . . intercepted . . . and gazed at as if they were rare specimens of wild beasts." Parker was unsure of how to solve the problem. To interdict visiting entirely, he believed, would not be proper or beneficial. Everyone, even the patients, liked "to see Gentlemen and Ladies strolling about" the grounds. The objectionable visitors were of the "low-bred class." But, as Parker admitted, it was no easy matter to discriminate between the two groups.[36]

To deal with these problems, the regents and physicians imposed various restrictions on visitors. The by-laws of 1850, for example, stated that no visitor would be admitted to the house without a permit from one of the regents. Residents of Columbia could only visit on Thursdays; nonresidents could come on any day but Saturday or Sunday. While in the building, visitors had to be accompanied by one of the officers or attendants and were prohibited from remaining long or conversing with the patients.[37]

The problems created by visitors sometimes aroused disagreement among the officers. The physicians tended to be more concerned about restricting visiting than the regents. In the 1840s, some of the regents pushed for a more liberal visitation policy. The proposal seems to have been aimed at Trezevant, whose limitations on visitation had been the subject of numerous complaints. The physicians, like their colleagues in other asylums, were particularly restrictive about visits to patients from friends and relatives. Trezevant claimed that he had found such visits so harmful that he always refused them as long as there was even the slightest chance of cure. Visits from family or friends often retarded the patient's cure because they revived thoughts of home and the associations that had led to the mental disease, turning "quiet, orderly, and well disposed patients" into "unhappy and violent maniacs." The patients sometimes misrepresented their treatment in the hopes of getting their friends to remove them, and the visitors went away with incorrect impressions of the asylum. Finally, as soon as the patient began to recover, his friends would report him well and want to remove him. If the physician demurred for the patient's good, it would "create unpleasant feelings in the family and neighborhood."[38]

In the face of the conflicting aims and desires of the officers, the visitation policy shifted periodically. In 1851, Parker reported that the asylum always welcomed visitors, including friends of the patients, to examine the interior of the building. Yet the following year, he argued that the visits of friends should often be prohibited for the patients' welfare.[39]

Rules were one way by which the asylum's officers sought to maintain an orderly and contented community. But rules alone, as they well knew, could not achieve their goals. They often lamented that they could not supply everything that was needed to make moral therapy effective. In 1842, the regents concluded that the asylum had not achieved many of its founders' expectations. The principles of moral treatment had nowhere received "*a more hearty approval*," and the patients were treated kindly and humanely. Yet the regents confessed to "some radical defects" in the asylum's management, including among these the lack of regular religious instruction, insufficient means to employ and amuse the patients, and an inadequate number of qualified attendants.[40]

The most easily solved of these problems was the provision of religious services. Religion formed an important element in the system of moral treatment in most antebellum asylums. At the York Retreat, the Tukes had placed strong emphasis on the role of religious instruction in aiding the patient's recovery. According to Samuel Tuke, religious precepts, where they had been strongly inculcated in youth, became almost part of the patient's nature, and they retained a power to restrain behavior even among the insane. In addition to their inherent value, encouraging the influence of these principles over the lunatic's mind was an important means of restoring self-control and aiding recovery. Some asylum authorities in Europe and America doubted the wisdom of presenting religion indiscriminately to insane persons, fearing that it might aggravate their condition. But most of them agreed with Tuke's view.[41]

Shortly after the South Carolina Lunatic Asylum opened, Davis recommended that religious services be introduced. The regents agreed and invited two local ministers to preach. In order to be admitted, patients were required to have tickets, which presumably they earned by good behavior. This system of guest preachers broke down periodically, and the regents had to reauthorize the practice in 1838 and 1842. Part of the problem, the regents argued, was that many people opposed religious instruction for the insane. Insanity often took a religious form, which led some persons to conclude that religion itself was the cause and that religious services would make the insane worse. But, the regents argued, religion itself never caused insanity. The true cause of so-called religious insanity was the frantic preaching of the revival meetings.

The regents also blamed the failure of previous attempts to introduce religious services into the asylum on lack of money, which had forced them to depend on the voluntary efforts of local ministers. These men lacked the time or inclination for the task, and the services they presided over had been irregular. Citing the authority of Luther Bell, superintendent of Boston's McLean Asylum, the regents suggested that the solution was to appoint a chaplain who could provide regular services and get to know the patients. Trezevant agreed. The regular presence of a clergyman, he claimed, could materially aid their therapeutic efforts. Religious sentiment was so strongly embedded in the human mind that it was one of the last vestiges of humanity destroyed by insanity. As such, a chaplain could employ it as a lever to help restore some patients to rationality. Daily contact with the patients would allow the chaplain to become familiar with their delusions, to gain their confidence, and to help them toward recovery.[42]

In 1844, the asylum engaged the Reverend E. B. Hort as a regular chaplain. In one sense, Hort was a strange selection. He was a Lutheran, and most patients belonged to other Protestant sects. But in some other respects he was a logical choice. For one thing, he needed the money. He had recently taken over Columbia's struggling Ebenezer Church, which as late as 1846 had only eleven members, and could not afford to pay much for his services. Also, the small number of his parishioners allowed Hort to spend a lot of time with the patients. Finally, he had suffered from some form of mental disorder in his youth, which gave him genuine empathy with the insane.[43] For about twenty years Hort preached every Sunday to the patients and, according to the physicians, worked hard to gain their trust and friendship. He had a difficult task, because the patients represented many modes of belief and unbelief. Parker and Trezevant nevertheless praised Hort for bringing consolation to many patients and promoting "moral order and quiet." In addition to those patients who attended Hort's services, a few were usually allowed to attend one of the local churches.[44] By 1844, the problem of providing religious instruction was largely solved to the officers' satisfaction.

The officers found it far more difficult to remedy other deficiencies in the asylum's therapeutic scheme, such as inadequate means of classification. The principles of moral therapy required that an asylum have the ability to separate the different classes of patients: the orderly from the unruly, the clean from the dirty, the respectable from the indecent, the rich from the poor, the women from the men, and the epileptics from the rest. The chances of cure, the regents claimed, were proportional to the degree such classification could be carried out. Experience confirmed that one of the greatest obstacles to recovery from insanity was the indiscriminate mixing of patients regardless of type or degree of disorder: "The ravings of the maniac destroy the hopes of the mere melancholy subject, the obscenity of the idiot drives the delicate and refined to despair. The educated and virtuous man or woman, is made more mad by contact with those whom ignorance and vice have made their equals."[45]

To devise a system of classification that would separate these various classes, in one small building in which the patients also had to be separated by sex and, after 1850, by race, was no simple matter. When the asylum had only a small number of patients, this was less problematic than later, when it became more crowded. During the first decade the officers seldom referred to problems of classifying the patients. Shortly after the asylum opened, the regents decided to segregate the unclean and epileptic patients by placing them on the ground floor (or basement, as contemporary documents called it). Excited or refractory patients were placed in strong rooms on the top floor. In 1832 the regents appointed a committee to superintend the classification of the patients, and after that said little more on the issue during the 1830s.

As the asylum became more crowded in the 1840s, however, its annual reports cited inadequate means of classification as one of the major therapeutic deficiencies of the institution. In 1842 a committee of the regents noted that there was an urgent need to improve the classification of patients, particularly to separate the refined and wealthy patients from the others. The insane needed social intercourse, but at the asylum, the patient who paid the highest rate was "doomed either to the society of his keeper, or to improper association." These evils needed to be speedily remedied, particularly in the case of the women. In describing the dangers of mixing women of the upper and lower classes, the regents exposed their class prejudices and fears, and no doubt those of the families of wealthy patients as well: "Can the society of the lowest women, whose lives have been lives of infamy, strengthen the virtuous impulses even of the youthful girl, who has been educated with the greatest care? Rather, will it not operate with the most destructive energy, and soon drive from the bosom the semblance even of that chaste and modest virtue, which once was so conspicuous?"[46]

Concern with classification may have intensified with the admission of increasing numbers of immigrants, especially Irish, in the 1840s and 1850s. Yet the officers of the South Carolina Lunatic Asylum, unlike their northern colleagues, never complained about the problems of dealing with insane immigrants. At some northern asylums, immigrants constituted a majority of the patients by midcentury. But South Carolina had a small immigrant population. In 1850 and 1860, less than 1 percent of the state's inhabitants were foreign born, most of them living in Charleston. The foreign born never made up more than a small minority of the total patient population at the South Carolina institution. During the 1850s, when the percentage of foreign-born patients was highest, they never exceeded 15 percent of the total in residence.[47]

Inadequate means of classification had important financial as well as therapeutic consequences. As the officers often emphasized, the asylum's inability to segregate the pauper and paying patients decreased its attractiveness to the rich. Because the fees of the paying patients covered a large part of the expense of maintaining the pauper patients, it was crucial to accommodate the sensibilities of the wealthy. If the asylum failed to provide enough suitable accommodation for the paying class, the regents warned, paupers would take over the institution and it would have to be supported entirely by public funds. In 1842 and 1848, the officers used these arguments to convince the legislature to fund extensions to the original building. By the early 1850s, they decided that proper classification was impossible within the existing structure and began a campaign to replace it with a new one.[48]

The asylum's officers also found it difficult to provide another central element of moral treatment: occupation and amusement. Soon after the asylum opened, Davis requested the regents to supply some means of employing and amusing the patients. In common with most asylum physicians of the time, he was convinced that the insane benefited, both mentally and physically, from vigorous exercise in the open air. He believed that the physical and mental condition of the patients was worsened by inactivity combined with the meat-heavy diet of the asylum. Farming, he argued, would help remedy this unhealthy combination by providing both exercise and vegetables.[49] Trezevant agreed that it was essential to involve the patients in outdoor exercise to promote the proper functioning of the bodily organs. Activity would help prevent diseases by stimulating proper perspiration, circulation, and digestion, and would help bring a restful sleep and increase the patient's chances for a quick recovery.[50]

The officers' efforts to provide the patients with outdoor employment and activity were inhibited by a lack of money and land. The original asylum land encompassed only four acres, most of which had been taken up by the main building, the outbuildings, and the courtyard. The regents were at first unable to purchase additional acreage for agricultural employ-ment; as they reported in 1832, they had to apply their meager funds to feed and clothe the patients. In 1833 they procured a few acres by convinc-ing the town council of Columbia to permit them to enclose a street next to the asylum. They established a farm on this small plot of land.[51] Piece-meal purchases of surrounding land during the following years increased the acreage under cultivation to about thirty in the mid-1840s and perhaps forty or more by the early 1850s.[52]

In the early 1840s, Trezevant got the regents to approve the creation of a garden on the grounds. But the full scope of the project was delayed for several years because of lack of space and reluctance to pay for a gardener. Trezevant was also disappointed with the results. Too much of the work, he complained, was being done by the gardener, instead of by the patients. He accused the regents of being more concerned with creating a beautiful gar-den in a short time than in providing occupation for the patients. His main object in establishing a garden, he told the regents, was to employ as many patients as possible, and he didn't care how long it took them to complete it: "To arrange those grounds in the order in which I wish to see them, would require at least ten hands, two years, constantly employed; but with such assistance as our people would render, it would take five times that period; but then employment is all I want, and the time they may consume in doing it is of no moment."[53]

For Trezevant, the main rationale for patient labor was therapeutic. But some of the patients' work also helped reduce the asylum's expenses, and in time this would become an increasingly important reason for encourag-ing employment. The officers sometimes encouraged patients to do work designed primarily to save the institution money. When the regents decided to run a drain through the garden in 1838, for example, Parker reported that he had inquired about the cost and suggested a less expensive plan using patient labor. In 1857, he announced that the women patients had produced almost two thousand garments and household linens for the in-stitution's use.[54]

Only a small minority of the patients engaged in agricultural or gardening work. Many lacked the inclination or skill for farming or gardening. Those who had been trained to a craft or were unused to outdoor work usually showed no interest in agricultural pursuits. Some wealthy patients spurned any physical labor. For those men willing and able to work, the only alter-natives to agriculture were sawing wood, grinding corn, and helping with repair and maintenance work. On one occasion, Trezevant permitted a patient who had been a blacksmith to work at a local smith shop during his convalescence, but he took advantage of his situation to escape, and it appears that the experiment was not repeated. The officers employed patients with particular skills around the asylum when they seemed willing. In 1842 a patient who had been in the asylum for nine years without speaking more than a few words suddenly began talking and requested employment in his trade as a bricklayer. Trezevant put him to work making drains and other things the institution needed. Patients also occasionally worked at crafts, such as making woodcuts or carving.[55]

Such ad hoc efforts, however, could benefit only a small number of patients. In 1842 Parker reported that twenty-five of the asylum's sixty-four patients were engaged in some form of employment.[56] The officers considered this to be unsatisfactory, and throughout the 1840s and 1850s they stressed the need to systematically diversify employments according to the social background, interests, conditions, and training of the patients.[57] Firsthand comparison with other asylums increased the officers' dissatisfaction with their achievements. One of the regents visited the Massachusetts Asylum at Worcester in 1844 and reported that the patients had the use of not only a farm but also various craft workshops. He praised the efforts of Dr. Samuel Woodward, Worcester's superintendent, to engage the patients in work and remarked that a "more striking picture of industry was never exhibited to his eye." Three years later, another regent, Francis Lieber, visited several northern asylums and reported that their facilities for employing patients were much superior to those at the South Carolina institution.[58] During the 1850s the officers repeatedly discussed the need to establish workshops, but lack of funds prevented them from achieving this aim before the Civil War.[59]

Financial difficulties also hindered their efforts to provide amusements for the patients. Soon after the asylum opened, the regents purchased a shuffle board, nine pins, and several card and board games. The keepers took some patients for walks in the neighborhood; friends of the wealthier patients sometimes took them for horse or carriage rides. During the 1840s, however, the officers repeatedly criticized the asylum's lack of facilities for amusement.

After his visit to northern asylums in 1847, Lieber reported that all the institutions he had visited provided far more opportunities for entertaining the patients than the South Carolina Lunatic Asylum. He was particularly impressed with the Pennsylvania Hospital and its superintendent, Dr. Thomas Kirkbride. Among the pastimes "Kirkbride's Hospital" provided were carriage rides, lectures, music, a wide variety of reading and instructional matter, a greenhouse, a circular railway, a bowling alley, shooting, billiards, and a variety of board and card games. New York's Bloomingdale Asylum and Boston's McLean Asylum provided many of the same attractions. Compared to these institutions, Lieber complained, the South Lunatic Carolina Asylum had little to offer its patients. He was particularly impressed with the advantages of providing carriage rides and a program of instruction for the patients. He recommended that the asylum purchase a carriage and horses, start a lecture series, and provide chess boards, a billiard table, maps, and books.[60]

Trezevant often criticized the institution's inadequate means of amusing the patients. Because of his concern about engaging the patients in vigorous physical exercise, he frequently recommended that they be provided with swings, seesaws, joggling boards, and skip ropes, and he encouraged gymnastics and children's games such as blind man's bluff, hide-and-seek, and battledore (badminton). The patients, he argued, had "become children a second time, and children's sports should be given to them. . . . [L]et us have a happy, though a noisy family."[61]

The officers were never able to supply the variety of amusements they believed the patients should have. The regents allocated five hundred dollars for the purchase of a carriage in the early 1850s but diverted the money to another purpose. Yet the asylum was somewhat more successful in providing amusements for the patients than in varying their occupations. Private donations, gifts, and occasional appropriations from the legislature provided some forms of amusement, such as newspapers, books, periodicals, a bowling alley, a billiards table, and a magic lantern. Despite many obstacles, the asylum was able to provide some variety of occupation and amusement for those who wished to take advantage of it.[62]

Many patients, however, showed no interest in occupying themselves with anything the asylum could offer them. Such patients often baffled all the efforts of the officers. The problem greatly troubled the physicians, who believed that the unoccupied patients would inevitably degenerate or be more difficult to restore to health. "Our greatest difficulty," Parker reported in 1855, "is with that class who take no interest in such occupation and amusement as this institution affords—who, passing their time in eating, sleeping, and walking listlessly about, with no pleasant object to fix their wandering minds upon, sink into a state of permanent imbecility, or, by brooding over imaginary or real ills, obstinately resist every effort on the part of the physician to give relief."[63] Some patients, according to Trezevant, could be bribed to work with treats of tobacco, sweets, or "a glass of toddy," but others resisted all incentives.[64]

During the asylum's first decade, its officers sometimes resorted to coercion as a means of overcoming a patient's refusal to work. The superintendents occasionally sent "idle" patients to their rooms, put them in the tranquilizing chair, or denied them a meal.[65] But the regents subsequently forbade the use of any form of coercion to compel patient activity. Trezevant strongly dissented from this decision on several occasions, arguing that it was better to use mild forms of coercion to encourage patient activity than to abandon one of the most important elements of the system of moral treatment. Because employment was one of the chief means of diverting the patient's mind from his insane delusions and initiating his cure, the institution had a duty to force them to work for their own benefit. No rational person, Trezevant declared, would object to making a child do his schoolwork or exercise his body. Why, then, "should there be any objection to the same course to a man, with whom accident has deprived of his judgment, and who stands before us in the relation of a child?" To compel the patients to work was better than to allow them to "sink into a state of helpless, hopeless imbecility."[66] Trezevant argued that the patients could be compelled to activity without the use of harsh or violent tactics. But the regents disagreed. So did Parker, at least from 1850, when he declared that attempts to coerce patients to work would generally "be unsuccessful and prejudicial."[67]

Most of the officers' discussion about the need to increase the variety of occupations and amusements centered on the men patients. The physicians complained that they found it much harder to occupy the men than the women. In 1857 only about one-fourth of the men patients engaged in any occupation. Most of the women, Parker reported, kept busy, but "with the male members of our family, circumstances are not so favorable."[68] Employment of the men was limited by lack of land, because men worked at agriculture, in the garden, and at other outdoor occupations. It was easier to supply women with work, because they did traditional female work, most of it sedentary and indoors: sewing, knitting, spinning, and cleaning.

In their efforts to provide employment for the women patients, the officers were limited by their acceptance of the Victorian patriarchal values. Trezevant, to be sure, dissented to some extent from traditional concepts of what were suitable activities for women. He argued that there was a need to get the women patients more involved in outdoor activities. The work many of them engaged in, though helpful in keeping them occupied and orderly, did not provide the exercise and fresh air he believed their minds and bodies needed: "We want something more than the dull routine of needle and thread. Something to divert the mind . . . to cheer up the spirits, is required. This is to be accomplished by amusement out of doors; not the mere walking out which they now do, for that, without object, becomes tiresome, but by employment in the garden, by sports, gathering together of an evening, reading, talking, singing and dancing."[69]

Some of the women patients themselves petitioned for more active and varied pastimes.[70] Trezevant supported their requests but was unable to provide them much outdoor activity, probably because the regents and Parker opposed his ideas. The things he was able to get for them tended to reinforce the existing relegation of women to sedate and cultivated pursuits. Parker was more complacent about the situation of the women patients. He reported in 1855 that the women were well supplied with the means of occupation and amusement: "Our females are not so much at a loss [as the men], having a superior piano and other musical instruments, a large and handsome bagatelle table for their amusement, and a garden filled with choice flowers and rare evergreens, which afford exercise and recreation. Many are busied in the ordinary routine of housework and seem to take an interest in their occupation. More room and *an occasional ride* are all they appear to require."[71]

The officers' efforts to engage the patients in work and amusement, indeed, the achievement of all their goals, were heavily dependent on the attendants. Moral treatment, as its proponents repeatedly stressed, required the active cooperation of a sufficient number of attendants who could carry out the orders of the physicians. The physicians at the South Carolina Lunatic Asylum frequently complained that they did not have enough attendants of the right quality to carry out their therapeutic program. It is not possible, except at a few points, to determine the exact ratio of attendants to patients for the antebellum period, because the annual reports did not normally provide that information. The original rules of the asylum required at least one attendant for every twenty patients. The annual report for 1831 listed four attendants for about 35 patients, a ratio of about 1:9. But this was not maintained as the patient population expanded. In 1842, the ratio was 1:15. A few years later, the regents changed the by-laws to require the asylum to provide one attendant to every ten patients; in 1852 there were 15 attendants for 135 patients, a ratio of 1:9. In 1860 the ratio was even better: about 1:7. But these figures may be somewhat misleading. Several of the attendants were normally assigned to the care of wealthy private patients; others had additional duties such as nursing the physically sick, laundering, ironing, mending, and sewing.[72]

Even more important than the number of attendants, the officers argued, was their quality. The "character of the Keepers," the regents asserted in

1842, was of fundamental importance to the patients' care and had been too much neglected. Many people mistakenly believed that anyone had the ability to care for the insane; the truth was that few attendants possessed the right combination of moral and intellectual qualities. Trezevant declared that moral therapy could succeed only if the physician had attendants who could understand and implement his aims. No one spent more time with the patients, and therefore no one had more opportunities to earn their friendship and esteem. If the physician were to gain the patients' confidence, it was essential to acquire attendants who were "kind, faithful, and intelligent" as well as "firm, polite, and obliging" in their behavior toward their charges.[73]

In practice, the South Carolina Lunatic Asylum, like similar institutions elsewhere, attracted few attendants who fully met these high standards. Low salaries and a lack of competent persons willing to undertake the work forced the asylum to hire applicants the physicians considered unsatisfactory. "It is deeply to be regretted," Trezevant complained, "that we have but little choice in our keepers, and that in the present state of society there is but little hope of doing better; the utmost we can expect from them is fidelity in what they consider the discharge of their duty."[74]

Most attendants had little education or refinement, and few had the capacity or the inclination to carry out the physicians' program in full. These deficiencies were exacerbated by the absence of any system of training for attendants and a high turnover rate. Nearly all of them came to the job as novices, and only a few remained long enough to learn more than its rudiments. In common with other antebellum asylums and hospitals, the South Carolina Lunatic Asylum sometimes hired former patients as attendants. During his gradual recovery in 1834 and 1835, Jonas Robertson served as a private attendant for another patient named Degraffenreid. According to Davis, Robertson took much pleasure in the responsibility and performed a valuable service. Trezevant, who replaced Davis about this time, was less certain. Trezevant agreed that Robinson had some of the qualities needed in a good attendant but doubted that he could do much to help the depressed Degraffenreid: "Robertson's mind is not active enough to get Degraffenreid to converse or to withdraw his attention from the object of his Hallucination."[75]

The officers were convinced that the northern asylums were more fortunately situated in respect to procuring the right kind of attendants. Trezevant attributed this to their location in the midst of a commercial society that both produced large numbers of educated persons and experienced periodic trade slumps that left many of them unemployed. Their misfortune allowed the asylums to hire many "well educated and gentlemanly persons" with "manners, intelligence and firmness." [76]

Trezevant exaggerated the ability of the northern asylums to attract a superior class of attendants. Those institutions had many of the same troubles with their staff as did the South Carolina Asylum. But when Parker visited the Pennsylvania Hospital in 1858 he was so impressed with the quality of the attendants that he asked Dr. Kirkbride to allow him to recruit a few to fill vacancies at the Columbia institution. Parker succeeded in getting several to come south and assured Kirkbride the following year that he had "been pleased with the attendants from your place." Nevertheless, he indicated that his staffing problems were hardly solved, by adding, "I am quite busy trying to do the best I can with very limited means." [77]

At times the asylum was badly understaffed because of the difficulty of procuring attendants. Parker reported in May 1852 that the institution was short four attendants because no suitable candidates had applied for the positions. His willingness to wait for competent help was the result of unhappy experience. Attendants were frequently reprimanded or dismissed for a variety of offenses against the regulations, especially drunkenness, insubordination, and mistreatment of the patients.[78] Parker discharged the night watchman in 1855 after having found him "beastly drunk" at five-thirty in the morning.[79] Dismissals would have been more common had it not been so difficult to find suitable replacements. The regents discharged an attendant for drunkenness in 1847, then told Parker that he might rehire him as a gardener—an insignificant change as gardeners worked with and supervised patients.[80]

The officers were disposed to be patient with the attendants because of the trying and sometimes dangerous nature of the work. A life spent caring for patients who were often dirty, abusive, and occasionally violent was not an attractive one. Attendants were required to reside in the asylum and allowed only one afternoon per week for recreation. Until night attendants were hired in the 1850s, they were potentially on duty around the clock. There were no holidays, although attendants were sometimes granted short leaves for illness. Slave servants did much of the heavy cleaning and scouring, but attendants sometimes had to perform these duties as well.[81]

Patients attacked and sometimes injured attendants. In 1848 a patient struck attendant Thomas Cullen on the head with a water pail, leaving him in critical condition. Most injuries were minor, but they were sometimes enough to provoke retaliation. Faced by a constant struggle to keep the patients and their rooms clean and orderly, to amuse and occupy them, and to patiently bear their verbal and physical abuse, even the most devoted and conscientious attendants sometimes lost their temper. In 1844 Parker reported that one of the female attendants, Miss Magee, had slapped a patient in the face after the patient had kicked her in the stomach. Parker told the regents that if he felt he could ever ignore such an incident, this would be the one. During her two years at the asylum, he noted, Magee had "been regarded by all who have had an opportunity of noticing her as very kind and attentive to the patients and while very efficient in the discharge of her duties is a decided favorite among the inmates."[82]

The salary and environment at the South Carolina Lunatic Asylum did little to improve the occupation's attractiveness. The regents set the salary for an attendant at two hundred dollars in 1828, and this remained the starting pay throughout the antebellum period. The regents were well aware of the inadequacies of the pay. The work, they noted in 1842, was "unpleasant, and wonderful indeed would it be if the small sum of two hundred dollars would command the services of fit persons."[83] That most of the attendants during the later antebellum period were Irish indicates the relative unattractiveness of the job among native South Carolinians. Moreover, most attendants seem to have left after a short time for other employment; several Irish attendants became saloonkeepers.[84]

Parker complained to the regents that his inability to raise the salaries of good attendants made it difficult to retain them and advocated paying more to those of proven ability and dedication. A few attendants did receive salary increases, either because they were especially able or because they had been assigned supervisory duties, but most remained at the same salary level throughout their employment.[85] Parker's efforts to attract surplus personnel from the Pennsylvania Hospital were marked by a sense of the inferior financial and other inducements the South Carolina Lunatic Asylum had to offer. On one occasion Parker wrote Kirkbride that he was reluctant to urge a woman attendant to leave "your delightful place, lest in our Institution she might not feel so well satisfied."[86]

In spite of these difficulties, the asylum managed to attract a few attendants who lived up to the physicians' expectations. Thomas Leavy, hired in the late 1830s, drew constant praise from the physicians. Trezevant cited him as an example of what an attendant should be: "[The patients] all yield to him without difficulty, and all look up to him as a friend and protector—of him none complain—and all are pleased when he is about. This is the effect of a certain kindness of manner, and of heart, for which they all love him." Leavy's ability was rewarded in 1850 when the regents created the position of head attendant and appointed him to it. The physicians strongly praised a few other attendants, mainly women. Trezevant referred to a Mrs. Jenkins as "the best that I have ever seen. . . . [H]er conduct towards [the patients] is uniformly kind and correct, and she manages to combine great firmness with affectionate manner."[87]

That the physicians singled out attendants like Leavy and Mrs. Jenkins for particular praise indicates the rarity of their qualifications. Most of the attendants, the physicians conceded, were good natured and willing to do what was asked of them, but they seldom understood exactly what was required or why it was necessary. Trezevant described the attendant corps in 1853 with a mixture of praise and dismay. Some of the keepers, he declared, "are incapacitated mentally and physically, yet they have strong moral qualifications, which induces us to retain them. Some are admirably adapted by temper and physical power for their occupation, but habitual indolence renders them indifferent ones, and some are not proper attendants, on account of their habits, yet the kindness and attention they bestow on the sick, render them at such times an acquisition."[88]

The attendant problem is another reminder that the context of life at the antebellum South Carolina Lunatic Asylum was not simply the working out of the therapeutic ideals of its officers. The nature of the asylum community reflected a constant, dynamic interaction among a variety of constituencies: physicians, regents, attendants, patients, families, government officials, and the wider society. Like their colleagues at similar institutions, the regents and physicians at the South Carolina Lunatic Asylum sought to model their institution on the patriarchal Victorian family. As advocates of moral treatment, they believed that such a community, headed by the benevolent father-figure of the physician, would maximize the patients' chances of recovery.

In their quest to create a well-regulated community, the officers had to confront daunting obstacles at every turn. Obstreperous patients, interfering relatives, insensitive visitors, and an inadequate corps of attendants undermined in various ways the physicians' ideal of a well-regulated community. Especially during the early years of its existence, the asylum community often seemed on the verge of revolution or anarchy. In time, the refinement of the asylum's rules increased internal order, but at the cost perhaps of monotony and regimentation.

Throughout the antebellum era, a preoccupied and unsympathetic legislature left the asylum without sufficient funds to provide the kind of accommodations and facilities the officers believed necessary to achieve their ideal therapeutic community. They bemoaned their inability to properly classify the patients according to type and severity of disorder, not to mention class and, after 1850, race. The officers also lamented their inability to engage enough patients in the occupational and recreational activities that constituted a crucial part of moral therapy. In their discussion of these problems, the antebellum officers revealed the limitations of their patriarchal conception of the asylum community. They were most concerned about the inactivity of the men patients, which they attributed to a lack of land and workshops. With the exception of Trezevant, the officers were complacent about the relegation of the women patients to indoor and sedentary pursuits. In spite of these problems, they came closer than their successors to achieving the ideal community of moral treatment.

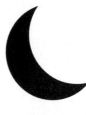

Six

AN OVERGROWN NUISANCE

THE STRUGGLE FOR A NEW ASYLUM

When the South Carolina Lunatic Asylum opened, its supporters believed that they had created an avant-garde institution. But within a few years, the asylum's officers began to criticize elements of its design and location. At first, they tried to solve these problems by extending and altering the structure and by adding more land to the original site. By the early 1850s, they decided that the original building had to be replaced with a new one. They could not agree on the best design and location for the new asylum, however; and their differences produced increasing friction between Trezevant and the majority of the regents. At the same time, Trezevant and Parker began to clash over their respective spheres of authority. For several years the conflict over the future of the institution and its internal administration raged with increasing acrimony until the regents forced Trezevant's resignation in 1856. Partly because of these divisions, only one wing of the new asylum had been built when South Carolina seceded from the Union in 1860.

Trezevant was the driving force behind the movement to construct a new asylum. His dissatisfaction with the original building went back to the mid-1830s. In 1835, he had urged the legislature to abandon the original building and construct one better designed to meet the needs of the insane. His pleas had no effect and, he lamented, the state had thrown away money only "to render an inconvenient building still more annoying to its inmates."[1] As the years passed and as he compared the facilities of the South Carolina Lunatic Asylum with those elsewhere, he became convinced that the state was falling farther and farther behind in its accommodations for the insane. At the time it was built, he conceded, the asylum was a legitimate object of state pride. But many newer asylums in the North and Europe now possessed superior facilities.[2]

To fully implement moral treatment in the existing building was impossible, Trezevant claimed. The facilities for classification, sanitation, bathing, and heating were totally inadequate, as were the arrangements for cooking, eating, laundering and ironing. There were no water closets or faucets inside the building. Patients had to go outside to use the conveniences or to get a drink of water from the well. The outhouses in the yard were offensive. The central heating system had never worked properly; it sent smoke rather than warmth into the rooms. The results were so intolerable that after fruitless attempts to repair the heating system, the officers had given up. The fireplaces and iron stoves that replaced it were inadequate and dangerous. The kitchen was poorly designed, dark and small, and ill-equipped to cater to the number of patients. The dining room was dark and gloomy, with small, heavily ironed windows and brick floors unadorned with rugs. The staircases were extremely deficient. The stairs in the new wings were made of wood, instead of the iron or stone the experts recommended. Those in the old wings were stone but were only about two feet wide and spiral in design. It was almost impossible for an attendant to carry a refractory patient up one of these without considerable strain and a high chance of injuring the patient.

Many of the patients' rooms were too small to provide adequate ventilation. The Association of Medical Superintendents recommended that no patient should be put in a room less than eight by ten, and twelve feet high. Some of the rooms in the South Carolina Lunatic Asylum were only six by nine feet, with eight foot ceilings. Those on the ground floor were unhealthy due to dampness and poor ventilation. Accommodations for the officers and staff were inadequate or wanting altogether. The superintendent's apartments were so unsuitable that the regents had allowed Parker to move out of the asylum in 1850. Trezevant himself had no regular office; he was forced to use a closet without a fireplace or any other comforts or conveniences. The matron, house-keeper, attendants, and servants also had no space of their own. These were not major deficiencies when the asylum had few patients. But when it became crowded, the absence of sleeping rooms, day-rooms, servants' halls, and storerooms was keenly felt. Some of these things had been added later in outbuildings, but others were still missing.

Indeed, Trezevant concluded, the whole arrangement of the building was ill conceived. He claimed, not entirely accurately, that the asylum's founders made security their first priority and gave little thought to the comfort or happiness of the insane. In the intervening years, the patients' comfort and happiness had become central to their treatment. But the building's design, featuring thick walls and arched ceilings, could not be altered to effect the needed changes. To add more wings to this "already overgrown nuisance," he argued, would be a waste of the taxpayers' money; the only solution was to replace it with a new structure.[3]

Trezevant also wanted to move the asylum to a new location. The existing site, he believed, was unsuitable for a lunatic asylum. From 1849 to 1855, his reports and letters to the newspapers repeatedly listed his objections to the asylum's location. The site was unhealthy: the asylum sat on the lowest part of the lot, so that water ran toward it and rested against the foundation. The inevitable result was damp rooms and rotten floorboards, and a higher than necessary incidence of disease. The site was too small: the space available was insufficient to provide the patients with adequate opportunities for outdoor exercise and amusement. Except for the forty or so acres used for farming and gardening, over one hundred patients had to take their exercise in the courtyards around the building, an area of one and a half acres. This tiny area, bounded on three sides by a ten foot wall and on the fourth by the building, could not provide the pleasant, cheerful prospect or the freedom of movement the patients needed. Their view consisted of a small spot of uncultivated and damp ground bounded by a high brick wall which blocked out any view of the outside world and increased their sense of being imprisoned. Enclosed within this small, depressing space, deprived of adequate means of employing and amusing themselves, it was not surprising that the patients became restless or sometimes acted like caged animals. It was an intolerable injustice to pen people up in such a small area when land was abundant nearby.[4]

The asylum was also too close to the business and residential areas of Columbia. Not only were the patients deprived of open space and vistas, they also lacked the privacy and quiet restful surroundings their condition required: "The noise and confusion of its busy population, the ringing of bells, the beating of drums, visitors, persons passing and re-passing, wagons, horses, etc., all induce the excitement of brain and distraction of mind."[5] Visitors from the town disturbed the patients by gawking, making insensitive remarks, and taunting them. The patients also disturbed the local community by shrieking, shouting, blaspheming, and preaching loudly. The town's proximity complicated the life of the superintendent as

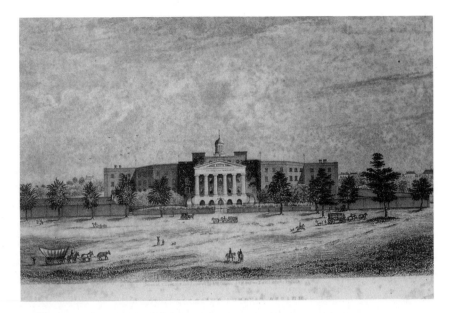

South Carolina Lunatic Asylum, Columbia, 1852.
(From Annual Report of South Carolina Lunatic Asylum, 1852*;*
courtesy South Caroliniana Library, University of South Carolina)

well. Patients constantly solicited him to be allowed to go for walks through town, to go shopping, and to attend local churches. Although the patients needed the exercise and stimulation of such excursions, both their friends and the townspeople objected to their appearance in the city streets. Treze- vant agreed; it was impossible, he vowed, to guarantee the safety of the public, and such excursions placed patients and attendants in the way of temptation and danger. The insane could "never be considered as safe; the slightest occurrence during their walk may prove a source of excitement, and their attendants may not be able to control them. The crowd and the dust of the streets annoy, and the appearance of the stores creates a feeling for possession, and . . . frets when it cannot be indulged, leads to acquain- tances that greatly injure, entices to frequent public places and to drink." On one occasion, a patient was severely beaten by a shopkeeper to force him to pay a debt contracted on one of these excursions. The trips through town also provided opportunities for the attendants to get drunk and bring alcohol back to their rooms.[6]

In support of his arguments for a country location, Trezevant cited nu- merous European and American authorities, including Conolly, Jacobi, Fal- ret, Kirkbride, and the Association of Medical Superintendents of American Institutions for the Insane (AMSAII). At its annual meeting in 1851, AMSAII had proposed that no asylum be erected less than two miles from a town or on less than one hundred acres of land. If South Carolina's legislature followed this advice, Trezevant declared, many of the asylum's problems could be eliminated and the objects for which it was created achieved. The officers would possess ample means for classifying and occupying the patients; the patients would enjoy fresh air, greater liberty, and improved health and comfort; and the end result would be a higher cure ratio: "I have no hesitation in saying one-third more cures will be effected, and ten times more comfort enjoyed by the unfortunate inmates."[7]

Trezevant brought many of the asylum's deficiencies to the attention of the regents in the 1830s and 1840s. But the depressed economy of the state and the antipathy of many legislators to publicly financed philanthropy made them reluctant to propose any major construction projects. By the early 1850s, however, he had become more optimistic about the chances of improvement. In common with many mid-Victorians, he had come to view progress as inevitable. In the treatment of insanity as in other aspects of life, he declared, it was man's destiny to advance, and opposition to that advancement must inevitably yield: "The age is that of improvement, and is with us; it is rapidly progressive and cannot retrograde."[8] His contact with people around the state convinced him that the old antipathy toward the asylum was fading, that the majority of citizens were now willing to support its work.[9]

Trezevant's optimism was not entirely unjustified. By the early 1850s, the possibilities of securing state appropriations for improvements at the asylum seemed greater than at any time since it was founded. The regents had decided that a new building was needed, and for a time their views and his seemed to coincide. An improving economic climate in the state helped generate more support than usual for the asylum's needs in the general assembly. So did visits to the state in 1846 and 1851 of the nation's most renowned asylum reformer, Dorothea Dix. As elsewhere, this energetic woman heightened legislative concern about the condition of the insane. Governor John Manning (1852–54) also joined forces with advocates of a major state commitment to improve the asylum.[10]

But proponents of a new asylum had many obstacles to overcome. Manning's support was encouraging, but the governor was a largely powerless figurehead. Political power was concentrated in the legislature, dominated by the large planters. Many of these men remained reluctant to provide state funds for public institutions and viewed reformers with apathy or antipathy, perhaps because the leaders of so many American reform movements had links to the abolitionist movement. Since the 1820s, many of the state's leaders had been absorbed by the conflict over slavery and federal powers.

The political environment frustrated the reform-minded. Men like Francis Lieber of South Carolina College, who served as one of the asylum's regents, and upcountry lawyer Benjamin Perry labored in vain for years in to secure penal and legal reforms. Perry complained that preoccupation with the states' rights and slavery issues had led the legislature to oppose reforms of all kinds. Dix reported to Lieber that she found South Carolina far behind any other state she had visited in its provisions for the insane and criminals. Its political leaders, she charged, were apathetic and ignorant about the need for asylum and penal reforms. The disillusioned Lieber considered their lack of interest perfectly natural. The leaders of South Carolina, he complained to a friend, lacked "the consciousness of belonging to a vast country, and of the hearty good will to join the great chorus of our times." Instead, they poured their energies into "eternal warfare with the general government . . . and . . . uninterrupted grumbling with all the world." The planter aristocrat, Lieber groused, prated endlessly about matters of honor and the relationship between the state and central governments, but roads, schools, and other hallmarks of progress meant little to him.[11]

Given these circumstances, securing an appropriation for a new asylum was a formidable task. But it was by no means hopeless. Contrary to Lieber's picture, South Carolina's leaders were not all chivalric buffoons blindly opposing progress. Some of them were sympathetic to the goals of asylum reform and conversant with recent innovations in the treatment of the insane. But they were unsure about the best means to achieve improvements. State legislators sought advice from outside experts such as Thomas Kirkbride, superintendent of the Pennsylvania Hospital and an acknowledged authority on the design and location of asylums. Kirkbride was the author of the influential propositions relative to the construction and arrangements of asylums passed by AMSAII in 1851, and he was soon to publish a book on the topic.[12] But even sympathetic legislators hesitated to take any decisive action without a clear consensus from the asylum's officers. This turned out to be impossible. As soon as they moved from a general conviction that a new structure was needed to deciding the particulars of its design and location, the officers' unanimity disintegrated.[13]

After investigating possible designs for an asylum, Parker and the majority of the regents settled on a design that Kirkbride had pioneered and promoted. The dominant feature of the Kirkbride Plan, which many American asylums of the period adopted, was its linear arrangement. It consisted of a central section to house administrative offices, kitchens, storerooms, chapel, lecture room, visitors' rooms, and staff quarters. From the central building, wings containing the patients' rooms extended out on each side. The design called for three sets of wings on each side, with each wing to be set back from the preceding one. Each wing contained a double row of rooms separated by a corridor.[14]

Trezevant adamantly opposed the Kirkbride model, particularly its use of the double row of rooms with a corridor between them. He was convinced that the "double-range system" could not provide adequate light and ventilation. Such an asylum, he feared, would be intolerably gloomy, hot, malodorous, and unhealthy, particularly in the South. Kirkbride, he argued, had designed for the cold winters of the North, not for the humid heat of the southern summer:

> But why should we copy after the North? Are our habits and climate the same? Do we not differ from them in every respect? They close up every crack, and try their utmost to exclude . . . the fresh and invigorating air. . . . This cannot be admitted in the winter, or their patients would freeze. Is it so with us? They build for the winter, and . . . we for the summer. . . . Can a building suitable for the one, really be advisable for the other? My judgment tells me that the more acceptable to the North, the less agreeable will it assuredly be to the South.[15]

Trezevant wanted a building with a single range of rooms, off a corridor lighted and ventilated by windows throughout its length. This design, he argued, would supply more light and a greater and more constant supply of fresh air. In defense of the single range, Trezevant cited the approval of several asylum superintendents, including Luther Bell, Isaac Ray, Pliny Earle, and John Conolly. Trezevant's views on the asylum's design became increasingly fixed as time went by. In 1854 Parker wrote Kirkbride that Trezevant would "go [to] his death for single rooms and an open corridor."[16]

Parker was equally convinced that the Kirkbride arrangement was superior to any other for convenience, economy, comfort, and ventilation. Parker's commitment to the double range is indicated by the fact that in 1854 he offered to pay Kirkbride fifty dollars from his own pocket for the plan of such a structure in order "to carry my views out." He also asked Kirkbride to help overcome Trezevant's opposition.[17] Kirkbride was already involved in the debate over the future of the South Carolina Lunatic Asylum; a few months before, he had written to the regents to defend the double-range plan against what he claimed were Trezevant's misstatements.

According to Kirkbride, the ventilation and lighting in his design was more than adequate for any asylum, north or south; since 1817, twenty-four of the twenty-seven asylums built in the United States had adopted it, including, most recently, one in Alabama. The single-range system, Kirkbride maintained, was suitable for small institutions, but in large hospitals it added greatly to the size of the building and increased costs by about 30 percent.[18]

Kirkbride's letter encouraged the majority of the regents to stand firm in their choice of the double-range system. Francis Lieber told Dix that Kirkbride's reply was "just the thing we wanted" and added mischievously that he could not say the same for Trezevant.[19] Indeed, Kirkbride's missive provoked Trezevant into a lengthy reply to the regents. He protested that his criticisms were not directed specifically at Kirkbride or his plan but at double-range designs in general. Although he admitted some errors of fact and judgment, Trezevant reiterated his commitment to the single-range system.[20]

Trezevant also came into conflict with the regents and Parker over the location of the new asylum. In 1851, the majority of the regents agreed with Trezevant that the long-term interests of the institution would be best served by moving it to a rural site. But after some shifting back and forth during the next two years, they decided that it would be more economical and advantageous to build a new asylum on the land belonging to the existing one.[21] In 1854, a committee of the regents reported that they could not find a reasonably priced tract of land equal to the land the asylum already owned within the town. The existing site, they argued, possessed several hitherto overlooked advantages over a more distant location. The asylum was close to market, in a healthy location, and provided with gas lighting and plenty of good water. They also questioned the therapeutic advantages of a country location. Trezevant considered the town overstimulating to the patients' minds; the committee feared that the country might not be stimulating enough: "Although deprived of reason, the lunatic and insane, in most instances, take a lively interest in what is going on around them. The locomotive whistle, the starting off or coming in of railroad trains, passing of carriages, people moving about on horseback or on foot, interest and amuse them. In all this, there is something cheerful and animating, and in most instances must be more beneficial to those unfortunates than the monotony of the forest."[22]

The patients' well-being, the regents' committee continued, was promoted by their proximity to the people of Columbia, who had always taken an active, intelligent interest in the management of the asylum. To remove it from the public eye might also remove it from the public mind and prove detrimental to its fortunes. Visiting the asylum would also be more difficult for the regents if it were moved to the country; the inconvenience might force some of them to resign. The majority of the regents agreed and voted to recommend the construction of a new building on the land already belonging to the asylum. The old asylum, they agreed, should be used only until the new one was finished.[23]

Meanwhile, Trezevant had won some prominent supporters. Robert Wilson Gibbes, a noted Columbia publisher and physician, promoted Trezevant's views through his newspaper, the *Daily South Carolinian*. In 1854 it printed a series of letters from Trezevant to Governor John Manning that detailed the deficiencies of the existing asylum. Gibbes also published the letters in pamphlet form.[24] Manning advocated Trezevant's arguments before the legislature, pleading with them to replace "that cheerless abode" in Columbia with a new asylum on a larger site out of town.[25] Dr. James M. Gaston, another Columbia physician, also defended Trezevant. In a pamphlet on the mind-body relationship in insanity, he referred to the ongoing asylum controversy and seconded Trezevant's condemnations of the existing establishment.[26]

The ultimate decision about the asylum's future lay with the general assembly. But with the asylum's officers so badly split, legislators could not agree on a policy. In 1854, the legislature appointed a joint committee to secure more information on the best design and location for a new asylum.[27] But the members of the committee were similarly divided into "town" and "country" camps and were unable to agree on a recommendation. The house members of the committee, led by Wade Hampton Jr., strongly supported Trezevant's call for removal to the country. The senate members agreed with the regents that the existing location was best. After more than four years of debate, the asylum's future seemed as unsettled as ever.[28]

The impasse was finally broken at the end of 1856. The legislature agreed to fund one wing of a new building on the existing asylum lands. The regents adopted Kirkbride's double-range design about the same time.[29] A few weeks later, they forced Trezevant to resign. During the course of the debate over the asylum's future, he had alienated most of the regents and many legislators. Francis Lieber told Dorothea Dix that Trezevant was rash, dogmatic, and so "unmanageable" that only "the strongest sense of duty makes me keep my place on the Board."[30] Trezevant had a tendency to characterize those who disagreed with him as parsimonious, ignorant, callous, or meddlesome. On several occasions, he implied that his opponents were motivated chiefly by a desire to save money, whereas he was concerned primarily with the good of the patients.[31]

In his reports, Trezevant sometimes lectured the regents, chiding them for not acquiescing to his opinions of what was best for the insane. They can hardly be faulted for resenting his tone: "I regret that our views do not correspond in these matters, but I must beg leave to say, that it is much more in my department than yours; that I have paid great attention to the subject, reflected, and read every work I could obtain; and most assuredly [I am] more fully acquainted with what is or is not for the advantage of my patients, than it can be possibly expected that you should [be]."[32]

Trezevant often implied that legislators who opposed his plans for the asylum were ignorant or uncaring. When he had gone to the legislature to "plead for the increase of the comforts" of his patients, he lamented, "the very rulers of the land have replied that it was unnecessary, and this, not from bad or parsimonious feelings, but from never having examined the condition of the insane, and from their utter ignorance of what is wanted for their successful management and cure."[33] At the end of his letters to Governor Manning he called upon God "to enlighten the minds of our legislators" concerning the needs of the insane.[34] Trezevant may have alienated some legislators by urging South Carolina to follow the example of Massachusetts in its policy toward the insane. Massachusetts had recently been involved in a debate similar to that taking place in South Carolina. The state asylum at Worcester, opened in 1833, was suffering from many of the same problems that Trezevant lamented in his institution. The Massachusetts legislature had voted to build a new asylum at Worcester, about two miles from the town, on at least 250 acres of land. By its decision, Trezevant declared, Massachusetts had become the exponent of advanced opinion in matters of insanity. South Carolina should follow its distinguished lead. Some members of the South Carolina legislature must have resented Trezevant's fulsome praise of abolitionist Massachusetts as a criticism of their own efforts on behalf of the insane.[35]

Trezevant also offended the regents and legislators by airing his views publicly. In addition to publishing his letters to Governor Manning, the *Daily South Carolinian* printed a poem, which Trezevant probably wrote, ridiculing the regents' decision to keep the asylum in Columbia:

> Nor must the Asylum be forgot,
> They have obtained the Taylor lot,
> On which the Regents will, they say,
> Build something grand for those who pay;
> That other nuisance overgrown
> Must still send forth its pauper moan, etc.[36]

Many of the leading citizens of the state capital became embroiled in the asylum controversy, and the discussion of the subject produced considerable acrimony within the town. The publications in the *Daily South Carolinian* led to a near duel between the editor, Major James J. Gibbes (son of Robert W. Gibbes), and Colonel William Wallace, whose father Andrew Wallace was president of the board of regents. A possible tragedy was averted when the sheriff arrested Gibbes on his way to the appointed rendezvous. The regents undoubtedly referred to this event as well as the general polarization of the town when they charged that the "protracted agitation" of the asylum question had "produced evil, and as far as we can perceive, evil only." [37] To the majority of the regents, Trezevant was the source of the trouble, and they decided that he had to go.

Trezevant's position as visiting physician and chief medical officer had long been an anomaly. By the 1840s most asylums in the United States and Europe were headed by a medical superintendent who resided in or near the institution and managed it full time. The South Carolina Lunatic Asylum had a resident medical man as superintendent in Parker, but he was not the chief medical officer. In the 1840s the regents considered changing the asylum's administrative structure to conform to that found in most other asylums but decided that the existing arrangement was working satisfactorily. [38] By the later 1840s, however, Trezevant and Parker began to clash openly over their respective spheres of authority. Parker became restive in his subordinate position. Trezevant, he believed, did not accord him the respect his experience entitled him to. Indeed, Trezevant seems to have viewed Parker as little more than a steward and apothecary, whose job was to purchase supplies, mix medicines, and keep the house in good order. Parker's resentment occasionally showed in his reports. In 1850, he prefaced an account of the patients' treatment with the remark that he was obliged "to trespass somewhat on the prerogative of the Physician" and would therefore "express *his views.*" [39]

Parker's dissatisfaction with his position was probably increased by his trips north in 1846 and 1851 to visit other asylums and attend AMSAII meetings. The men he met on these occasions were the unquestioned medical chiefs of their institutions, and the comparison with his own position must have rankled him. Moreover, unlike Trezevant, they treated him as a professional equal. His participation at these meetings undoubtedly increased his professional self-esteem and consequently his discomfort with his subordinate and unusual position at the South Carolina Lunatic Asylum. [40]

In 1850 the regents made several changes in the rules of the asylum that increased Parker's authority. The disagreement between the regents and

Trezevant in the early 1850s over the asylum's future may have encouraged Parker to further challenge the visiting physician's position. As the regents became increasingly angry with Trezevant's public criticism of their policies, some of them began to see the more amenable Parker as a suitable alternative. Although Parker initially agreed with Trezevant that removal to a new site was best for the asylum, the superintendent later endorsed the regents' decision to stay in Columbia. Parker also, again in agreement with the majority of the regents, supported the Kirkbride double-range design.[41]

By the mid-1850s, the two physicians were clashing constantly over various issues, such as the admission of visitors and the treatment and discharge of patients.[42] By the end of 1855, relations between the two men had become so unpleasant that the regents decided to merge the offices of physician and superintendent.[43] But Trezevant and Parker continued in their respective roles throughout 1856. Then in November the regents suddenly asked for Trezevant's resignation, after receiving his annual report. In it, he accused the regents of systematically undermining his authority over Parker and the asylum staff and making his position intolerable. Trezevant dismissed the regents who opposed him on the issue of the new asylum as reactionary or incompetent and insultingly referred to Parker as a mere steward or apothecary. If Trezevant had sometimes antagonized people by careless remarks in the past, on this occasion his words seemed calculated to offend.[44] He resisted the regents' efforts to force his resignation, but they abolished his position by electing Parker as superintendent and chief medical officer.[45]

After serving the asylum for almost thirty years as regent and physician, Trezevant left it with great reluctance. The bitterness of his last report was tempered by an obvious sadness at ending his long connection with the institution. For him, the asylum was "like a loved child. I have been identified with its interests so long, that I have looked upon it as having a special claim, not only upon my sympathies, but upon my time and utmost exertions. I have struggled long and cheerfully to raise it to a high standard of excellence, and thought it was advancing to that state I so anxiously sought to give it."[46]

Trezevant may have been overzealous in promoting his concept of what was best for the asylum. Certainly, he had offended people needlessly and been oversensitive himself. It would also be a mistake to accept his characterization of his opponents as unenlightened cheeseparers. Some of them may have been. But others were as concerned as he for the insane. Francis Lieber kept himself well informed concerning the latest ideas about the care of the insane and the design and governance of asylums. He visited northern asylums and corresponded with leading asylum reformers such as Dix and Samuel Gridley Howe. Lieber's criticism of the backwardness and ignorance of the planters who dominated South Carolina's government was even more caustic than Trezevant's, although he kept his opinions confined to private letters.

Trezevant predicted that his departure would inaugurate a period of decline for the asylum, and he was right. Despite its problems, the institution had probably come closer to meeting the expectations of its founders during his twenty years as physician than at any period of its existence. Yet it would not be fair to blame the decline that followed his removal on the inadequacies of his successors. Other asylums experienced a similar deterioration in their position after 1850, and in South Carolina the causes that led to this retrogression were to be exacerbated by the destruction of civil war, the upheaval of Reconstruction, and the long-term economic malaise of the state.

Parker, like Trezevant before him, was frustrated by his inability to secure the facilities he felt his patients needed. Whatever his differences with his old colleague, Parker shared with him a sense of the inadequacies of the asylum. His monthly and annual reports to the regents form a litany of laments about problems of overcrowding, substandard facilities, and lack of money to do anything about them. A visit to several other asylums in the summer of 1858 sharpened his conviction that the South Carolina Lunatic Asylum was not keeping up with the advances in the care of the insane. South Carolina had done much for its insane, but he was "surprised to find so much more doing elsewhere, in perfecting arrangements, and in adding to their accommodations." The Pennsylvania Hospital was erecting a new building for males at a cost of $300,000. The Virginia State Asylum at Staunton, containing 400 patients, possessed a large area of well-cultivated land and every modern improvement. This institution alone cost the state of Virginia $45,000 a year, yet it also supported another large asylum at Williamsburg and was erecting a third at Western. The new asylum at Raleigh, North Carolina, was also "fully up with the age." Built for 250 patients at a cost of $250,000, it contained excellent and complete facilities for every need. Without actually saying so, Parker implied that his own state's efforts on behalf of the insane were niggardly by comparison.[47]

The blame for this failure, he felt, lay partly with the regents and partly with himself. In his report for 1860, Parker claimed that the "intelligent members" of the legislature were always ready to provide liberally for the needs of the insane whenever they had been persuaded that humanity and the interests of the asylum demanded it. But the general assembly needed to be fully informed in order to act correctly. Many of its members, along "with a large and intelligent proportion" of the public, were still ignorant of the true needs and nature of the insane, and the regents had not done all that they could to enlighten them.[48] In letters to Dix, however, Parker blamed his own tendency to rely on the regents to accomplish needed improvements. When Dix promised to aid him, he told her that she had inspired him with the confidence to take more initiative to secure the asylum's needs.[49]

It was to Dix that Parker now looked as his greatest hope of achieving his goals. By the 1850s this frail Massachusetts woman had become the preeminent asylum reformer in the United States and had traveled thousands of miles working to help found and improve mental hospitals. Where others had failed, she seemed to have the ability to convince male-dominated legislatures to vote substantial appropriations for the insane. Her successes had earned her a reputation as something of a miracle worker. Her indomitable energy and single-minded devotion to her cause had captivated people wherever she went, and South Carolina was no exception. As a reformer from abolitionist Massachusetts, she initially aroused suspicions and some hostility in the South. After Dix's trip to South Carolina and other southern states in 1851, Lieber wrote to newspapers in the region to explain her work and to dispel the antinorthern prejudice he felt was hindering it. Yet Dix gradually won the support and confidence of many southerners because she refrained from connecting asylum reform with abolition. By the late 1850s she could boast, accurately, that she was "much beloved by my fellow citizens" in the South.[50]

Lieber believed that Dix could obtain concessions from the South Carolina legislature no one else could. "You do not excite the same opposition," he wrote her after her first visit to the state in 1846. "No one can suspect you of ambitious party views and you can dare more because people do not dare to refuse you many a thing which they would not feel ashamed refusing to any one of our sex."[51] After Dix visited South Carolina in the spring of 1851, Lieber sang her praises to a friend: "Miss Dix has been with us again. . . . What a wonder! What a hero! . . . [W]here she steps, flowers of the richest odor of humanity are sprouting and blooming as on an angel's path."[52]

Lieber was not a native South Carolinian, and his views were often at odds with those of his fellow citizens; but others in the state accorded Dix the same adulation. When she visited Charleston at the beginning of 1859, a citizen who accompanied her on a visit to the insane wards of the city hospital recorded that he felt "it a great privilege and a solemn lesson to be almost daily with one, whom Mrs. D. Holbrook has justly described as 'a good woman upon an awful scale.'"⁵³ Several months later, when Dix returned to present the needs of the state asylum before the South Carolina legislature, she received a public ovation from the citizens of Columbia. The house Committee on the Asylum, before whom she had testified, proclaimed that her efforts on behalf of the insane entitled "her to be placed scarcely second to the great and good Steward."⁵⁴

Parker shared this saintly view of Dix and called upon her to aid him in bringing about needed improvements at the asylum. The most pressing task for which he needed her help was the completion of the new building. The first part of it, a section of the south wing, was completed and opened in October 1858. The male patients were transferred to it and to nearby wooden structures constructed a few years earlier, leaving the old building exclusively to the females. The asylum was finally able to achieve the complete separation of the sexes in distinct structures. The patients were no longer overcrowded, and it was now possible to provide an improved system of classification and more room for exercise. By the end of 1858, however, Parker reported that all the sleeping apartments were already filled, and that there remained patients in frame houses who needed to be removed to safer and more adequate structures. In order to accommodate both these patients and new admissions, it was imperative to finish the remaining parts of the building. Once this was completed, he claimed, the asylum would probably not need to again ask for aid from the state.⁵⁵

The legislature refused additional appropriations in 1858. The senate Committee on the Asylum acknowledged the defects of the existing plant, but insisted that the state was currently unable to afford to fund another extension. They predicted that the legislature would aid the asylum as soon as the financial situation improved. In the meantime, they recommended that the asylum's officers try to fund additional building from its surplus revenue. But this, Parker contended, was impossible, given the already overcrowded situation. According to law, preference in admission had to be given to pauper patients, so that the asylum was once more in the invidious position of refusing the admission of wealthy paying patients and in danger of losing its self-supporting status. The only way to prevent that, Parker argued, was to complete the rest of the new asylum immediately. He estimated that this would require an appropriation of $150,000, but the regents decided to request only $80,000 to erect the center building and another section of a wing. Fulfilling a promise made on an earlier visit, Dix aided the lobbying effort before the legislature. The legislative committees on the asylum seemed convinced of the genuineness of the need, but they proposed and the legislature granted an appropriation of only $35,000.[56]

The regents decided to use this money to construct another section of the south wing. The bitterly disappointed Parker urged them to go ahead with the rest of the building and lobby for additional money the next year. But the appropriation was inadequate even to complete the wing, and in November 1860 the regents applied to the legislature for another $10,000. Parker wanted to ask for more than that. But when the legislature convened, the state was on the verge of secession, and the regents decided that at such a critical juncture it would be unwise to seek a large appropriation. The needs of the asylum would have to be postponed.[57]

Parker refused to give up. He appealed to Dix to work her magic once more on the South Carolina legislators. She was in Mississippi when the call came. According to her own account, she left immediately, traveled for three days and nights on trains, and reached Columbia early in November. As soon as she arrived, she went straight to see the legislative committees on the asylum, and "reasoned, explained, persuaded, urged, till I secured a unanimous report from these parties to their respective bodies in favor of extension by new wings, etc. of the state hospital." On December 19, she reported triumphantly to a friend that "My Bill" had passed both houses by a large majority, and the asylum would receive $155,000 for extensions, repairs, back debts, and general support.[58]

The victory celebration was premature. The following day a state convention passed the Ordinance of Secession. A few weeks later Parker wrote Dix that the legislature had in fact appropriated only $10,000—the amount the regents had asked for—to complete the section of the south wing then under construction. By the fall of 1861 the section was completed, and South Carolina was at war. The rest of the new asylum building was not to be completed for more than twenty years.[59]

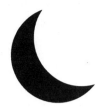

PART THREE

Beyond the Asylum

1828–1915

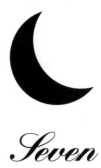

Seven

BOUND WITH CORDS AND CHAINS

DOMESTIC CARE OF THE INSANE

Dorothea Dix, the most prominent asylum reformer of antebellum America, visited South Carolina for the first time in 1846. There, as in other states, she claimed that she had found the insane "in pens, and bound with cords and chains." One patient had been in jail for twenty years before coming to the state asylum; another spent years chained to a log; a third had been confined naked in a hut ten feet square. The family of one young girl had kept her "in a dismal cabin, filthy and totally neglected. Her hair was matted into a solid foul mass; her person emaciated and uncleaned; nothing human could be imagined more utterly miserable, and more cruelly abandoned to want."[1] Dix undoubtedly drew her examples from the records of the South Carolina Lunatic Asylum. The asylum's annual report of 1842 cited several similar cases in greater detail.[2]

Publicizing such examples of mistreatment and neglect of the insane in the community was largely a matter of educating the public about the advantages of asylums. As Superintendent John Parker put it, they helped to "point out to the community the errors into which they have fallen" in withholding the advantages of asylum care from the insane. Such stories illustrated "very forcibly, the evil of confinement in jails and private prisons, and demonstrate the value of Institutions of this character."[3]

Beyond their obvious propaganda value, one must ask how typical cases such as those Dix mentioned were. The actual number of instances of abuse and neglect of the insane that nineteenth-century asylum reformers cited was not large, which might lead one to conclude that they were rare.[4] This would probably be a mistake. One can find similar examples throughout the nineteenth century in state and local government records as well as those of the asylum. But it would be equally mistaken to assume that abuse or neglect of the insane in the community was universal or even typical. The nature of the records makes it virtually impossible to declare with any confidence what constituted "typical" community care. Little evidence has survived concerning the care of the great majority of the insane outside asylums. The evidence that does exist is sketchy and ambiguous; it reveals concern and sympathy as well as neglect and abuse on the part of those caring for the insane. As in the eighteenth century, varying perceptions of the insane and how they should be handled coexisted. Wealth, race, gender, and type of disorder could influence where and how the insane were cared for in the community; so could the attitudes of families, neighbors, local officials, and in the case of slaves, owners.

In order to understand the significance of community care in the nineteenth century, it is important to recall that the opening of the South Carolina Lunatic Asylum in 1828 had little immediate impact on the circumstances of most of the insane. The patients in the state asylum during the antebellum period constituted a small minority of the total number of insane in the state. According to the notoriously flawed census of 1840, the first census that enumerated the insane, there were 513 lunatics and idiots in South Carolina, 376 whites, and 137 blacks. Of these, only about 60, all white, were in the South Carolina Lunatic Asylum. Ten years later, only about 120 of the 597 lunatics and idiots enumerated in the census were in the asylum. The census returns almost certainly understated the numbers of insane in the community.[5]

There were several reasons why large numbers of the enumerated insane remained in the community despite the existence of a state asylum. First, the asylum virtually excluded black patients until after the Civil War. Second, many white families long remained reluctant to avail themselves of asylum care or could not afford its cost. Third, until 1871 financial responsibility for the care of most of the insane poor lay with local government authorities, who often chose to save money by keeping them in the community instead of committing them to the asylum.

In the 1870s, the state's assumption of financial responsibility for pauper patients, combined with emancipation of the slaves, greatly increased recourse to asylum care. But for much of the nineteenth century, the majority of South Carolina's insane could be found living at home with their families (or their owners in the case of slaves), boarding out at private or public expense, lodging in jails or poorhouses, or simply wandering about. The purpose of this chapter and the two that follow is to shed some light on the world of the insane who lived, often for many years, sometimes for their whole lives, beyond the asylum. This chapter investigates the insane under "domestic" forms of care: those who were cared for at home by their families or owners or boarded out. The following two chapters deal with the care of insane under the care of local government and with the medical treatment of the insane in the nineteenth-century community.

The opening of the South Carolina Lunatic Asylum in 1828 offered the state's white families burdened with an insane relative an additional care option, as did the proliferation of corporate and private mental institutions in the North. For example, there were at least forty-eight psychiatric admissions from South Carolina to the Pennsylvania Hospital between 1810 and 1874. South Carolina families also sent insane relatives to asylums in New York, Maryland, and other states to the north.[6]

Yet many families preferred for various reasons to keep the insane at home. Distrust of asylums, reluctance to part from a loved one, fear of exposing a family disgrace, inability or unwillingness to bear the expense, the advice of physicians—all kept down asylum admissions. The asylum was often a place of last resort, to be tried only when home care had clearly failed or the patient had become unmanageable. In the 1850s a Charleston man named Condy adamantly refused to send his wife to the state asylum despite the advice of two physicians that it was the best place for her. Instead, he cared for her at home, nursing her and cooking her food himself for several years until she recovered. Family physicians themselves sometimes counseled domestic care of the insane, particularly in the case of women and patients who required little restraint.[7]

Asylum physicians, however, routinely condemned home care. The physicians of the South Carolina Lunatic Asylum were no exception.[8] Doctors Davis, Trezevant, and Parker repeatedly argued that the insane could never receive anything but improper treatment if kept at home. The community, Trezevant wrote, rightly refused to tolerate the extravagant and potentially dangerous behavior of the insane in their midst. To keep the insane at home, therefore, inevitably meant keeping them in close confinement, deprived of exercise and fresh air. When a patient was kept at home, Trezevant claimed, he was placed "under the strictest and severest restraint—manacled, tied to the bed post, his doors and windows closed and barricaded, the very light and air of Heaven excluded." Home care was particularly inappropriate for the master of a plantation accustomed to rule as lord and patriarch of his domain. For such a man, confinement at home resembled the world turned upside down: "You can easily imagine the feelings of a man, with sensibilities morbidly acute, and judgment so far gone . . . to find himself opposed by his wife and children . . . and watched and controlled by his own slaves. It is sufficient to drive him to madness, and make him resist (even to the destruction of those around him) all those attacks upon his liberty."[9]

Trezevant's rhetoric was not exaggerated. Home care, especially if the patient were violent, often meant confinement in a dark room or hut or the use of chains or ropes. In the seventeenth and eighteenth centuries, many writers had popularized the conception of the madman as an irrational brute who could only be mastered by close confinement and brutality. This idea persisted into the nineteenth century in some quarters and is reflected in romantic novels such as *Jane Eyre*, in which the animalistic Bertha Rochester is caged in the attic. Some home medical manuals perpetuated the image of the animal madman, as in this description of maniacal fury in Simon Abbott's *Southern Botany Physician*:

> In furious madness, the complaint often commences with severe pains in the head, redness of the face, noise in the ears, wildness of the countenance, rolling and glistening of the eyes, grinding of the teeth, loud shouting or roaring, violent exertions of strength, absurd, incoherent, or obscene discourse, unaccountable malice towards certain persons, particularly the nearest relatives and friends, a dislike to such places and scenes as formerly afforded particular delight, and withal, sensation is so much impaired, that the unhappy patient will often bear, to a most astonishing extent, the effects of cold, hunger, and want of sleep.

Abbott advised placing the violent patient "alone, in a dark and quiet room, so that his mind may have a better chance of being composed, and thus become more readily disposed to sleep." The author added, however, that great care should be taken to confine the patient so as to minimize the chances of causing injury or uneasiness.[10]

Novels and medical advice literature may have encouraged some families to resort to close confinement, but so did simple necessity. Faced with violent and outrageous behavior on the part of a relative, many families, especially those living in isolated rural areas, probably did not know any other solution than to secure the lunatic in some way and hope for the best. The records of the South Carolina Lunatic Asylum contain many cases of patients who had experienced long periods of close confinement prior to their commitment. Andrew Stephenson, brother of Colonel Hugh Stephenson, a Fairfield planter, was confined for three years in a log cabin before his admission in 1829. David McMillan, admitted in the same year, had been similarly confined for eight or nine years, and because of his attempts to escape, was eventually chained up as well.[11]

Decades after its opening, the asylum continued to receive similar cases. The family of John Wells, a Greenville farmer, had kept him chained and handcuffed for ten years before his commitment in 1859. Mrs. E. C. James, who was admitted in 1857 in an "exceedingly filthy condition," had been shut up for more than a year in a "close room, every crack stopped, and from her appearance had not washed herself or changed her clothing during that time."[12] Many patients admitted to the asylum between the Civil War and World War I had been chained, tied up, handcuffed, or kept in close confinement at home prior to admission. Several patients had been tied or chained to trees. One patient's family had nailed her up in a room before sending her to the county jail. The parents of a feeble-minded adolescent sent to the asylum in 1895 revealed that they "had to whip him in order to manage him."[13]

Court records reveal similar cases. In 1835, a judge in Barnwell County revealed that the husband of Elizabeth Platts had confined her "to a small chamber of nine feet by ten in hot weather, with the door and windows closed; in a state of accumulated filth . . . utterly disgraceful to humanity. . . . When she was permitted, for fear of actual suffocation, to breathe the pure air of heaven it was in chains like a beast fastened round her body and to a tree."[14] In 1852 the grand jury of York District implored the court to do something to improve the situation of William Miskelly, who was chained in an open log house near the public road leading from York to Chester. The unfortunate Miskelly had apparently become something of a local attraction, a kind of Bedlam in miniature. The jurors claimed that he was very "uncomfortably Situated" and his disorder "Much Aggravated by the Curiosity which prompts Travelers to Stop and Talk to him."[15]

A recital of such cases might lead one to assume that mistreatment and neglect was the inevitable result of home care. But we know too little about the conditions of most of the insane under domestic care to make such a judgment. The case history of Agnes Allen, who had been "partially insane" at home for eight years before coming to the asylum, is typical of many in the asylum's records. It says nothing specific about her care at home, except that during the last few months she became "so ungovernable that it was necessary to keep her constantly confined."[16] Mary Allston, member of a wealthy planting family, was alleged to have been insane for thirty years before her family committed her in 1848, but her case records do not reveal anything about her situation during that time. Other evidence indicates that Allston's care at home is unlikely to have been harsh. The family's correspondence prior to and during her commitment reveals a strong concern to provide her with comfortable accommodations and humane treatment. Allston's own letters from the asylum, although critical of her commitment and the asylum, never accuse the family of mistreating her while at home.[17]

That home treatment did not necessarily mean harsh treatment receives indirect support from the objections asylum physicians sometimes directed against it. Trezevant, for example, condemned home care not only because families might mistreat or neglect the deranged but also because they might be too indulgent: "Which will offer the best chance of success, the care of friends who will humor him, or the kind control of those who know well what he ought to have, and will compel him to do that which is necessary for his comfort and restoration? . . . No private house can possibly furnish the means for properly regulating the Insane—no friend is duly qualified for exerting a controlling influence. . . . Friends will interfere, they will plead, and will often counteract the very best efforts which the Physician can make."[18]

Families sometimes exhibited a strong solicitousness toward the feelings of relatives who became insane. John C. Calhoun initially opposed sending his brother Patrick to the South Carolina Lunatic Asylum in 1838 because Patrick would feel it "to be a great cruelty." At first, the anguished senator counseled the family to give home care a try before trying the asylum: "I do hope that Dr. Richardson may be able to relieve [Patrick]. I cannot but think the case is within the reach of medicine and good treatment. It would be much, if he should be even so far relieved, as to supersede the necessity of sending him to the Asylum, which I have always believed, from his sensitive nature, would be fatal to him."[19]

Family members occasionally went to great lengths to humor a relative who became deranged, in the hope that it would bring about a recovery. An example is the case of Mrs. Georgia Robert, who became insane in May 1844 after giving birth to a child. According to her husband's history of the case, the family acceded to her every whim for weeks before sending her to the asylum. While she suffered from melancholy and periodic "fits of Hysterics," her husband and other members of the family nursed her, consoled her, and tried to divert her from her preoccupation with gloomy religious thoughts. In order to cheer her up, her husband brought friends to see her. When she asked to be removed to her father-in-law's house eight miles away, the family complied. When she expressed a fear of being seduced by her husband or other males in her sleep, they brought her sister to stay with her at night.[20]

The case of Susan Simmons is similar. Her uncle, Dr. William Read, provided the asylum with a history of her care prior to commitment. Her treatment at home, Read claimed, was "gentle" and "mild." Her friends had tried to divert her mind by providing her with "a change of air, and . . . the advantage of sea bathing." They had tried to humor her in an effort to avoid aggravating her condition, but nothing had helped. Although Simmons was occasionally furious, Read did not indicate that she was shut up or physically restrained in any way. He did note that she had to be coerced to take medicine and was denied the use of scissors because she used them to cut up her clothing.[21]

One of the most poignant descriptions of the domestic care of an insane relative is found in the autobiography of writer John Andrew Rice. Growing up in the late nineteenth century, Rice frequently stayed with his grandmother and aunts, who lived a marginal matriarchal existence on a former family plantation. There he discovered, in time, that one of his aunts was "touched." He noticed that Aunt Mollie never went to church with everyone else but always stayed at home in the kitchen; when he asked why, he was sharply rebuffed. One day when he was in the kitchen with Aunt Mollie, she discovered that there were maggots in a pot of ham. She began acting strangely, crying and repeating over and over, "I can't help it. I can't help it if there're maggots in the ham. . . . It's all my fault. I shouldn't have stole that money. I know. I'm guilty." Rice was initially terrified by Mollie's strange talk and appearance, and no one would tell him what was the matter with her. For days he avoided the kitchen, and

was finally calmed only by the matter-of-fact way in which the others treated her. At first they did not speak to her; but as the tension rose and even the toughest could stand it no longer they began to argue with her. "You didn't steal any money—well, when did you steal it?" Then Aunt Mollie's voice got shrill—I had never heard it so before—and she shrieked at them, "I tell you I stole it," and burst into tears. Then came long silences, as she puttered about the cooking, letting the tears fall on the stove and disappear in a puff of steam. But silence itself became intolerable; taut nerves snapped and madness entered into the rest. Then they began to jibe, to tease her into relieving speech. "What about that money you stole," they would ask, and find comfort in the torrent of noise. Aunt Jinny and her four children, even Aunt Lou, joined in the hateful sport; all except my grandmother, who sat silent in her corner.[22]

When nineteenth-century families decided, for whatever reasons, that they could not keep an insane relative at home, they did not necessarily opt for an asylum. They might resort to the time-honored practice of boarding out. Although records dealing with actual cases of boarding out are rare, references to it indicate that it was common. Mary Allston's family seriously considered boarding out before finally deciding to send her to the asylum in Columbia in 1848. Some of the persons who boarded the insane in their homes did so on a regular basis and had experience in their care. Archibald Beaty, who served as superintendent of the state lunatic asylum from 1828 to 1832, had boarded patients in his home. In the 1820s, the family of Susan Simmons boarded her for eight years with "a lady who had been accustomed to the care of persons in her unfortunate state of mind."[23]

Families resorted to boarding out for a variety of reasons. Simmons's family decided that her condition was being worsened by her remaining at home and decided to see if a change would help. Some families chose boarding out to avoid sending a relative to an asylum. In the 1840s, James White of Charleston boarded out his insane sister until she became unmanageable and then paid for her care in the lunatic wards of the city poorhouse. When the Charleston commissioners of the poor decided that she would be better off at the asylum, he opposed her transfer there and announced that he wanted to board her again.[24] Other families boarded out merely because they did not want the insane person at home. In 1838 Trezevant asked the relatives of a patient in the asylum to remove her when he became convinced that she could not benefit by further asylum treatment and was sufficiently improved to function at home. Her family adamantly opposed her return home but eventually agreed to board her out at Trezevant's suggestion with a family at Platt's Springs.[25]

Some families chose boarding out over the asylum for economic reasons. Many of the insane came from families sufficiently well off to put them above the pauper class but not wealthy enough to afford the expenses of long-term care in an asylum. Boarding could cost considerably less than asylum care.[26] In 1846 the relatives of Isaac Lindsey, a lunatic under the supervision of the equity court, petitioned the court for permission to board him out. Lindsey had previously been in the asylum and been discharged as cured but had relapsed. He was currently living at home, but the family wanted to move him elsewhere because they considered him "to be dangerous when with them." The family did not want to return him to the asylum, however, because they claimed that they had found it difficult to meet the expenses out of his estate. Lindsay's property consisted of a farm with some stock "barely sufficient for the use of the farm" and one negro boy of eleven. The court granted the family's request to board Lindsay, but his relatives later returned him to the asylum. By 1853, payments for his care were more than eight hundred dollars in arrears.[27]

Inability to afford asylum care probably induced the family of John Miller to board him with William Little of Union District in the early 1840s. In return for caring for Miller, Little was to receive the proceeds from his estate, but these turned out to be insufficient to cover the expenses of caring for him. Miller was no pauper, but neither was he rich. The inventory of his property included sixty acres of land along with "one negro man, one cow and calf, one bed, two Jars, one oven, one smoothing Iron and one Kittle."[28]

Distrust of asylums and lack of money were not the only things that kept the insane at home: race could too. The South Carolina Lunatic Asylum could not legally accept black patients until after 1848 and only about thirty were admitted between then and the Civil War. Only after emancipation was the asylum fully opened to black patients. The Charleston poorhouse hospital accepted some insane blacks into its lunatic department during the antebellum decades. But for most blacks who became deranged prior to 1865, domestic care was the only option. Most of them were slaves, but a small number were free blacks.

Any attempt to assess the situation of insane slaves is complicated at the outset by two major problems. One is simply a lack of information. The fate of individual insane slaves seldom became a matter of public concern, so there are few records from which to make a judgment. Moreover, although many historians have investigated the health and medical care of slaves, few have examined the psychiatric aspects of the subject in more than a cursory fashion.[29] The second problem, which may help explain the first, is that the situation of insane blacks was not simply a medical issue—it was a political and cultural one. Antebellum apologists for slavery often claimed that insanity among slaves as (opposed to free blacks) was extremely rare. Proslavery propaganda attributed the alleged immunity of slaves to mental disorders to the supposedly happy and carefree life of the bondsman, whose master supplied his every want. According to the proslavery argument, blacks were mentally unsuited to a life of freedom because their nervous systems were allegedly more primitive than those of whites and thus less capable of coping with the stresses and temptations of civilized life. The cocoon of slavery sheltered blacks from the anxieties and vices which afflicted whites, and kept the black insanity rate low. If this protection were removed by emancipation, blacks would succumb to mental disorders in much larger proportions than whites.[30]

Proslavery writers found ringing confirmation for their argument in the census of 1840, which seemed to show that free blacks in the North suffered from a much higher incidence of insanity and other health problems than either southern slaves (or southern whites, for that matter). According to the census, there were only 137 black lunatics and idiots in South Carolina, a proportion of 1 to 2,477 of the black population. In Maine, where all the blacks were free, the proportion was said to be 1 to 14, and for South Carolina's whites it was supposedly 1 to 689. Dr. Edward Jarvis, a northern alienist, demonstrated in 1844 that the insanity statistics were riddled with errors, but his efforts to get the census revised were blocked by Secretary of State John C. Calhoun of South Carolina, who found the data too useful to the proslavery argument. In 1844, for example, Calhoun cited the census in justifying to the British government the decision to add Texas to the Union as a slave state. To Calhoun, the census showed that slavery was beneficial, freedom detrimental, to blacks. In states in which blacks had been freed, he claimed, they had "invariably sunk into vice and pauperism, accompanied by blindness, insanity, and idiocy—to a degree without example; while in all [the slave states] they have improved greatly in every respect."[31] Proslavery writers repeated Calhoun's arguments throughout the 1840s and 1850s, predicting an unprecedented onslaught of black deviance should the benevolent discipline of slavery be removed.[32]

The need to present slavery in a positive light encouraged southern apologists to minimize the extent of mental disorders among slaves and to ignore evidence to the contrary. When the English writer Harriet Martineau visited South Carolina in the mid-1830s, she was puzzled by whites' apparent lack of knowledge and concern about the condition of physically and mentally disabled slaves. "I was beset by many an anxious thought about the fate of disabled slaves," she recorded later; "while there are many [slaveholders] who abuse the authority they have over slaves who are not helpless, it is fearful to think what may be the fate of those who are purely burdensome." As she traveled about the state, she was particularly struck by the absence of insane slaves; except for an occasional idiot, she had seen none. She visited the South Carolina Lunatic Asylum only to learn that there were no slaves confined there. A physician, possibly Davis or Trezevant, took her and a group of local citizens on a tour of the asylum. Surveying the patients from the roof promenade, Martineau remarked on the absence of black patients and asked if "negroes were as subject to insanity as whites." The physician answered that given "the violence of their passions" they probably were, "but no means were known to have been taken to ascertain the fact." None of her companions remembered having seen any insane blacks. "Where were they then?" she asked. No one seemed to know. Finally, the physician said that "he had no doubt that they were kept in outhouses, chained to logs, to prevent their doing harm."

Coming from England, where the state of the insane had recently become a matter of considerable public interest and investigation, Martineau was appalled to learn that "no member of society is charged with the duty of investigating the cases of suffering and disease among slaves, who cannot make their own state known." Such slaves, she concluded, were "wholly at the mercy of their owners."[33]

Not surprisingly, Martineau's remarks about insane slaves, published in 1837, offended her former hosts. Although she mentioned that the few idiot slaves she had seen "were kindly treated, humored and indulged," she implied that many masters were prone to mistreat "useless" slaves. She also insinuated that South Carolina's white citizens neither knew nor cared about the mental state of their black bondsmen. Finally, and most damagingly, she cited a local authority on insanity who admitted that many insane slaves were indeed probably neglected.[34] Charleston writer and plantation owner William Gilmore Simms quickly leapt to the defense of slavery and the honor of his state and region. In an essay on "The Morals of Slavery," Simms ridiculed Martineau's remarks about slavery and insanity. She had seen few insane blacks, he countered, because there were few to be seen, thanks to the advantages of the slave system:

> The absence of all care for the morrow, for the future, for their own support in age, and the support of their children, together with the restraints of labor, tending to the subjection of those intense passions of which Miss Martineau speaks, and which are not in consequence so active, I am inclined to think, in the negro as in the white man, must greatly abridge the tendency to insanity; and it may be that the general inferior activity of their minds, is one cause of their freedom from this dreadful malady. Certain it is, that we have few or no madmen among the negroes. . . . [I]n truth, there is little or no madness in South Carolina, whether among black or white.

Simms scorned Martineau's implication that masters mistreated or neglected insane slaves. A suffering slave, he replied, was not at the mercy of his owner. Slaves were seldom reticent about complaining; a brutal slaveholder would soon become known and the courts would punish his transgressions. Besides, the slaveholder had an economic interest in protecting the health and life of his slaves that made any formal public supervision of his management unnecessary. The notion that slave owners chained up lunatic slaves in outhouses was "ridiculous." Necessity might force one to employ such restraint in an emergency, but it would only be temporary: "A madman, chained in an outhouse, would be a sufficient source of disquiet to all the country round; and the neighborhood would soon rise, *en masse*, and compel his removal to a place of safe-keeping."[35]

Simms's arguments were not necessarily an opportunistic fabrication for northern consumption. Thoughtful southerners such as Simms may have believed what they said, because they seldom saw or heard about insane slaves. Most slaves lived on rural and often isolated plantations. Despite what Simms said about public vigilance, as long as a slaveholder kept an insane slave under close control, his existence was unlikely to attract much public attention. Moreover, it is likely that slaveholders often failed to recognize the existence of insanity in a slave. Diagnosis was complicated by owners' or overseers' tendency to suspect slaves of feigning illness to avoid work. Writers on plantation management and the medical care of slaves warned slaveholders and physicians to be wary of the slaves' proclivity to malinger. In 1818, Charles Cotesworth Pinckney listed among his slaves not working in the fields one named Old Sambo who "Pretends to be Crazy."[36]

The ability of slave owners to employ slaves who were only mildly or temporarily disturbed undoubtedly further diminished the number of slaves that were reported as insane. The English actress Fanny Kemble, who spent some time at one of the Butler plantations in Georgia, recalled meeting a slave, "a poor, half-witted creature, a female idiot, whose mental incapacity, of course, in no respects unfits her for the life of toil, little more intellectual than that of any beast of burden, which is her allotted portion here."[37] Many slave owners probably mistook some cases of mental disorder for wilful misbehavior and resorted to whipping, jail, or the trading block instead of the physician. When Will, a slave belonging to Mrs. W. B. Blythe, became "violent and unmanageable," the family pressed her to sell him and then sent him off to jail.[38] Sarah, one of Pierce Butler's slaves, told Kemble that she once became mad and ran off into the woods. After being recaptured, Sarah claimed, "she was tied up by the arms, and heavy logs fastened to her feet, and was severely flogged."[39]

Slaveholders and physicians may have attributed some forms of insanity among slaves to overactive imaginations or superstition. One southern physician argued in the 1850s that many of the slaves' diseases and much of their unhappiness were the result of "purely imaginary causes" such as belief in witchcraft.[40] Whites were sometimes mystified by slaves who claimed that they were conjured, possessed, or poisoned, or kept jumping into water. Some of these symptoms may have been the result of pellagra, a deficiency disease that can produce severe depression and bizarre behavior in its advanced stages.[41]

Some antebellum physicians believed that the incidence of some forms of mental disorder among slaves was underdiagnosed. Daniel Drake, for example, argued that slaves exhibited a high incidence of hysteria and epilepsy.[42] Dr. Samuel Cartwright of New Orleans claimed to have discovered mental diseases that were peculiar to blacks. Cartwright, a strong advocate of both slavery and a distinctive southern (or states' rights) medicine, argued that blacks exhibited diseases and conditions that only a properly (i.e., southern) trained physician could recognize and treat. Cartwright labeled one of these disorders drapetomania, the disease that caused slaves to run away. The chief diagnostic symptom of drapetomania, "absconding from service," was well known to planters and overseers. But medical writers, who had not paid enough attention to blacks' diseases, refused to see it for what it was: a disease of the mind. Slaves who suffered from drapetomania had become so irrational that they tried to flee from the position that God and nature had designed them to fill.

Cartwright attributed another peculiar form of mental illness to blacks, which he called "Dyaethesia Aethiopica, or Hebetude of Mind and Obtuse Sensibility of Body . . . called by Overseers, 'Rascality.' " This disease, he claimed, was much more common among free blacks than slaves; it attacked slaves whose owners allowed them too much freedom. The symptoms of dyaethesia included mental lethargy and a partial loss of sensibility in the skin. The victims of the disorder tended to do a lot of mischief that seemed to be intentional but was in reality due largely "to the stupidness of mind and insensibility of the nerves induced by the disease." Dyaethesics tended "to break, waste and destroy everything they handle." They "tear, burn rend their own clothing, and paying no attention to the rights of property, steal others, to replace what they have destroyed. They slight their work. . . . They raise disturbances with their overseers and fellow servants without cause or motive, and seem to be insensible to pain when subjected to punishment." Cartwright noted that northern physicians had observed the symptoms of dyaethesia but wrongly attributed them to slavery and ignored their greater prevalence among blacks who had been free for generations. The disease was "the natural offspring of negro liberty—the liberty to be idle, wallow in filth, and to indulge in improper food and drinks."[43]

It is difficult to judge how much influence Cartwright had on the diagnosis of insanity among blacks. Many southern physicians agreed with his general conclusions about the uniqueness of the Negro constitution and the need for a distinctive southern medicine but dissented from some of the extremes to which he pushed the idea. Reviewers in the *Charleston Medical Journal and Review* argued that Cartwright had overstated his case out of his desire to buttress the political cause of the South and the institution of slavery, and that some of his arguments were absurd. James Smith, a Louisiana physician, dismissed Cartwright's arguments contemptuously as an attempt to medicalize vices "which shall no longer be treated by the Penitentiary, but by calomel, capsicum, etc."[44] Whatever the effects of Cartwright's article, it is doubtful that many slave owners or physicians tried to control obstreperous slaves by labeling and treating them as insane. The institution of slavery would seem to have usually provided all the control that was necessary. On the other hand, some slave owners may have felt better by diagnosing an unhappy or difficult slave as insane.[45]

Just how problematic the diagnosis of insanity in slaves could be is indicated by some entries in the journal of planter Thomas B. Chaplin of St. Helena Island. In December 1848, Chaplin recorded in his journal that his slave Peter had been unable to work for some time and commented, "God knows what is the matter with him, I do not." Chaplin's physician neighbor, Dr. John Scott, sent over some "powders" for Peter, but the slave only got worse. Scott came to see Peter himself in January but was also mystified by the slave's condition. At first he thought that Peter was suffering from some form of "strain," then he attributed the problem to an overactive imagination. Chaplin reported that Scott "thinks [Peter's] mind is worried by Negroes putting notions in his head that he is tricked, etc." A few days later, Scott confessed that he was unable to diagnose the source of the problem. When he returned in March, he decided that Peter's "mind was diseased." A few days later, Scott added that he thought that Peter's liver was diseased.[46]

The fate of slaves diagnosed as insane varied considerably. With one eye on northern opinion, slaveholders often proclaimed their concern for the health and welfare of their slaves; and treatises on the management and care of slaves stressed that humanity and self-interest demanded that slave owners care for their diseased or disabled bondsmen. It was not all rhetoric. Slave owners often expended considerable effort and money to provide care and medical treatment for their slaves. Large plantations sometimes featured well-equipped slave hospitals; others provided regular medical service through a contract with a physician. More often, the master or overseer called in medical help as needed or sent sick slaves to a physician for treatment. Physicians in Charleston, Columbia, and Savannah operated slave hospitals during the antebellum period, and they seem to have been well patronized.[47] When Joe, a slave on a plantation near Charleston, became insane in 1846, his owner brought him to town and placed him under the care of Dr. W. T. Wragg. Joe's treatment, which lasted for two months, must have cost his master a sizable sum.[48] Some slaveholders were able to place insane slaves as pay patients in the lunatic wards of the Charleston poorhouse or in the city's Roper Hospital, which took over the poorhouse's psychiatric functions in 1856.[49]

But not every owner was willing or able to provide extensive and expensive care for an insane slave. Many slaveholders, particularly the less affluent, tried to do without physicians or turned to them only after trying and failing to cure a sick slave themselves. One planter wrote that he avoided "sending any [of his slaves] down to the Doctor as much as possible. I know how extortionate [physicians] are."[50] Experience convinced some slaveholders that calling in the doctor rarely did the slaves much good. James Henry Hammond took a great interest in the medical care of his slaves, and he initially employed physicians regularly. But the high mortality rates on his plantation eroded his faith in regular practitioners and he turned to home remedies and to irregular medical practices such as Thomsonianism and homeopathy.[51]

Plantation hospitals, where they existed, were sometimes little more than shacks with dirt floors and an aged slave to attend the sick. Fanny Kemble was shocked by the condition of the slave hospitals on the Butler plantations in Georgia, in one of which she found a "half-witted" young woman: "So miserable a place for the purpose to which it was dedicated I could not have imagined on a property belonging to Christian owners. The floor (which was not boarded, but merely the damp hard earth itself) was strewn with wretched women, who, but for their moans of pain, and uneasy, restless motions, might very well each have been taken for a mere heap of filthy rags."[52]

Slaveholders might view an insane slave as simply a nuisance, especially if he seemed to be incurable. Pierce Butler listed one of his slaves in the 1840s as "deranged unfortunately and in the way."[53] Some owners tried to sell or send away mentally disordered slaves. One wrote in 1835 that he had sold a slave who was "*nearly* an idiot" for six hundred dollars, which he thought "an excellent price for her."[54] Given these attitudes and actions, it would hardly have been surprising if some slave owners simply chained insane slaves up in outhouses or turned them loose. Admittedly, there is not much evidence that owners often treated insane slaves in this way. But if white lunatics sometimes suffered abuse and neglect, it would be myopic to think that insane slaves fared better; the probability is that they generally fared worse.

Some evidence supporting this assumption comes from slaveholders themselves. William Gilmore Simms, who ridiculed Harriet Martineau's insinuations about the neglect of insane slaves, wrote an article a few years later that advocated opening the state asylum to blacks. In it, he argued that insane slaves should not be "suffered to be left in the hands of owners . . . either kept in outhouses, perhaps chained, or roaming at large, mischievous and troublesome—and without any prospect of being relieved, save by death, from their misery."[55] In 1847, a legislative report on the colored insane concluded that "even the kindest and best" owners could not provide insane slaves with the kind of attention and comfort that their situation and humanity demanded.[56]

Many owners probably felt at a loss when confronted with an insane slave. In 1857 Adele Petigru Allston wrote to her husband that one of their slaves, Lizzie, was showing signs of mental disorder. "I do not know what is to be done with her," Mrs. Allston confessed. Slaveholders may occasionally have practiced a rudimentary form of moral treatment by shifting a disturbed slave to a different environment or type of work. Mrs. Allston speculated that if Lizzie was not provided with "some regular employment . . . suitable to her . . . she will lose her senses from these tempers. . . . If she was in a house next to Old Thomas, perhaps he would acquire some influence over her."[57]

Slaves themselves may sometimes have influenced their care. When Dr. John Scott decided that the mind of Thomas Chaplin's slave Peter was diseased, he advised Chaplin to give him a change of scenery. Scott recommended sending Peter to the mainland. But Chaplin decided instead to send Peter to the home of another neighbor, Frank Capers, who offered to try to cure him for free. Chaplin's motivation may have been a desire to save money (he had chronic financial problems), but he recorded that Peter had expressed "a willingness to go with Frank and unwillingness to go to the main[land]."[58]

Most insane blacks during the antebellum period were slaves. But a small number were free. Despite legislation restricting and then virtually halting manumission of slaves, the free black population of South Carolina (which included many mulattoes or "browns") grew from about three thousand in 1800 to nearly ten thousand in 1860. The majority of free blacks lived in or near Charleston, where they made up nearly 20 percent of the black population in 1860; in the state as a whole, only 2.4 percent of the blacks were free. The great majority of free blacks were extremely poor, though some of them, particularly members of the mulatto elite of Charleston, were artisans or merchants who possessed considerable property. A few owned slaves.

The legal position of the free blacks within the antebellum state was anomalous; they existed in the margins between the whites, who had full citizenship status, and the slaves, who had no rights. The state government accorded free blacks the status of "denizens" who had rights to life, liberty, and property but not political rights. The rights of the free blacks were always insecure. Many whites feared them as a threat to the slave system and as a source of conspiracies, or, as in the case of white labor in Charleston, as economic competition. The fears of whites increased after the Denmark Vesey conspiracy of 1822 and produced numerous proposals designed to control, deport, or enslave the free black population. Paternalistic white aristocrats successfully resisted the most draconian of these efforts, at least until the eve of the Civil War. But from the 1820s, the law required adult free blacks to have a white guardian and restricted their movement in and out of the state.[59]

Free black families, in contrast to slave families, could theoretically choose the form of care for their insane relatives. But poverty and discriminatory laws conspired to narrow the free blacks' options. The state lunatic asylum could not legally admit blacks before 1850 and admitted only about thirty between then and 1865.[60] Unlike wealthy whites, free blacks were not able to send insane relatives to asylums out of state. Few antebellum asylums, north or south, accepted black patients, and those that did accepted very few. The Eastern Virginia Lunatic Asylum at Williamsburg was exceptional among American asylums in that it accepted many free black patients during the antebellum period. But it was a state institution that accepted few nonresidents; in 1856, the Virginia state legislature banned out-of-state patients.[61] Very few free blacks would have been able to afford care in northern private asylums, and it is doubtful that any of these institutions would have accepted them. Dr. Thomas Kirkbride, superintendent of the private Pennsylvania Hospital for the insane, spoke for most of his colleagues when he condemned the idea of "mixing up all colors and classes" in asylums.[62]

As we will see in the next chapter, Charleston's antebellum poorhouse admitted some free blacks to its lunatic wards, as did the city's Roper Hospital after 1856. But most free blacks who became insane were probably cared for at home. How they fared is a mystery on which the records of the time shed little light. Their families may have derived some assistance from other members of the free black community. Charleston's free people of color supported several benevolent societies that aided those of their number who were in sickness and distress.[63] Free black lunatics without friends or family to care for them sometimes ended up wandering about the country. A legislative committee that favored opening the state asylum to blacks argued that the safety of the community and humanity demanded that "Lunatic Free Negro[es]" should no longer be permitted "unrestrained freedom to roam when they may and where they may."[64]

Although asylum physicians in South Carolina as elsewhere repeatedly condemned domestic care of the insane, there was little they could do to end it. Local officials were reluctant to interfere in the case of a lunatic who was under the private care of his or her family. Public intervention generally occurred only when a lunatic was considered a public nuisance or danger or when his family could not or would not take care of him. Communities sometimes forced the authorities to intervene because the lunatic's condition had become a matter of public scandal or a nuisance. For example, after the York County grand jury complained about William Miskelly's confinement in his roadside hut, the equity court ordered his family to send him to the asylum.[65] In 1856, the grand jury of Union County demanded that something be done about the wanderings of Ann Rodger. The jurymen complained that she was an "annoyance and disturbance to the community," and that her husband obstinately refused to send her to the state lunatic asylum. Public opinion prevailed, and the court ordered her committal.[66]

In the absence of such community protests, local authorities sometimes left insane persons at large for years. William Ryan of Marion County allegedly became insane during the Civil War yet was allowed to wander about and live off local charity until he was committed in 1878.[67] The phenomenon of the wandering lunatic has often been viewed romantically, but the evidence about the condition of such persons should caution us against it. One such man, found in the swamps of Horry County in February 1880, was almost dead from cold and hunger, having been "without food or fire for several days and nights."[68]

Sometimes the insane were allowed to go at large for long periods of time because neither their families nor the public authorities would accept responsibility for them. Harriet Bounds, who wandered rural Marlboro County in the 1820s, is an example. Harriet was born in Marlboro, but had married Reuben Bounds, who lived in nearby Richmond County, North Carolina. She became deranged about 1823 or 1824. Her husband allegedly went to "great trouble and expense" to control her and bring about her recovery, but she ran away several times and returned to her childhood home in South Carolina. Her father, Robert Purnell, returned her to North Carolina a couple of times, but he died in 1825. Purnell's death brought Harriet a small legacy. The executors gave her husband most of it in return for his promise to "keep and use her well." Harriet soon escaped again, however, and returned to the old homestead. At this point James Purnell, a relative, agreed to board her in return for the rest of her legacy. But after getting the money, Purnell decided, in the words of a neighbor, to "get clear of

Harriet." He carted her to the North Carolina line, set her free, and quickly "removed out of the District."

For several more years, Bounds wandered the area between her homes in North and South Carolina, living off charity. Although local people clothed her, she was often found naked. At this point she was clearly a pauper, without family or property in the district, but the Marlboro commissioners of the poor refused to do anything for her. By her marriage to Reuben Bounds, they argued, she had lost her right to a settlement in Marlboro and was entitled to one only where her husband resided. Responsibility, they claimed, lay with her husband or the poor-law authorities in North Carolina.

Nevertheless, the Marlboro commissioners contributed to Bounds's support beginning in October 1829. They were moved to do so by the plight of John Woodel, a former tenant of her father. During Harriet's sojourns near her old home, Woodel frequently supported her, a burden he could ill afford, because he was a poor man with a large family. In October 1829 the Marlboro commissioners agreed to assist Woodel in supporting her, but they later claimed that they had done this out of "pure pity to Woodel and not Harriet," for whom they continued to deny any responsibility. In July 1830 the commissioners finally sent her to the asylum in Columbia. But they claimed she was a transient pauper and therefore the responsibility of the state. The asylum's regents took the dispute to the legislature, which ruled that she was a resident pauper of Marlboro and the responsibility of the commissioners of that district.[69]

As the Bounds case indicates, nineteenth-century local authorities, like their eighteenth-century predecessors, tended to see the care of an insane person primarily as a family responsibility. Many families shared this view. For a variety of reasons, families often preferred to keep their insane relatives at home rather than to send them to an asylum. This was particularly true before the state accepted financial responsibility for the care of the insane in 1871. Local authorities seldom interfered with family arrangements for the care of the insane, for to do so would only increase their own fiscal and administrative responsibilities. But sometimes, as in the Bounds case, the family was unable or unwilling to provide the required supervision; or the lunatic had no family in the area. In such cases responsibility for the insane often devolved upon the local authorities, such as commissioners of the poor or the sheriff. The fate of these public charges is taken up in the following chapter.

Easy generalizations cannot encompass the experience of the insane who came under domestic care in nineteenth-century South Carolina. No doubt, as asylum advocates charged, the insane kept at home were sometimes "bound with cords and chains," neglected, abused, or left to wander. But equally, domestic care might mean the devoted care of sympathetic, kind, and (as asylum physicians lamented) even indulgent relatives and friends. The quality of care an insane person received at home varied for many reasons, not least of which was the severity of their symptoms. Those who were calm and tractable tended to fare better than the violent and outrageous. Moreover, we must remember that the insane were not only mentally disordered. They were also rich, middling, and poor, men and women, white and black, slave and free. Some insane came from families who had the wealth and power to care for their lunatic relatives as they wished; the families of others lacked the resources or the autonomy to do so. Finally, we must continually remind ourselves that the extant evidence about home care reveals little about a small minority of the mentally disturbed. The fate of the great majority is, and probably will always remain, unknown.

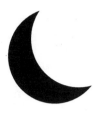

Eight

THERE IS NO DISCOUNT ON BEING CRAZY

LOCAL GOVERNMENT AND THE INSANE

In 1829 the *Charleston Mercury* pre-
dicted that the recently opened South Carolina Lunatic Asylum could not
"fail . . . to become the chosen habitation to which all southern unfortunates will be sent for cure."[1] South Carolina's asylum reformers shared
the *Mercury*'s confidence. They did not anticipate that the new institution
would encounter difficulty in attracting patients. Soon after it opened, the
legislature required counties to transfer lunatics there from the jails and
poorhouses. But the laws provided no penalty for noncompliance, and
local officials often ignored them. County and city governments continued
to maintain the insane in poorhouses, jails, or private homes throughout
the nineteenth century and beyond. Some patients experienced all these
modes of care in addition to asylum care as families, local officials, and asylum authorities shuttled them back and forth in an attempt to help them,
secure them, or merely get rid of them.

It is difficult to assess the condition of these unfortunate persons, for the
sources rarely discuss specifics of their care and treatment. The state asylum
records reveal occasional examples of terrible neglect and abuse but tell us
little or nothing about the situation of the great majority of patients prior
to commitment. Local government records are usually even less informative
on details of care and treatment. But they occasionally provide a certain
balance to the generally negative picture of the asylum records. They show
that some local officials took their responsibilities seriously and tried to as-

sist the insane within the limitations set by their economic, political, racial, and medical environment.

Why did local authorities sometimes choose to retain insane paupers in the community rather than divest themselves of a troublesome and unrewarding task? Asylum officials had no doubt as to the reason: to keep down local taxes.[2] During the antebellum period, a pauper lunatic could usually be maintained in the community for about half what it would cost to keep him in the asylum.[3] In 1871 the state assumed financial responsibility for pauper patients at the asylum. Although this legislation took away much of the economic incentive for community care of the insane poor, it did not entirely remove it. By keeping a pauper lunatic in the county, the commissioners avoided the expense of transferring him to the asylum, which could run as high as seventy-five dollars for transportation, a guard, and a medical examination. Given these costs, local authorities were often reluctant to commit someone to the asylum, especially if the insanity was believed to be temporary or easily manageable.[4]

Asylum officers frequently complained that local officials kept the most manageable insane paupers under their care and removed the most troublesome and dangerous to the asylum, irrespective of the chances of cure. Undoubtedly, this was often the case. The lunacy committee of the Charleston poorhouse reported in 1853 that most of the insane inmates were "civil and easily managed, except during violent paroxysms of excitement."[5] In 1869 the York County commissioners declared that the proper place for a pauper lunatic who was manageable was the poorhouse; a lunatic who was not manageable should be sent to the asylum.[6] In the case of poorhouses, an added element working against commitment might be the usefulness of the inmate to the institution. In arguing against the commitment of five poorhouse inmates in 1842, the Charleston commissioners of the poor noted that they were all "inoffensive persons, with sufficient intelligence to perform the household duties which they are directed to do."[7]

The decision to keep a lunatic in the local poorhouse or jail was often experimental, an attempt to see if he or she could be managed without resort to the asylum. In 1882 the Anderson physicians who examined Yancey Smith recommended that he "be confined in the County Poor House for the present and if there are not sufficient means to restrain him then he be sent to the Lunatic Asylum." Several weeks later the commissioners sent him on to the asylum because the superintendent of the poor farm could not control him.[8]

From these cases one might conclude that local officials sent the insane to the asylum to be managed rather than cured. But local officials often did not explain the reasons for such transfers. Sometimes they provided several reasons, and which reason was most important is not easy to determine. That poor-law officers did not always ignore patients' prognoses is evident from some cases in the Charleston poorhouse records. In January 1844 the Charleston commissioners sent Mary Hanahan to the asylum on the recommendation of the physician of the poorhouse. In a letter to the Board, Dr. Henry W. Desaussure reported that Hanahan's mental condition was deteriorating because he was "reluctantly obliged to keep her confined to her Cell." But, he argued, she might get better if removed to the asylum: "You would give her in my opinion, her only chance of recovery, which her youth and previous good health also render more probable, while the longer she remains here the less her prospect of ultimate recovery. [By removing her] you would be conferring a signal benefit, on a poor and nearly friendless young woman."[9]

In 1850, the commissioners sought permission from the city council to transfer Sarah Waters to the asylum, arguing that she might "be restored to her right mind under the skilful care of that establishment." Waters was admittedly a difficult patient, and the description of her case indicates how difficult it is to determine exactly why local authorities sent a patient to the asylum. She was not violent, except for "kicking at the privates of men." But she was in the habit of passing feces on the floor and smearing them on the walls. She also "exhibited venereal propensities, throwing herself on a female lunatic who is similarly disposed."[10] The Charleston commissioners sometimes cited a poor prognosis as a reason for not transferring a pauper lunatic to the asylum. In advising the Charleston poorhouse board not to send five inmates to the asylum, the board's lunacy committee argued that the effort would be fruitless: "they have all been a long time in the House, one of them nearly twenty years, and your committee think that there is not the smallest prospect that they could be restored to their right senses in the best regulated Asylum."[11]

Public opinion could also affect the authorities' decisions in such cases. Although keeping pauper lunatics in the community might keep down local taxes, neighbors sometimes demanded their removal to the state asylum. In 1846, citizens of Charleston succeeded in getting the commissioners of the poor to remove Matthew Giannini from the poorhouse to the asylum as "a nuisance to the neighborhood."[12] In 1859 the grand jury of York County reported that Robert Brakefield, a pauper, was a dangerous lunatic wandering about "mostly and at times entirely Nude." The court ordered the commissioners of the poor to have Brakefield removed to the asylum in Columbia and to pay for his care there.[13]

The families and friends of pauper lunatics sometimes influenced the local authorities' decisions about commitment. In 1833 the Charleston poorhouse commissioners agreed to send Samuel Miller to the asylum at the request of his mother, although they considered him incurable. A few years later, the wife of Robert Carr petitioned the Charleston commissioners to have him sent to Columbia on the grounds that he had a better chance of receiving proper treatment there and might be able to recover his reason. The commissioners granted her wish even though they considered Carr to be "a confirmed lunatic with no prospect of his ever being better."[14] During the later nineteenth century, after the state assumed financial responsibility for the pauper insane, county officials often committed patients to the asylum on the grounds that their families were unable to provide proper care and treatment at home.[15]

Family preferences also influenced local officials not to send a lunatic to the asylum. When the Charleston commissioners decided to remove Thomas Casey to the asylum in 1840, his mother wrote to request that he be allowed to remain in the poorhouse. Citing "the natural anxiety of a Mother to avoid a Separation from her Son," she pleaded with the board not to remove him "to a distant place." In order to encourage a favorable reply, she proposed to pay for his food and clothing. The commissioners agreed to let Casey remain in the poorhouse at a charge of one hundred dollars a year.[16]

Poor-law officials may have even consulted the wishes or needs of the insane themselves in deciding whether or not to commit them to the asylum. In 1842 the Charleston commissioners decided not to send two poorhouse inmates to the asylum after the lunacy committee reported that "they themselves think they ought to be retained in the House." The commissioners also decided to keep five other inmates, who were said to be "contented with their situations, and . . . perhaps happier than they would be if restored to their wits."[17] A few years earlier, the commissioners took familial bonds into account when they sent two sisters, Angelica and Louisa Bunuel, to the asylum. Angelica, the commissioners declared, was a "confirmed lunatic." Louisa had been insane but "was not now labouring under mental derangement." The commissioners nevertheless decided to send Louisa to the asylum as well, because her affection for her sister was so strong that they feared that separation would "render her [insane] in a short period thereafter."[18]

In some cases, the removal of a lunatic to the asylum was inhibited by the sheer force of bureaucratic inertia. The committal of a lunatic in nineteenth-century South Carolina involved setting up an examination by two physicians, a hearing before a judge, filling out the necessary forms, and making arrangements for transporting him to Columbia. Because the vast majority of South Carolina's population lived in rural areas, bringing an alleged lunatic together with the doctors and judge might prove a time-consuming and troublesome task. Unless the person was perceived as manifestly dangerous, local officials might prefer to avoid or put off commitment. An example is the case of Harriet Bounds, cited earlier.

In 1830, Marlboro's commissioners of the poor decided to remove Bounds to the asylum. It took them several months to secure the necessary commitment papers. In April, the commissioners arranged a time for her to be examined before a justice and physicians and directed the man then caring for her to bring her to the courthouse. On the appointed day the man, John Woodel, appeared and announced that Bounds had run off and he could not find her. The commissioners then turned the job over to their clerk, Nathan Thomas. In May, a stranger found her naked on the banks of the Pee Dee River, clothed her, and brought her to the courthouse. She was lodged in the jail for a few days, then Woodel came and took her to his home. Nevertheless, her examination did not take place until two months later. The exasperated clerk reported that he had "repeatedly requested the physicians and Justice to go and examine her but never could have it done till the 15 of July." Thomas then had to arrange for Woodel to take Bounds to Columbia. More trouble followed when the Marlboro commissioners refused to pay for her care in the asylum.[19]

Poor-law officials did not always retain pauper lunatics in the community by choice. During the later nineteenth century, with the advent of state support of pauper or beneficiary patients in the asylum, local authorities became more willing to divest themselves of responsibility for insane paupers. The consequent influx of pauper patients resulted in severe overcrowding at the asylum and complaints from its officers that the counties were dumping paupers on them who would do better in the poorhouse or at home. To relieve the congestion, the asylum's officers periodically sent some of these "harmless incurables" back to the counties for care. As a result, many pauper lunatics in the community, especially during the later nineteenth century, had already made one or more trips to the asylum. In 1881, Georgetown County authorities committed Christian Hartliss to the asylum because he was violent, threatened people at his boardinghouse, and took a hatchet to bed with him. He remained in the asylum for three years and was then removed to the Georgetown County Poorhouse as harmless. A few months later, the county sent him back to the asylum claiming that he had assaulted the poorhouse nurse and that the keepers there could not "prevent him from running at large and exposing himself in the streets."[20]

Evidence about the condition of the insane under the care of local government is neither abundant nor detailed. Local records provide few specifics about their care. The records of the state asylum occasionally provide some of this information, mostly uncomplimentary to the local authorities. Pauper patients often arrived at the asylum showing signs of severe neglect or abuse.[21] One of the physicians recorded the following account of a patient admitted in 1885, who had been boarded out by Berkeley County officials: "She was very weak and exhausted and in a most foul, offensive, and neglected condition. Numerous and large surfaces of her body were denuded of skin . . . and these [sores?] were very offensive and infected with maggots. All that was possible was done for her, but she died within twenty hours after her admission."[22] This was admittedly an extreme example; the physician noted that it was the worst case of neglect he had ever seen. But other patients were received in conditions almost as bad. The situation of those who remained in the community is unlikely to have been enviable.

One reason for this was purely economic. The strong antipathy of South Carolina's local communities to tax increases militated against attempts to provide even basic care for the insane poor. At the beginning of the antebellum period, few counties possessed a poorhouse, much less one equipped to accommodate the insane. Most counties supported their pauper lunatics on outdoor relief, if at all. As in other states, local officials sometimes auctioned off the care of insane paupers to the lowest bidder. The state encouraged counties to build poorhouses during the antebellum period, and many did. Most possessed a poorhouse of some sort by the later 1870s. But several counties still did not have one at the end of the 1890s.

In any event, the establishment of a poorhouse did not necessarily mean the abandonment of outdoor relief. Counties often used a mixture of indoor and outdoor relief or moved back and forth from one to another according to local circumstances and the attitudes of those in control of poor relief.[23] Spartanburg County supported several "distracted" and "foolish" paupers on outdoor relief between the 1790s and 1820s. In 1826, Spartanburg opened a poorhouse. But by the 1870s the county had resumed supporting lunatic paupers on outdoor relief. Lancaster County built a poorhouse in the early 1830s but abandoned it after a few years on the grounds that outdoor relief was cheaper and more beneficial to the poor than indoor relief. During the 1850s, the Lancaster Commissioners of the Poor boarded out lunatics. But by the late 1860s, they were requiring the pauper insane to seek relief in the poorhouse.[24]

Local authorities sometimes granted outdoor relief to the pauper insane as the result of family requests or community pressure. In 1890, citizens of Garvin Township in Anderson County successfully appealed to the board of county commissioners to provide outdoor relief for the support of a pauper lunatic. In other cases, however, local authorities rejected such appeals and required the insane to enter the poorhouse. In 1869, the York County Board of Commissioners rejected a petition for outdoor relief for an alleged lunatic. At the same time they redefined the term "pauper" to mean someone who was sick or insane. Persons "having no bodaly or Mental diseas[e]" were discharged from the poorhouse. In 1871 the board agreed to readmit a former poorhouse inmate who was now said to be insane.[25]

Most poorhouses provided their insane inmates with little more than bare lodging and subsistence. To judge by the grim reports of the county grand juries, poorhouses were frequently unable to supply even these. The Greenville grand jury complained in 1854 that the poorhouse buildings were "too small for the convenience, comfort or health of the inmates," who lacked clothing, bedding, and shoes.[26] Barnwell County grand juries repeatedly condemned their poorhouse for its unsanitary conditions and inadequate diet. In 1847 they reported that two old women were "literally lying in filth, and one of them was in a bed of Straw very badly provided with covering. She complained that she didn't get clean clothes but once a week." Later reports noted that paupers were forced to drink from a puddle due to the lack of a proper well. The sick were not given sufficient nourishment or care. In the 1870s the grand jury declared the poorhouse so dilapidated as to be unfit for human habitation. Inmates were not receiving adequate food, medicine, or clothing and were periodically forced to depend on private charity to survive. Similar conditions existed in other poorhouses.[27]

Poorhouses sometimes provided medical care for sick and insane inmates on a contract or case-by-case basis.[28] But the best poorhouses lacked special facilities or personnel for the care of the insane. The typical poorhouse consisted of a few cabins or a farmhouse with no outer walls or secure rooms. The physician to the Spartanburg County poorhouse reported in 1899 that he could not do anything with an epileptic boy who constantly ran away, because the building had no enclosure. Poorhouses could seldom provide adequate supervision or medical treatment. In the 1840s, Trezevant claimed that the poorhouses usually appointed as keeper "some wretched old crone, half-crazed herself, or unable to move about . . . and the effect of their injudicious parsimony is very speedily made obvious, by the wanderings of the maniac, the trouble he occasions in the neighborhood, or the injuries inflicted on him, by those who, ignorant of his misfortune, deem him an impudent and troublesome vagrant." Sometimes, he added, the pauper arrived at the asylum "with the skin literally roasted from his limbs by the fire, for the want of proper attention."[29] Trezevant was not exaggerating. Cynthia Peach, an inmate of the Kershaw County poorhouse, arrived at the asylum in 1829 near death from the effects of dirt eating and a severe scalding on her legs. Fire was a particularly great danger in the usually wooden poorhouses. Insane inmates often burned themselves or others or tried to burn down the institution itself.[30]

The poorhouses often found themselves unable to control violent or wandering inmates. A Sumter County physician recommended that a pauper lunatic be committed to the asylum in the 1870s because the poorhouse staff found it impossible to handle him: "They can do nothing with him—cannot manage him at all, and have no one to attend him."[31] In 1885 the staff of the Georgetown poorhouse was unable to prevent an inmate from roaming at will and exposing himself. He assaulted the poorhouse nurse and resisted all attempts to control his behavior.[32] An insane inmate of the Abbeville poorhouse killed a small child in 1898.[33]

During the antebellum period, Charleston's poorhouse was the only one in the state that provided special facilities arranged for the care of the insane. The lunatic department of Charleston's poorhouse had its origins in the later colonial period. It consisted of a separate building or buildings behind the main poorhouse that usually housed between twenty and forty insane patients during the antebellum period. The commissioners of the poor provided the insane inmates with a special keeper who resided on the premises and medical attendance from the poorhouse physician.[34]

The insane inmates of the Charleston poorhouse were a heterogeneous group. They included white paying patients, slaves, and free blacks as well as the white paupers for whom the institution was ostensibly intended.[35] They were committed by their families or friends, their owners in the case of slaves, or by the city authorities. In 1795, the legislature granted the Charleston commissioners of the poor the power to confine "Strolling Beggars" found in the city's streets. An ordinance of 1819 gave the city authorities the power to send "persons laboring under insanity or other mental malady . . . found wandering or strolling about the streets" to the "Asylum for Lunatics" at the poorhouse.[36] The lunatic department was apparently an object of particular attraction for locals and tourists alike. In 1821, the commissioners forbade anyone to visit the insane wards unless accompanied by the physician, the master of the poorhouse, or a commissioner.[37]

The lunatic department was not a purely custodial operation. During the early antebellum period, to be sure, the physicians may have made little effort to treat the insane inmates actively. A report of 1829 listed 20 lunatic inmates as incurable and only two under treatment. But the therapeutic optimism of antebellum asylum reformers eventually infected the poorhouse physicians. In 1851, a report noted that 5 of the 19 insane patients in the house had been discharged cured. The following year, the physician claimed that 15 of 22 recent cases were cured.[38] Over the 1841–56 period, 30 percent of the patients admitted to the department were discharged as cured or relieved. Most stays were short. Of the 121 admissions during the period, 95 remained in the lunatic wards for less than a year, and most for only a few days or weeks.[39] The physicians tried to implement some aspects of moral therapy. They encouraged patients to work at such things as tailoring, needlework, cooking, and general labor. During the early antebellum period, the patients were sometimes subjected to mechanical restraint. By the 1850s, however, the poorhouse was emulating the trend of the state asylum away from the use of mechanical restraints. The house physician reported in 1853 that the only coercion the staff used was solitary confinement, "seldom extending beyond twenty four hours."[40]

Nevertheless, the officers of the Charleston poorhouse frequently questioned its suitability for the care of the insane. Lack of space for recreation and occupation was a constant problem, as was the proximity of the various classes of insane to one another and to the other inmates of the poorhouse.[41] The poorhouse officers often complained about the insufficient number of "cells" for the patients; the poor condition of the walls, which made escape relatively easy; and the problems of housing patients of different sexes, races, and classes in close quarters. Providing sufficient and competent staff to care for the insane inmates, as in the state asylum, was a perennial problem. Several keepers and nurses left suddenly or were dismissed for drunkenness or breaking the house rules (for example, selling liquor to the inmates).[42] One keeper resigned in 1840 when the board was considering cuts in pay for the staff, complaining that "the Salary I receive for charge of the Maniac Department is entirely not enough." The poorhouse committee on retrenchment agreed: "$250 per Annum to one who has to sleep in one of the Cells of the Maniac House, is with Maniacs day and night, ministering to their wants, subjected to their violence, and shut out from all Society; can hardly be imagined by any one too much. Neither can he be supposed to have too many Nurses, when we have but one for the Male Hospital, one for the Female, and one for the Maniac Department and we give them but $6 a month." [43]

Chronic economic depression during much of the antebellum period worsened conditions in the poorhouse lunatic department. The commissioners of the poor faced constant demands to reduce the burden of poor relief. The state legislature cut its grant to Charleston for the transient poor by two-thirds between 1825 and 1828, from twelve thousand to four thousand dollars. During the same period, the amount spent on the poor in Charleston dropped from almost twenty-four thousand dollars to a little over ten thousand dollars. The annual expenditures hovered slightly above or below this latter figure for the duration of the antebellum era, hitting their lowest point in 1845, at seven thousand dollars. During these decades, the number of recipients of relief was increasing. In order to keep costs down, the commissioners cut down on grants of outdoor relief, reduced the salaries of the staff, and tried to shift the burden of the paupers' support to their relatives or other jurisdictions. In 1828, for example, the commissioners determined that persons responsible for six of the lunatic paupers could pay the costs of their care in the institution.[44] The commissioners also became more determined than before to exact payment for the pauper insane who came from outside the city or to send them back to their place of origin. In 1842, they returned Charles Toelkin to his home in Augusta, Georgia, because he had relatives there and "it is not improbable he was sent to Charleston by the Rail Road, in order to get rid of the expense of supporting him." [45]

The insane patients suffered, perhaps more than most of the poorhouse's inmates, from the Charleston commissioners' economizing measures. In 1832 a committee of commissioners reported that the lunatic department was in such poor condition that it could provide "neither security for the safety of the persons confined, nor comforts for their accommodation." The department had become so overcrowded that many of the inmates had to sleep in the corridor.[46] Twenty years later, the commissioners noted that many of the insane had "remained too long in an institution quite unsuited to their unfortunate situation." [47] Dr. J. F. Prioleau, who took over as poorhouse physician in 1851, found most of the inmates, especially the insane, suffering from scurvy as a result of defective diet. In 1854, the superintendent of the state lunatic asylum, Dr. Parker, complained that three patients he had recently admitted from the Charleston poorhouse arrived in a filthy and verminous condition.[48]

The Charleston commissioners would have preferred to relinquish the job of caring for the insane. They often complained about the difficulties of administering an institution that combined the functions of an almshouse, a house of correction, a hospital, and a lunatic asylum.[49] By the 1850s, they had decided that the presence of the insane and vagrants was giving the institution a bad reputation among the respectable white poor. In 1853, they complained that the lunatics disrupted the discipline of the house and disturbed the sick with "their unearthly whoopings and halooings."[50]

The commissioners had another reason for wanting to remove the insane from the poorhouse: many of them were black. Insane blacks had been admitted to the lunatic wards since late colonial times. Between 1841 and 1856 they accounted for about 40 percent of the total psychiatric admissions.[51] Black lunatics arrived at Charleston's poorhouse by several routes. Masters sent their insane slaves to be cared for. Free black families brought their deranged relatives. City officials sent both slave and free black lunatics who were considered a public danger or nuisance. In 1820, city council decided that the lunatic department was the best place to send "Insane Persons of Color" who were going at large and presenting a public nuisance.[52] Some of the free blacks were paying patients; a few had incomes or legacies of their own that paid for their care. Nancy Pencil, whose mulatto husband William was a slaveholder, was supported for a time in the lunatic department by a legacy he left her. The expenses of Aaron Thompson, another free black inmate, were defrayed by money he inherited from his master.[53]

The commissioners frequently protested the admission of black lunatics into Charleston's poorhouse, whether as pay or pauper cases. The poorhouse, they repeatedly stressed, was intended for whites only. The commissioners were uncomfortable trying to run a biracial institution in a society highly sensitive to situations in which the races were even apparently mingled on an equal footing. The presence of blacks also complicated the administration of the lunatic wards because white staff refused to attend black inmates. In 1816, the board of commissioners reported that it had lately received many applications for the admission of insane blacks but had rejected them because the house had "no one to clean up their dirt and nastiness."[54] As an interim measure, the commissioners demanded that whoever was responsible for the black inmates should pay for their maintenance and provide servants to care for them. In 1820 the city agreed to pay for the maintenance of insane blacks it sent to the poorhouse and for the employment of as many "Coloured persons [as] Nurses as are necessary to attend the unfortunate of this class." The commissioners normally required the owners of lunatic slaves to meet the same conditions.[55]

In practice, the commissioners found it difficult to enforce their regulations. On several occasions, they agreed to admit free black lunatics without charge; in effect, to accord them de facto white pauper status. In 1821, the board agreed to let Nancy Pencil remain in the lunatic wards at the request of city council, although her husband William could no longer pay for her care. Pencil was resident in the poorhouse for more than twenty years, much of the time as a pauper patient. About the same time, the commissioners approved a petition from Thomas Inglis, another free person of color, to be relieved of paying for the care of his wife in the insane department. His petition also had the support of the city council. The Pencil and Inglis families were members of the respectable free brown elite, many of whom had close connections with the city's white aristocracy. William Pencil won the gratitude of the city's white leadership in 1822 by helping to expose the Denmark Vesey conspiracy, an abortive slave uprising.[56]

The commissioners rarely bent the rule about payment in the case of slaves, even when their owners pleaded poverty. In 1846, Mrs. M. E. Toomer petitioned to have her lunatic slave Buck, who was then in the poorhouse, kept free of charge because he was "one of the few slaves upon whose wages she depends for support; and as her circumstances are very limited, she begs you will take her case into consideration." The board refused her request and required her to conform to the rule about payment.[57] Nor was the board willing to accept another argument that the masters of insane slaves sometimes employed: the city derived a substantial revenue from taxes on slaves and should therefore provide for their care when insane. The commissioners strenuously resisted this reasoning, and their reply to it provides an interesting commentary on proslavery claims that insanity among slaves was rare: "If ever this institution is opened for the reception of Lunatick Slaves free of charge, our Cells will be filled to overflowing." [58]

On at least one occasion, however, the commissioners agreed to keep a lunatic slave without charge. In 1820, Archibald Lord, who had sent his slave Beck to the poorhouse, fell behind in his payments for her care. The commissioners resolved to dismiss her unless he agreed to pay for her keep and sent a servant to clean out her cell and attend to her. After several months of negotiation, the board agreed to exonerate Lord from the back payments because Beck had recovered and was "of great use to the Institution in washing the Clothes of the Maniacs." He agreed to let her remain for a time to work off the debt. Beck subsequently relapsed, however, and Lord once again fell behind in his payments for her care. In 1828 the commissioners resolved to sue him.[59]

The commissioners tried to restrict black admissions to the lunatic department by hedging them about with various restrictions and generally making them as difficult as possible. In 1824, the board resolved that blacks would be admitted only if their insanity was certified by a physician. They sometimes discharged blacks on the grounds that they had been admitted through an irregular procedure or were not seriously or dangerously deranged.[60] The commissioners also restricted admissions to slaves whose masters were resident in the city. In 1843, Robert Miller asked the board to admit his mother's deranged slave to the lunatic department. They refused the request on the grounds of nonresidence, although Miller's mother agreed to pay all the slave's costs and Miller pleaded that the family was "nearly worn out by their constant attendance upon her."[61]

Periodically, the commissioners proposed that insane blacks should be provided separate accommodations, either within the poorhouse or in connection with the city workhouse. The workhouse had long functioned as a house of correction for unruly slaves and free black vagrants; its punishments included whipping and the treadmill. City council approved the idea of moving the city's insane blacks to an "asylum" within the workhouse on at least two occasions, in the late 1820s and the late 1830s, but for reasons that are unclear never implemented it.[62]

Some of the city's white leaders probably opposed the idea out of a sense of paternalism, especially toward the free brown elite. Prominent whites often worked to protect the rights and privileges of this group. Political concerns may also have influenced the decision not to send the insane blacks to the workhouse. During the 1830s and 1840s, South Carolina's leaders were increasingly concerned with defending slavery. They often framed public policies relating to blacks with an eye to its effects on northern opinion. Charleston's leaders apparently decided that removing the black insane from what was ostensibly a welfare institution (the poorhouse) to a clearly punitive one (the workhouse) would supply antislavery forces with propaganda. In 1842, a committee of Charleston's poor-law commissioners argued that the city's free blacks had a right to poor relief and that by recognizing that right, "we can best and most effectually repel and refute the calumnies of our fanatic Enemies, who misrepresent our domestic system, traduce our character, and invade our peace."[63]

In the absence of an acceptable separate facility for black lunatics, the city's leaders had little choice but to send them to the poorhouse. To leave insane blacks at large or in the hands of owners or families who could not or would not control them was unacceptable. During the antebellum period, whites' fears of black deviance were continually aroused by real and imagined conspiracies, waves of arson, and the emergence of the abolitionist movement. Living as they saw it on the edge of a racial volcano, the city's leaders were determined to control the black population. They feared that deranged blacks might commit crimes and perhaps act as catalysts for wider attacks on the established order.[64]

These concerns were reflected in discussions about the city's policy toward the black insane. In 1838 Mayor Henry Pinckney confessed that he regretted having to send black lunatics to the poorhouse, because it was "an institution whose benefits were specifically intended for destitute whites." To allow the admission of blacks into the poorhouse was "contrary to the true spirit of our policy" and "repugnant to my feelings." But it was the only humane alternative to allowing "them to go at large at the imminent hazard of the commission by them of murder, arson, or any other crime."[65] The determination of the city's authorities to keep insane blacks in a secure place sometimes coincided with the desires of slave owners to rid themselves of troublesome servants. In 1850, a master successfully petitioned to have the poorhouse receive his insane and badly disfigured slave Agnes, who had an "uncontrollable fondness for the streets."[66]

In 1856 the Charleston commissioners succeeded in getting the poorhouse moved to new quarters in an abandoned cotton factory and renamed the Alms House. Determined to make the new institution attractive to the respectable white poor, the commissioners convinced city council to leave the insane, the sick, and the vicious behind. The city contracted with the trustees of newly completed Roper Hospital, which was next to the old poorhouse, to care for the sick and insane poor. The trustees (the Medical Society of South Carolina) were granted the use of the poorhouse's hospital wards, which they remodeled and managed until the end of the Civil War. The main part of the old building was renovated to serve as a house of correction.

After the Civil War, Roper's trustees were financially unable to fulfill their contract with the city. Charleston authorities, aided by the Freedmen's Bureau, resumed direct care of the sick and insane poor. They established City Hospital, which incorporated the workhouse (rebuilt in 1850–51 and formerly used to discipline unruly slaves) and the house of correction. In 1873, the city secured additional room by leasing Roper Hospital from its trustees, who had been forced to close it due to inadequate funds. In 1886, most of these buildings were severely damaged or destroyed by the great Charleston earthquake. The patients were transferred to temporary facilities in the Agricultural Hall until a new building was opened in 1888 at another site.[67]

City Hospital admitted the insane, both black and white, until the early twentieth century. The number of mental patients it accommodated in-

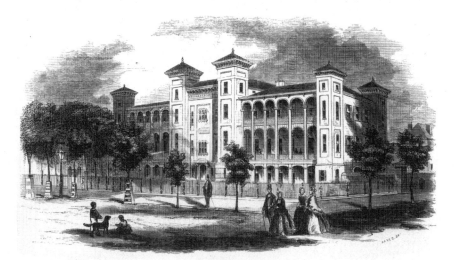

Roper Hospital, Charleston.
(*From* Ballou's Pictorial Drawing Room Companion, *August 8, 1857;*
courtesy Waring Historical Library, Medical University of South Carolina,
Charleston, S.C.)

creased after the Civil War, then declined by the 1890s. Census reports listed twenty-three patients in City Hospital's insane wards in 1870 and thirty-seven in 1880. Between 1899 and 1905 the average number of insane patients resident at the end of each year was seven, and admissions never exceeded forty-five in any year.[68]

In the late 1850s, the Charleston authorities contemplated providing long-term care of the insane poor in a city facility. But a bill introduced in the state legislature to allow them to do so received an unfavorable report in committee and was not acted upon.[69] For the rest of the century, City Hospital functioned primarily as a center for short-term psychiatric care and treatment. Its commissioners declared in 1880 that the institution functioned as "a temporary asylum" that received and treated the insane "in their incipient stages." Most of the patients were discharged "convalescent to their friends" or, if found incurable, transferred to the state asylum.[70] To judge by the scattered records that survive, most patients seem to have been discharged back into the community or committed to the state asylum within a few weeks or months. In 1870, 55 lunatics received treatment in the insane department; 28 of them were discharged or sent to the state asylum. Between 1899 and 1905, 172 patients were admitted to the insane wards. Of these, 90 were subsequently committed to the state asylum and

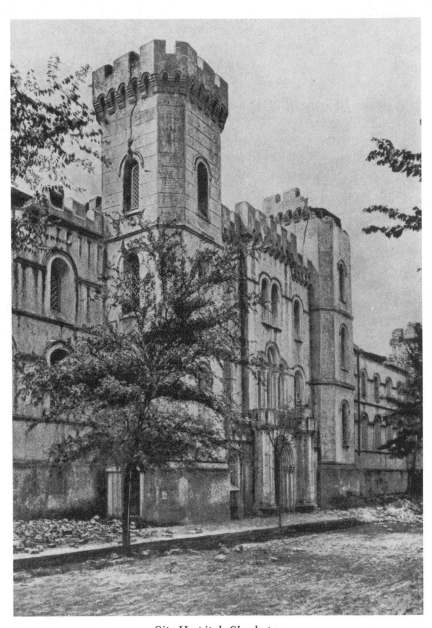

City Hospital, Charleston
(formerly the workhouse for unruly slaves), showing damage from earthquake of
1886. (From Ninth Annual Report of the United States Geological Survey
[Washington, D.C.: Government Printing Office, 1889], p. 268)

66 discharged.[71] Yet some psychiatric patients remained in City Hospital for years. This was partly the result of attempts by state hospital authorities in the 1880s and 1890s to reduce overcrowding by returning chronic "imbeciles" to the city's care.[72]

Conditions at City Hospital discouraged long-term psychiatric care. In 1867, Francis P. Porcher, the hospital physician, reported that "new, airy, and well-ventilated Cells and Wards" had recently been built to accommodate the insane patients. But the following year, his successor, S. Chatham Brown, claimed that the hospital's facilities for treating and housing the insane were unsatisfactory.[73] In 1880, the commissioners of City Hospital declared that the insane wards "were in shocking condition and a subject of mortification to the Board and attending physicians." The wards were crowded and dirty, and some patients lacked adequate clothing and shoes. The commissioners' dissatisfaction with the wards was increased by "the mingling therein of the white and colored patients," a problem that was soon solved by fixing up another hospital room as a ward.[74]

City Hospital's staff was not well equipped to handle the more violent and obstreperous patients. The records of patients sent to the state asylum frequently mention their uncontrollable behavior; destruction of furniture, doors, clothing, and bedding; and attacks on staff and other patients. References to mechanical restraints are common. The staff placed patients in straitjackets and foot straps and sometimes tied them up or confined them closely in their "cells." The physicians described one patient as having "several times attacked the keepers of the Insane ward. . . . [He] is with difficulty overcome and we are obliged to keep him tied." Another patient broke down the door and destroyed the radiator of the "wild insane room."[75] Around 1903, one of the inmates set the insane ward afire, and in the ensuing blaze, several patients were killed. For about two years thereafter the insane were lodged in the jail or the police station until they could be transferred to the asylum in Columbia.[76]

In 1906, a new Roper Hospital opened and Charleston once again contracted with its trustees to care for the city's sick poor. The new hospital provided a psychiatric ward, but it was designed for emergency care and diagnosis rather than long-term care or treatment. Most of the patients were either transferred within a short time to the state hospital or discharged.[77] The facilities for the insane at the new Roper Hospital seem to have been little better than those at earlier hospitals. The head of the psychiatric wards described them in the early 1930s as "in many cases woefully inadequate."[78] A Charleston probate judge recalled in the 1980s that Roper's old psychiatric wards used to be known as "the Black Hole of Calcutta."[79]

The county poorhouses and the Charleston hospitals were not the only local institutions that housed the insane. Throughout the nineteenth century some of the insane resided in county and city jails. Some were criminal lunatics, that is, persons accused of crimes who were found insane on arraignment, were acquitted on the grounds of mental disorder, or became insane while serving a sentence. But many insane persons sent to jails had never been formally charged with a crime. The local authorities simply considered them to be too dangerous, troublesome, or unmanageable to be handled in any other way. According to his own account, John Adams was sent to jail because he frightened his neighbors. Upon entering the asylum in 1831 he told the physician that "he has at times been a hard drinker and that when he drinks he goes crazy. . . . He says when he is crazy he is not violent . . . but that he runs about and haloos and whoops and scares the people."[80] One of the more bizarre cases involved a Colleton County man sent to jail in 1876 and formally charged as a lunatic in the county court.[81]

Before the state lunatic asylum opened in 1828, lunatics sent to jail might remain there until they died or were considered sufficiently well to be released. Several of the first patients admitted to the state lunatic asylum had been in jail for years.[82] In 1829, the legislature passed a law that required county authorities to transfer lunatics in jails to the asylum. For the balance of the antebellum period, long-term care of the insane in jails seems to have been unusual.[83] But jails continued to receive the insane throughout the century and sometimes held them for extended periods.

After the Civil War the number of the insane sent to jails increased. In the 1870s, the superintendent of the state asylum charged that many of the insane were "thrust, often in chains, into the damp, cold gloomy cells of the county jails, without medical attention."[84] The case records of at least 142 persons admitted to the state asylum between 1893 and 1913 noted that they came from the county jails. The increased resort to jails in this period was partly the result of emancipation. More than 80 percent of the patients admitted from jails were black.[85] Poverty may account in part for the blacks' higher rate of incarceration. Fewer black than white families had houses where they could secure a violent relative even for a short period of time. But white local government officials were also clearly more comfortable sending black than white lunatics to jail.

Gender as well as race affected the chances that an insane person would be sent to jail. White women were much less likely than men or black women to be sent to jail previous to being committed to the state asylum. Of the 142 patients admitted from jails between 1893 and 1913, 62 percent were black men, 19 percent were black women, 15 percent were white men, and 2.8 percent were white women. Local government authorities apparently viewed the jail as an appropriate receptacle for insane black men, and an acceptable one for black women and white men. But the authorities' concept of southern chivalry would rarely permit them to jail deranged white women.[86]

Yet jail officials were not necessarily eager to keep any of the insane, whatever their race or gender. The insane were generally unwelcome in jails because they disrupted the normal routine and discipline (such as it was) and because they were often violent, destructive, or noisy. The jailer of Florence County went to court to have a female prisoner removed to the asylum in 1903. His affidavit claimed that she was "the worst case he has ever had in jail . . . she curses and laughs nearly all the time . . . she is exceedingly filthy and her talk is the most vulgar he has ever heard . . . she beats her pans and buckets all to pieces . . . [and] spends most of her time dancing, singing, crying, etc."[87] The sheriff of Barnwell County made plain his distaste for caring for an insane inmate in a 1903 letter to the asylum superintendent: "I send my special deputy with papers and O. There is no discount on his being crazy, violent, and dangerous. . . . [I]t is not part of my duty to care for the insane."[88] Another sheriff begged the asylum to take a "crazy" prisoner off his hands "at once," even offering to pay the costs of a telegram to speed up the commitment process.[89]

In many counties, however, the jail was the only public facility in which violent or dangerous lunatics could be lodged. Even if a poorhouse existed, it might not be considered secure enough to hold a violent or outrageous person. The commitment papers of many patients state that they were sent to jail for safekeeping or simply to be examined by physicians. Some of the insane who ended up in jail were strangers or had no family; others were alleged to be too violent or destructive to remain at home or in the poorhouse. Sumter County authorities sent a troublesome vagrant to the asylum in 1879 because there was "no place here he can be kept, except the jail."[90] In 1872 the Newberry Board of County Commissioners ordered that a lunatic who had previously been an inmate of the poorhouse be confined in the county jail for safe keeping.[91]

Local authorities sometimes kept an alleged lunatic in jail for a time in the hope that the insanity might turn out to be temporary or not insanity at all. Laurens County officials kept an apparently deranged man charged with fraud under observation in the jail in 1898 in the belief that he was feigning insanity. After a week, they decided that he was really insane and needed to be sent to the asylum for treatment. The asylum authorities decided that he was indeed a malingerer and returned him to the sheriff a few weeks later.[92]

In 1874 the Williamsburg County commissioners had Gadsden Gamble examined by two doctors with the instructions that if he were found to be dangerously deranged he should be sent to the asylum. The doctors reported that they considered Gamble to be temporarily insane and predicted that he could be cured without having to be sent to the asylum. Upon hearing this report, the commissioners ordered Gamble confined in the jail for a few days and given medical treatment. A few months later, the Williamsburg commissioners sent Paul Cooper to the county jail and put him under medical treatment after the examining doctors declared that he could be cured there, with a considerable savings to the county.[93]

The cases of Cooper and Gamble indicate that local authorities sometimes provided medical treatment for jailed lunatics. But local officials do not generally seem to have viewed the jail as a proper place to treat insanity. More often, they justified committing an inmate to the asylum on the grounds that he could not receive proper treatment while in jail. In 1884 the physician to the Richland County Jail refused to provide an inmate with medical care because he was a lunatic and therefore belonged in the state asylum.[94]

Most state and local records reveal little or nothing about the situation of the insane in jails. To judge by reports about jail conditions in general, it can hardly have been good. County grand juries often complained that the jails were so poorly constructed and maintained as to imperil the health and lives of the inmates.[95] In 1837 the Greenville grand jury cited their jail as "a General Nuisance." The floors were covered with excrement and the prisoners were "in an intolerably bad condition."[96] The jails were often woefully insecure. The Barnwell jail was so poorly built, according to an 1839 report, that prisoners were continually escaping. Nearly twenty years later, Barnwell jurors complained there was a "very large hole" in the jailhouse through which two prisoners had escaped.[97]

The insecure state of many jails meant that insane inmates were often chained or tied up in some way. Two Spartanburg physicians who examined a lunatic in the county jail in 1896 noted that they had found him shackled in his cell and explained that the sheriff had to keep him this way in order to manage him. In another case in Georgetown a few years later, the physicians found the inmate lying on the floor of the cell with his hands and feet tied. In 1885 a patient arrived at the asylum from the Edgefield County Jail with a wire muzzle over his mouth, ostensibly to prevent him from biting.[98] A legislative investigation of 1909 reported that sheriffs or their deputies routinely brought patients to the asylum in iron shackles and handcuffs.[99]

Conclusions about public care of the insane in the community of nineteenth-century South Carolina must be tentative and guarded. We know too little about the condition of the vast majority of the insane who became the responsibility of local authorities to justify sweeping generalizations. That poor-law and other local officials often neglected and occasionally abused their insane charges is undeniable. Even a casual reading of the relevant records is likely to erode romantic conceptions about the virtues of public care outside the asylum walls. But it does not follow that the insane in the community were inevitably brutalized or left to rot, or that those responsible for them were unfeeling monsters or callous bureaucrats. The records also reveal local authorities who showed genuine concern for the plight and prospects of their irrational charges. The quality of care that local officials provided for the insane was impaired by their lack of knowledge about insanity, by the racial attitudes and perceptions of the dominant white community, and by inadequate financial and institutional resources. But within these limitations, some local officials may have done their best to deal with complex problems whose solution eludes us to this day.

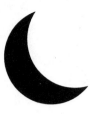

Nine

HOW VARIOUS AND CONFLICTING

THERAPY IN THE COMMUNITY

Nineteenth-century asylum physicians routinely opposed community care of the insane on the grounds that their disease might go untreated and become chronic and incurable. But they had another concern: the insane might receive the wrong kind of treatment. As asylum doctors moved away from a reliance on heroic therapies in the 1840s and 1850s, they often complained that the therapeutic efforts of community practitioners jeopardized the lives and chances of recovery of insane patients. "Talk of madness," Trezevant lamented, "and you have the lancet, drastic cathartics, emetics, etc., etc. instantly presented, and lamentable are the effects constantly produced by their injudicious use. . . . It is a very mistaken idea that Insane Patients bear the extremes of treatment with impunity. There is no mistake more generally made, and unfortunately for them none more fatal."[1] The heroic treatments Trezevant denounced were commonly inflicted upon the insane, especially during the antebellum era. But regular therapies varied, and they tended to become more moderate over time. Moreover, throughout the century numerous irregular practitioners offered various cures of their own, and many people resorted to domestic or self-help medicine.

To determine how insane persons were treated in a community setting is a formidable task involving analysis of a diverse body of sources. Medical treatises and journals, domestic medical manuals, and the writings of some irregular practitioners are helpful in establishing the general outlines of therapeutics but rarely tell us what happened in practice. Most local records relating to community care of the insane do not reveal what treatment, if any, they received for their mental disorder. The patient records of the South Carolina Lunatic Asylum rarely provide detailed information about treatment previous to commitment.

From the late 1870s to the early 1890s, the commitment form used by the asylum specifically asked if the patient had received any treatment for his mental disorder prior to admission. But the responses to this question varied enormously. Some respondents provided no information about treatment; others wrote vague or confusing answers. In many cases, we learn only that the patient had received some form of unspecified treatment. Some responses mention specific therapies, but not who provided them, or where; others state that the patient had been treated by a physician, but not how.[2] Many of the patients may have received no treatment, or at least no treatment from a physician. In 1884, 1889, and 1894, less than 40 percent of the commitment forms indicated that the patients had received medical treatment prior to admission. This percentage was probably somewhat low, however, because many of the persons filling out the commitment papers did not know if the patient had received treatment or did not answer the question. The answers may also have been influenced by the respondents' concept of what constituted treatment. Some respondents may have discounted any treatment but that carried out by a regular physician.[3]

Why an insane person received a particular form of treatment—or no treatment—is not easily explained. Therapeutic decisions were not the reflexive result of medical theories or principles but the outcome of a complex interaction of medical, economic, cultural, and social variables. Physicians and their ideas and experiences often played a dominant role in these decisions. But irregular healers, families, friends, caregivers, public officials, and the insane themselves could all influence what therapies, if any, might be selected in a given case.

Even when a family called in a medical man, they or the patient could influence the therapeutic approach he took. Family members, friends, or patients might be skeptical about the physician's diagnosis or remedy. They might not share his physicalist explanation of the disorder. An example is the case of a woman who fell prey to religious melancholy. The family called in a physician, who attributed her mental trouble to "sympathy with her physical condition." But a friend disagreed and diagnosed the trouble as fundamentally spiritual or psychological: "I fear the case is beyond the reach of any but the Great Physician. You know what a nervous, energetic woman she is, and you can understand the vehemence with which she would crave the evidence of the Spirit of God present in her heart."[4]

The insane themselves often played a role in determining the degree and types of treatment they received. Most of the time they probably acquiesced in or grudgingly tolerated the treatments prescribed for them, but not always. Patients sometimes refused to submit to bleeding or drugs and frustrated the therapeutic aims of physicians or families. One patient admitted to the state asylum had refused to take any medicines because Jesus Christ told her not to. Another arrived announcing that Jesus would provide his physic.[5] Some people diagnosed with insanity believed they were victims of possession, spells, or curses that could not be influenced by medical treatment.

Faced by a patient who adamantly resisted medical treatment, many physicians may have hesitated to use force for fear they might aggravate the disorder. The author of a medical thesis on mania warned that "whatever creates excitement tends to increase the disease; we are therefore to avoid forcing the patient to take our medicines, as the excitement thus created would be more than sufficient to balance the good derived from their operation."[6] A determined patient could sometimes avoid medical treatment even when confined in an institution like the Charleston poorhouse. The poorhouse physician reported in 1850 that the medical treatment of Terry Moore had been "thwarted in consequence of his refusal to take any medicine prescribed for him."[7] Inadequate or uncooperative nursing sometimes abetted a patient's opposition to a particular therapy. An exasperated physician reported in 1885 that his attempts to treat a patient had been "entirely unsatisfactory as he refuses to take any medicines and the nurses [are] unable to use force [and] cannot follow directions." Another physician noted that his attempts to treat a hysterical patient were frustrated, "as she would not submit to it and [I did not have] a nurse who would carry out directions."[8] Patients who had consulted physicians sometimes lost faith in them and turned to self-medication or irregulars. One man with incipient symptoms of general paralysis went to a physician, who treated him with potassium iodide, strychnine, and trichloride of mercury. The patient (perhaps not surprisingly) got worse and started treating himself. His physician later reported that "he used one thing and then another without any medical direction that I know of."[9]

The case of Mrs. Georgia Robert, mentioned earlier, provides a detailed example of how the dynamic interaction of patient, family, and physicians influenced therapies in particular cases. According to her husband's account, Mrs. Robert had been troubled by "religious doubts and fears" for several months before the onset of her mental disorder, which manifested itself shortly after she gave birth in May 1844. She became feverish and chilled and was greatly excited, "thinking she was going to die." Noticing a "bilious appearance about the tongue," her husband "administered a large dose of Calomel and Rhubarb." Two days later, Dr. F. H. Harris, the physician who had attended her during her labor, examined her. By this time, her "menstrual discharge had already stopped or turned into a whitish secretion which was very offensive."

Harris bled and purged her. She improved but soon became excited again about dying and called for the family to come to her bedside. Mr. Robert decided that "it was a fit of Hysterics and refused to comply with her request." Her gloomy religious thoughts came and went during the next two days, and her husband brought her company to cheer her up. Harris returned during this time but prescribed nothing but pleasant company. A few days later, her fits returned. At this point, Mr. Robert's brother arrived on a visit. His arrival added another medical adviser to the scene, for although he was a clergyman, he was also a former physician. After visiting with Mrs. Robert, he suggested to Mr. Robert that "her brain was affected, and should be attended to."

Mrs. Robert now began to take part in her treatment. She begged her brother-in-law to cut her hair and to be moved to her father-in-law's house a few miles away. The family complied, and she seemed to get better. That night she refused to take her medicine. On the day after the move, Dr. Harris reappeared and decided to bleed, "but she would not consent to have anything done to herself." Two days later, Mr. Robert called in Dr. Sidney Smith to consult with Harris. Smith cut the patient's hair short and "induced her to take a large dose of Calomel and Rhubarb." After this, she began to cry "that she was God's chosen daughter and would have to suffer as Christ had done." But she did not accept her fate meekly; once again she refused to be bled. The doctors returned the same evening, but she remained uncooperative.

Family members now became more adamant than the doctors about the need for an active therapeutic approach. Mr. Robert recorded that the doctors "would not be prevailed upon to bleed her by force." Instead, "they left a lancet for my brother to bleed her with as they thought he had more influence over her than anyone else." The doctors returned the next day more determined; they now used force to bleed the patient, continuing until she fainted. The bleeding made the patient more cooperative, at least for a time: "She was then considerably relieved and was rational, begging to be treated as a little child for she knew not what was for her own good when her mind wandered so much." The following day, the doctors bled her again, but had only removed a couple of ounces of blood when "she appeared to faint and they desisted." During the next few days the family was able to bleed her several times and get her to take small doses of medicines, but they frequently had to force them down her throat. They also made "Bold applications" of cold water and ice to her head, gave her warm baths, and put "her feet in as hot water as she could bear." [10]

The Robert case shows how family members and the insane themselves could influence both the types and the extent of therapeutic measures physicians used. Indeed, nineteenth-century general practitioners were often in a weak position when called in to deal with a case of insanity. Few of them had much knowledge about insanity or experience in treating the insane. Many physicians, especially in the early part of the century, had not received any formal medical education but were trained by the apprenticeship method, if at all. Others had attended one of the many inferior medical schools that emerged during the antebellum period. Until the last part of the century, the curriculum of even the better medical schools did not provide regular or systematic instruction in psychiatry. At most, interested professors or visiting specialists occasionally lectured on insanity.

Faced with an insane patient, the community practitioner was not totally at a loss. He could consult colleagues for advice or turn to a medical treatise or journal for help. Many general texts provided a section on insanity, and the number of specialized treatises on the subject proliferated during the nineteenth century. A physician determined to keep abreast of the latest medical thought on insanity could buy the works of European and American authors or read summaries of their works in the medical journals. Charleston's antebellum bookstores regularly advertised standard treatises on mental and nervous disorders. A student who wrote a medical thesis on insanity at the Medical College of South Carolina in 1845 cited most of the leading specialists in psychiatric thought, including Pinel, Rush, Esquirol, Bayle, Prichard, Haslam, Broussais, and Foville. But not all practitioners would have taken the trouble to read the books and journals; some would have been unable to afford them. Moreover, the assistance received from these sources was often contradictory and as likely to confuse as enlighten. "How various and conflicting are the directions which [the general practitioners] meet!" Trezevant declared. [11]

The gamut of directions was wide indeed. During the early nineteenth century, it ran from Benjamin Rush's bloody medical interventionism to the "masterly inactivity" of Philippe Pinel, which emphasized psychological treatments and a limited role for medicine. The two approaches were not mutually exclusive. Rush advocated moral remedies such as occupation and amusement, and Pinel saw value in the occasional use of purges and sedatives. But the advice of Rush and Pinel represented the extremes of therapeutic practice.

Pinel's less activist approach commended itself to many antebellum asylum superintendents, but they had the option of subjecting the patient to moral management within the confines of an institution designed for the care of the insane. The community practitioner had no such advantage. He was often faced with a violent patient who was tied down in bed or shut up in a small room. A medical professor like Eli Geddings of Charleston might exhort his students to imitate the "bright example" of Pinel and anoint "the poor Lunatic's sorrowed heart" with "the healing balm of your tender sympathies."[12] But met with a family's demand to do something effective quickly about a severely disturbed patient, the community physician was likely to opt for drastic medical action of some kind. On the other hand, if the patient was suffering from one of the milder mental disorders, or was not difficult to control, the general practitioner might be more inclined to suggest some form of psychological or moral therapy, such as a trip, exercise, or cheerful pursuits.

The therapies that community physicians inflicted upon insane patients altered subtly and slowly during the course of the nineteenth century. These changes, which involved a gradual retreat from the heroic therapeutics that held sway at the beginning of the nineteenth century, reflected broader developments in medical therapeutics in general. During the first third of the nineteenth century, most physicians in South Carolina, as elsewhere in America, employed depleting therapies in insanity as well as many other diseases. The influence of Benjamin Rush was at its height, and his system of medicine had numerous devotees in South Carolina. As we have seen, Rush's theories attributed most diseases, including insanity, to vascular inflammation, for which he invariably prescribed drastic bleeding and purging with calomel and jalap. Rush advocated particularly massive bleeding in acute mania, followed by vomiting, purging, blisters, and a low diet consisting of the "least nutritious" vegetables.[13]

Many South Carolina physicians may have used such drastic therapeutics to treat insanity. Dr. Thomas Y. Simons, a prominent Charleston physician who wrote a short treatise on insanity in 1828, recommended bleeding to lessen "vascular action," followed by a course of alteratives to "restore the organs to their appropriate and healthful functions." Simons noted that he often used the "powerful combination" of calomel and tartar emetic in cases in which calomel alone did not have a strong enough effect.[14] Thomas Moore, a student at the Medical College of South Carolina where Simons taught, recommended a similar approach in his 1829 thesis on mania. He claimed that the "first remedy" in cases of insanity was bloodletting, followed by cathartics and a low diet. Other useful remedies included emetics, warm and cold baths, blisters, issues, and large doses of narcotics.[15]

It would be misleading to conclude from these examples, however, that community practitioners of the early nineteenth century invariably combatted insanity with massive bleeding and drastic purging. Medical treatises usually advised the practitioner to reserve the most drastic treatments for the most acute, severe, or furious forms of insanity. Physicians who urged the effectiveness of heroic remedies often hedged their advice about with various limitations and cautions. Much of the therapeutic literature of the time warned that it was necessary to consider the nature of the malady, the condition of the patient's system, and the constitutional idiosyncracies of the patient before deciding upon the exact course of treatment to follow.

Moore stressed these caveats in his thesis. The wise physician knew that "in insanity, as well as every other disease, medicines are not to be used indiscriminately; but with caution and due attention to symptoms." Before commencing his treatment, the medical man should investigate every aspect of the case. If the patient's pulse was "full and pretty strong" and he possessed a "sanguineous temperament," bleeding was strongly indicated. But care was necessary; heroic measures could be taken to extremes. Insanity might result from "diminished as well as increased action." As a general rule, the physician should cease bleeding after three repetitions if no improvement occurred in the patient. Discrimination was also necessary in the use of other remedies. An active cathartic like black hellebore should be used in the early stages of the disease, when the pulse was full and strong and the patient was furious. But when it was necessary to use cathartics for some time, it was best to choose ones that were not too violent in their action. Such cautions were standard features of many medical treatises of the early nineteenth century.[16]

Moreover, for the treatment of milder nervous disorders, such as hypochondriasis, treatises usually advised physicians to employ a more moderate version of the traditional therapies. Henry Holland, who wrote his medical thesis at the Medical College of South Carolina in 1829, followed eighteenth-century tradition in advising psychological remedies for hypochondriasis: cheerful company, a change of scene, travel, amusements, outdoor sports, and horseback or carriage rides. The purpose of these was to divert the mind from its "morbid association of ideas" by supporting a "continued train of associated impressions of superior force." Mental therapy was not enough, however; Holland argued that hypochondriasis was a physical disorder, with its seat in the gastrointestinal system, and it could only be fully cured by medical measures, including emetics and cathartics, magnesia for stomach acid, and mercury as an alterative. Holland also recommended the use of tonics and bathing in tepid water. Opium, used with "much precaution," should be used to attack the "Spasmodic pain or the high irritation which is supposed to exist here." Friction should be applied to the skin with brushes or fresh flannels, the patient should be kept warm and provided with exercise, and his diet should be light but nutritious.[17]

Rush undoubtedly had a great influence on the treatment of insanity in the early nineteenth century, but his therapeutic ideas did not command universal respect. Many American physicians questioned the single-mindedness (as well as the bloody-mindedness) of his medical system. South Carolina, too, had its dissenters. "I have long since *sheathed my lancet*" in yellow fever, Charleston doctor J. L. E. W. Shecut wrote in 1819. He also announced that he had largely abandoned mercury, for "fatal experience" had taught him that it was "a dangerous remedy." Shecut did not completely give up traditional therapeutics, but he became a proponent of other methods, including electric therapy. Following the ideas of some eighteenth-century physicians, he posited that many diseases were the result of an imbalance of "electrical excitement" within the body. Electrical therapy, he argued, was of great advantage in diseases that were caused by a deficiency of electrical excitement. Among these disorders, he included melancholia, hysteria, hypochondriasis, and epilepsy. Electric therapy was of little benefit in mania, Shecut held, because it was caused by an "excess or superabundance of the electric fluid."[18] Apparently, for Shecut, mania still required traditional depleting therapies. Other physicians followed Shecut in advocating electrical therapy.[19]

Antebellum physicians uncomfortable with Rush's more drastic psychiatric therapies could have found some justification for moderation in other medical systems. An example is the work of French clinician F. J. V. Broussais. In 1831 Thomas Cooper, the president of South Carolina College, translated Broussais's *On Irritation and Insanity* into English. Broussais held that disease was generally the result of irritation, primarily of the gastrointestinal tract, brought on by overstimulation of the bodily functions. To reduce the stimulation and consequent irritation, Broussais recommended a low diet and bleeding by leeches.[20]

Broussais's influence on psychiatric therapy was probably ambivalent.

He condemned drastic treatments of the sort associated with Rush. It was a mistake, Broussais argued, to wear out the strength of the insane "by enormous bleeding, to torment them by dashing of cold water, and the dread of immersion, or to inflame their digestive organs by violent cathartics." But he was equally critical of fellow French physicians like Philippe Pinel for virtually abandoning active medical therapy in insanity. Pinel and his followers had been too "sparing of the blood of insane patients." Broussais opted for a medium between these therapeutic extremes. Insanity, like other diseases, was an irritation, which had to be fought by a depleting therapy consisting of bleeding, abstinence in diet, soothing drinks, and the application of cold. He opposed the use of drastic purges and emetics but conceded that a mild purgative might be useful once bloodletting had put the digestive organs into a state that could support its action. For physicians seeking a way to justify some moderation of psychiatric therapy, Broussais's approach could be appealing. Those wedded to Rush's more draconian measures, however, probably agreed with Cooper that Broussais's therapeutics seemed somewhat "feeble." The southern climate, Cooper declared, seemed to require a "more bold and decisive practice, than the northern climate of Paris or London." [21]

It is difficult to determine the influence Broussais or any of the medical systematizers had on community physicians' prescriptions for the insane. As John Harley Warner has pointed out, substantial gaps often existed between the medical theories individual doctors held, and their therapeutic principles and practices. Moreover, early-nineteenth-century physicians increasingly rejected systems altogether and adopted a self-consciously empirical stance. But whether physicians embraced a system or not often made little difference as to the types of therapies they employed. The medical systems varied in their explanations of disease but all shared an assumption, going back to the ancients, that disease was a general state of the body, a disequilibrium or imbalance of the circulatory, biliary, or nervous systems. All the systems attempted to restore proper bodily functioning through regulation of the secretions, which in practice meant recourse to some version of traditional therapeutics. Whatever their attitude toward medical systems, most physicians remained loyal to the old standbys of bleeding, purging, and the rest. They might differ, however, in the specific remedies they used in a given case or the severity with which they pursued a particular type of treatment. [22]

By the 1830s and 1840s, some American physicians were openly questioning the efficacy of the more drastic therapies. The skeptics were influenced by experience and by the work of Pierre Louis and the Paris Clinical

School. Physicians such as Boston's Jacob Bigelow wrote of "self-limited diseases" and argued for a more supportive therapeutics that would assist the "natural" process of recovery. But the growing skepticism about the theory and principles of traditional therapeutics did not lead American physicians to suddenly abandon traditional remedies in practice. For practical and professional reasons, most American practitioners continued for decades to rely to a greater or lesser extent on the old therapies. Many physicians may have moderated their use of traditional therapies, but few abandoned them.

Change was cautious, gradual, and uneven. Country practitioners, often poorly trained and isolated from new ideas, were generally slowest to change. Frontier physicians in the South and West were notorious for their heavy reliance on calomel, which they justified on the grounds that the region's climate was particularly conducive to biliary diseases. But physicians everywhere were reluctant to abandon heroic measures totally, partly because they had nothing so impressive to put in their place. To trust to nature, rest, diet, and tonics alone seemed too feeble a regimen to command the respect of the public.

As Charles Rosenberg has argued, traditional therapeutics appealed to physicians and laymen alike because both groups tended to share the ancient concept of the body and its functioning upon which they were based. According to this concept, disease was not so much a specific entity as a general state of the body, a lack of internal balance or equilibrium. Medicine was largely a business of attacking symptoms and restoring internal harmony, and it did this mainly by regulating the secretions through drugs, bleeding, counterirritants, and so forth. The continuing appeal of these measures lay in their visible and measurable physiological effects; they seemed to "work" in the sense that they altered bodily states, often in dramatic and predictable ways. It was difficult for physicians to abandon such powerful weapons, especially as so many of their patients or their patients' families expected or demanded them. The medical man who gave up traditional therapeutics entirely did so at his peril.[23]

Even asylum physicians, among the most critical of heroic medicine, did not advise the wholesale rejection of traditional therapies. In 1854, Pliny Earle, superintendent of New York's Bloomingdale Asylum, wrote a lengthy article in the *American Journal of Insanity* that summarized the views of scores of specialists in mental diseases. Earle concluded that bleeding was seldom required and was often prejudicial in mental disorders. But he added that mania and conditions sometimes associated with insanity, such as inflammation or apoplexy, might require bleeding. Moreover, he was far from advocating the abandonment of other traditional therapies, including depletive ones. In many cases in which bleeding might seem appropriate, he argued, it would be better and safer to "treat by other means, equalizing the circulation and promoting the secretions and excretions."[24]

The same moderate, gradual approach to therapeutic innovation in the treatment of insanity is evident in the work of a leading South Carolina physician, Samuel Henry Dickson. A highly respected professor at the Medical College of South Carolina from the 1820s to the 1850s, Dickson trained many of the state's antebellum physicians. He also wrote substantial medical texts such as *Pathology and Therapeutics* (1845) and *Elements of Medicine* (1855), in both of which he discussed the treatment of insanity. Dickson recommended most of the traditional therapies, and issued the traditional cautions about the need to prescribe according to the state of the patient's general system. Bleeding and purging, he argued, should be confined to acute cases in which the patient's constitution was robust; in chronic cases or where the patient was in a weakened state, bleeding and purging were more harmful than beneficial. In both works, Dickson showed little enthusiasm for mercurials but extolled the benefits of opium to combat the sleeplessness, restlessness, and agitation that characterized many insane patients. In the earlier work, he also claimed that he placed a heavy reliance upon tartar antimony as a means of restoring the maniacal patient to tranquility. His therapeutic recommendations, like those of many other American physicians, tended to become more moderate over time. In 1845, he noted that some physicians considered general bleeding in insanity to be useless or even harmful, but that he "should not hesitate to bleed freely" in acute cases marked by a flushed complexion, rapid pulse, headache, and outrageous behavior. In 1855, he declared that bleeding was "much less frequently and energetically employed now than formerly, and is not often, perhaps, requisite or beneficial." In cases of insanity in which the patient was in a low or weakened state, Dickson stressed the importance of supportive measures designed to build bodily strength. The patient should be kept warm and given a nutritious and agreeable diet, along with a moderate use of tonics and stimulants.[25]

Community practitioners followed Dickson in gradually moderating their therapies. But many of them were more cautious about changing their methods than he. Evidence concerning the medical treatment of the insane in the antebellum community indicates a continuing reliance upon traditional therapeutics throughout the period, with a gradual trend toward moderation evident by the 1850s. The case records of antebellum state asylum patients seldom discuss their treatment before commitment. But when treatment is mentioned, it is usually depletive and drastic. Allen Griffin, who came to the South Carolina Lunatic Asylum in 1829, had been "largely bled" by a physician prior to his admission. When Stephen Monk arrived at the asylum in 1836, Dr. Trezevant noted that "he had been bled freely and kept low and much prostrated." Another patient had "been treated very actively, bled rather . . . too much."[26] Most of these patients came from affluent or middling families. But the poor sometimes received the same treatments, if not the same degree of attention. When Walter McKlintock was admitted to the asylum in 1838, Trezevant reported that he had been "freely bled" while an inmate of the Charleston poorhouse.[27]

Insane slaves received similar treatments. One of the most detailed histories of community medical care to survive from nineteenth-century South Carolina is the case of a slave named Joe, who resided on a plantation near Charleston. When Joe became insane, his owner brought him to town and placed him under Dr. W. T. Wragg's care. In a published report of the case, Wragg noted that he had subjected Joe to repeated bleeding, blistering, purging, hot foot baths with mustard, and other depleting therapies. These methods were repeated for nine days. They succeeded in calming Joe's excitement and procuring him rest and a restored appetite. But they did not restore his reason. Wragg then inserted a seton (a piece of thread or cloth designed to produce inflammation) in the back of Joe's neck, where it remained for fifty-eight days. Once it began to discharge pus, the patient's delirium began to subside, and by the time the seton was removed, his mind was "perfectly clear and his physical health completely restored."[28]

It is difficult to know how typical Joe's treatment was, because few descriptions of the medical treatment of insane slaves have survived. Other physicians asked to treat a case of insanity in a slave may have been less — or more — heroic in their approach than Wragg. An influential school of antebellum southern medical thought held that blacks possessed certain physical "peculiarities" that required a distinctive approach to therapeutics, and that treatments that worked well on whites might be ineffective or positively dangerous in the case of blacks. Some advocates of a "negro medicine" argued that the black man, in consequence of his "underdeveloped" nervous system, did not require and did not bear bleeding and other drastic therapies to the same extent as the white man. But other physicians claimed that the "inferior" organization of blacks meant that they needed and could tolerate larger dosages of some medicines than whites.[29]

By the middle of the century, community practitioners in South Carolina seem to have been gradually reducing their use of drastic depleting measures and making greater use of supportive and sedative means. The physician to the Charleston poorhouse reported in 1853 that the medical treatment of the pauper lunatics was confined to the maintenance of "a strict supervision over them, and an attempt to preserve their Physical health."[30] After 1856, when the city's insane poor were transferred to the care of Roper Hospital, this less drastic approach to treatment appears to have continued. Case records from 1859 to 1862 reveal that the physicians used traditional treatments for insanity, including calomel, blisters, cold showers, and opiates. But as far as one can judge from the sketchy nature of the records, they applied these remedies moderately in comparison to earlier times. None of the patients was bled; some received no medical treatment. Mary Brennan, an Irish immigrant, was "subjected to no particular treatment, was simply kept quiet in the cells, treated kindly, and allowed to walk in the Cell yard."[31]

The gradual abandonment of bleeding was the most radical change in the treatment of insanity in the late nineteenth century. During the later antebellum period, physicians began to use it less often and less drastically, and by the 1880s they had virtually given it up. A measure of the change of sentiment about venesection is revealed in the commitment paper of a patient admitted to the asylum in 1884. According to her physicians, one of her delusions was that "[she] fancies the only way to relieve her condition is by bleeding."[32]

Other traditional depleting therapies lingered on longer than bleeding, especially among rural practitioners. A Barnwell County physician reported in 1880 that he had given an insane patient "blistering and antiflogistic treatment."[33] The physicians who treated "R. E." for mania before his commitment in 1891 discussed his case and treatment in ways that would have been familiar to a physician of the 1820s: "He is a hard working man and has been exposed very much to the sun. His habit is one of constipation and there has been considerable torpor of the liver, but his mental faculties have not perceptibly improved under the action of mercuries."[34] In 1878 a physician combatted religious monomania in a young Oconee man with regular doses of calomel, a blister, warm baths, and the cold douche. Except for the absence of bleeding and the use of chloral hydrate to help him sleep, the treatment was little different from that followed by eighteenth-century practitioners.[35]

The decline of bleeding was to some extent balanced by an increased use of drugs, especially sedatives and pain-killers. During the late nineteenth century, community physicians (like their asylum colleagues) were calming patients by dosing them with the wonder drugs of that era, the bromides, chloral hydrate and morphine. These were often followed by tonics containing iron, quinine, and alcohol. General practitioners of the late nineteenth century often combined old and new therapies in an eclectic fashion, hoping that something would work. Blisters might be used with bromides, mercury with morphine, chloral with calomel, setons with strychnine. One physician used the following on a patient: ergot, bromides, mercury, potassium iodide, chloral, morphine, suppositories, iodoform, cannabis, indica, belladonna, hyoscyamus, conium.[36]

Regular physicians were not the only ones who treated the insane. For numerous reasons, families confronted by insanity did not always call in medical help, especially in the early stages of the disorder. Although the proportion of physicians grew considerably in relation to the population during the antebellum period, poverty, poor transport, and isolation limited access to professional medical care. Charleston residents might have to fight off the doctors when sick. But in rural areas, the nearest regular medical man might be many miles away, and his fees would often increase with the distance he had to travel to reach the patient. Many people tried to avoid the cost and trouble of consulting a physician if they could.[37]

A lack of confidence in regular medicine also sometimes inhibited recourse to the physician. During the antebellum era and beyond, regular practitioners were often on the defensive, as growing skepticism about the efficacy of traditional heroic therapies united with the antielitism of Jacksonian democracy. Physicians themselves contributed to the public's doubts by questioning heroic medicine while having little to put in its place. The triumphs of modern scientific medicine lay well in the future. Many nineteenth-century doctors were poorly trained, and they faced increasingly stiff competition from a legion of irregular practitioners. South Carolina, along with most other states, abolished its already weak laws against unlicensed practice during the Jacksonian era.

Distrust of the ability of regular medical men was reflected in many letters to the newspapers. One to the *Charleston Courier* in 1843 stated that "the practice of physic is little more than the making of experiments. Hence the frequent failures in medical practice . . . and the longstanding suspicion that doctors *kill* sometimes."[38] Planter James Henry Hammond employed regular physicians for some years, but the high mortality of his slaves eroded his faith in their ability, and he tried various forms of domestic practice. He wrote in 1861 that "observation . . . and experience lead me to throw all physic to the dogs. Every drug in the apothecary shop *is poison*. I have see hundreds die of Doctors and scarcely a week passes that I do not hear of a case."[39] Public confidence in and recourse to regular physicians may have declined even further in the later nineteenth century.

Postbellum South Carolina was not a fertile field for physicians, because many people were too poor to afford their services. The state's poverty discouraged many men from a medical career and encouraged the ambitious to leave for more profitable locations. The training and general quality of physicians in the state declined in the later nineteenth century, while their numbers did not increase greatly.[40]

After 1865, insane blacks were probably even less likely than before emancipation to receive regular medical treatment in the community. Emancipated blacks no longer had masters to provide medical care, and most were too poor to afford it themselves. Freedmen were sometimes able to obtain care from a regular practitioner. A few were sufficiently wealthy to pay a physician, or they received medical assistance as a charity, as in Charleston City Hospital. Former owners or employers sometimes took an interest in the fate of an insane black. One man wrote to the asylum superintendent about a recently admitted patient: "She and her husband have been in my employ for about three years and they are two of the best colored people I ever knew. I write this to kindly ask you to see that this unfortunate woman shall receive as good treatment as if she were white."[41] The family of one black patient admitted to the asylum in 1879 had consulted several different physicians over a period of four or five years in an attempt to cure him at home. The attention he received from local physicians may have been partly a reward for being politically correct. One of the physicians who treated him wrote the superintendent of the asylum that "the said Harvey Jackson is a colored man of good character and respected by the good men of the neighborhood, has always favored good government." In the political lexicon of the time, this meant that Jackson had supported the Democrats in their overthrow of Reconstruction in 1876–77.[42] In any case, it is unlikely that many emancipated blacks were able to command this level of medical attention.

Out of choice or necessity, many families faced with insanity resorted to home remedies or irregular practitioners of various kinds. Help and advice from these sources was abundant but, like that emanating from the physicians, often contradictory and confusing. The number of domestic medical manuals proliferated during the nineteenth century. In addition to old standbys such as William Buchan's *Domestic Medicine*, families could purchase John Gunn's *Domestic Medicine* or James Ewell's *Medical Companion, or Family Physician*, all of which went into numerous editions. Several medical advice books were written or published in antebellum South Carolina, such as (Anon.), *The Medical Vade-Mecum*, Alfred Folger, *The Family Physician*, J. Hume Simons, *The Planter's Guide and Family Book of Medi-*

cine, and Simon Abbott, *The Southern Botany Physician*. The popularity of home medical manuals continued into the later nineteenth century. An example is *The Cottage Physician*, which billed itself as "A Complete Hand Book of Medical Knowledge for the Home." [43]

Few of the manuals provided advice on the treatment of severe mental disorders such as mania and melancholia, but most discussed milder nervous conditions such as hypochondriasis, hysteria, and "weakness of the nerves." Several devoted sections to the diagnosis and treatment of conditions that were often related to or confused with insanity, such as epilepsy and delerium tremens or *mania a potu*. Buchan had a section on melancholy; Ewell discussed puerperal mania; Abbott provided a chapter on "insanity or madness," which he also referred to variously as "derangement," "mania," and "craziness." The treatments the manuals recommended included both moral (psychological) and medical remedies. Several manuals advised the importance of gaining the patients' confidence by a mild demeanor and by diverting his thoughts through agreeable exercise, employment, or travel. Buchan and Ewell generally advocated a light, easily digestible diet, which avoided fatty meats and most alcoholic drinks. Abbott, a Thomsonian, emphasized botanical rather than chemical remedies. "In prescribing medicine for lunatics or crazy persons," he claimed, the best results would be obtained from repeated courses of the nervine powder in a strong tincture or tea, along with bitters. He also recommended the favorite Thomsonian remedy, the emetic lobelia, especially in the case of "furious fits, which it might possibly put a speedy end to." [44]

Some manuals recommended supportive measures such as tonics, nourishing diet, and stimulants for weakened patients, hysterics, or hypochondriacs. But several manuals prescribed only drastic depletive remedies. When faced with a patient furious from "Inflammation of the Brain, or Phrenzy" Simons advised:

> Bleed immediately, and let the blood flow until the patient is sick at his stomach. If he is not relieved by one bleeding, bleed again and again, from time to time. Cut the hair short, or shave the head, and apply a bladder half full of cold water, with a piece of ice in it, if it can be had. . . . If he is a grown person, give him 10 grains of Calomel, and four hours afterwards, a dose of Epsom or Glauber Salts—less for a child etc. Cup the temples, or put leeches to them. Remember the bowels must be kept open. . . . Put a blister on the back of the neck, and keep putting them on as soon as the place heals, throughout the course of the disease. . . . Be careful to keep the room dark and quiet. [45]

For puerperal mania, Ewell counseled "shaving and blistering the head, keeping the bowels open by cooling laxatives, determining to the surface by diaphoretic powders or mixture, and afterwards allaying irritation by the camphorated mixture in their usual doses."[46] Folger's favorite remedy was calomel, which he recommended for almost everything. He also urged the use of various "antispasmodics" and stimulants (such as camphor) for mania, and assafoetida, sulfuric ether, and hartshorn (ammonia) for hysteria.[47]

The remedies the manuals prescribed were often similar, and many changed little over long periods of time. In the 1890s *The Cottage Physician* recommended a therapeutic regime for insanity similar to that found in eighteenth-century manuals such as Buchan's. Where there was excitement and inflammation, *The Cottage Physician* prescribed mild antiphlogistic measures, simple purgatives (such as rhubarb or castor oil), and a spare diet. In cases marked by debility, the author advised a nourishing diet; for sleeplessness, opium; for all cases, exercise, fresh air, and cleanliness. The regimen for hypochondriasis differed little from that advocated by physicians a century before: keep the bowels open and provide cheerful society, a change of scene, tonics, and exercise.[48]

The domestic manuals were not the only written sources of medical advice. Just as today, journals and newspapers were filled with articles on health care. The Charleston editors of the *Southern Botanic Journal*, for example, announced that their aim was to provide a work of reference for planters and others who had purchased the right to practice the Thomsonian system of botanic medicine. Planters concerned with issues of slave health could also consult the numerous journal articles by physicians who had studied "negro diseases."[49] Most of this literature did not deal with mental diseases, for other illnesses presented a far greater threat to planters' investments. But articles by Dr. Samuel Cartwright of Louisiana provided some advice on the treatment of mental disorders he claimed were unique to blacks. (For his descriptions of these disorders, see chapter 7.)

For drapetomania ("the disease causing negroes to run away"), Cartwright prescribed a form of moral or psychological treatment. To prevent or cure this disorder, it was essential to elicit "awe and reverence" from the slave toward the white men who were his natural superiors. The master and overseer had to impress on the slave that his intended lot, decreed by Scripture, was submission. They should treat the slave graciously, supply his physical needs, and protect him from abuse. But they should never allow him to be anything but "the submissive knee bender." If a slave began to be restless in his position, to become "sulky and dissatisfied," Cartwright warned, it was a sign of incipient drapetomania. The causes of dissatisfaction should be investigated and removed. If no cause could be detected, the best remedy was the traditional one of "whipping them out of it." Probably many masters and overseers did not need this advice.

The other mental disorder unique to blacks, dyaethesia aethiopica ("rascality") was readily cured "if treated on sound physiological principles." The great need was to stimulate the skin, which was "dry, thick, and harsh to the touch," and the liver, which was inactive. The patient should be scrubbed with warm water and soap, then covered with oil, which should be slapped in with a "broad leather strap." Then he should be required to do some hard work in the fresh air and sunshine, to force him to expand his lungs. After resting from the labor, the patient should be fed "some good wholesome food, well-seasoned with spices and mixed with vegetables." After more work, rest, and lots of liquids, he should be washed and sent to a clean bed in a warm room. Repeating this treatment each day would soon "effect a cure in all cases which are not complicated by chronic visceral derangement."[50] How many planters or physicians followed Cartwright's advice is a mystery. As we have seen, his work aroused considerable interest, though not necessarily admiration, among South Carolina physicians.

People trying to cope with mental disorder at home without a physician were not restricted to manuals and other written advice. Numerous irregular practitioners stood ready to help. Lobbying by regulars had convinced the state legislature to outlaw unlicensed practice in 1817, but the act was not very effective and was virtually repealed in 1838.[51] The absence of effective licensing allowed irregular practitioners of all kinds to flourish in South Carolina throughout the nineteenth century and beyond.

During the antebellum period, the parade of irregulars was joined by medical sects such as the Thomsonians and homeopaths. The Thomsonians derived their name from Samuel Thomson (1769–1843), a New Hampshire farmer. As a young man Thomson had developed a distrust of the harsh therapies of the regulars, particularly their use of calomel and other mineral remedies. He became interested in botanical medicine and established himself as a local herb doctor. In time, he developed a medical system of his own and began selling the right to practice it along with his manual. Although he intended that his system would be used by laymen, it soon gave rise to a body of Thomsonian practitioners who practiced botanical medicine as an occupation. He also inspired many imitators who developed botanical preparations of their own.

Thomson violently attacked the therapies of the regulars as useless and murderous, but his own methods were in some respects remarkably similar to theirs. He theorized that disease resulted from cold and sought to restore the body's natural heat. He did this by sweating his patients with steam baths and cayenne pepper and scouring out clogged digestive systems with botanical emetics and purgatives, such as lobelia. The aim, as one disciple put it, was "to infuse fresh vigor into the system, remove obstructions, and promote healthy secretions."[52]

Thomsonians used these methods to treat insanity as well as physical disorders. In 1839 a Virginia correspondent of Charleston's *Southern Botanic Journal*, published by Thomsonians, described how he had successfully treated a maniac slave with lobelia. He had consulted a physician who told him that the only remedy was solitary confinement and the application of constant irritation to the spine with tartar ointment. Rejecting this advice, the writer tried Thomsonian remedies and the patient recovered. He communicated his results to the *Journal*'s readers in the hope that it "might be useful to . . . those who might possibly have similar cases in their family."[53]

The Thomsonians had strong popular support in South Carolina during the 1830s and 1840s. Thomson's vocal condemnations of the regular physicians, and his cry that every man could be his own physician, appealed to the antielitist sentiments of the Jacksonian era. In 1835, the Medical Society of South Carolina charged three Thomsonian practitioners with illegal practice of medicine, but the grand jury refused to issue an indictment. Thomsonians were soon practicing with impunity throughout the state. One of them, Simon Abbott, operated a Thomsonian infirmary in Charleston that provided separate rooms for blacks and "female attendants for the ladies."[54] In 1845 an irate South Carolina physician complained that the country was filled with Thomsonians and "Botanic Doctors" who were taking advantage of the popular prejudice against calomel to peddle their own noxious preparations.[55] By the late 1840s Thomsonianism began to decline as a movement, but the vogue for botanical medicine remained strong for decades, as can be seen from advertisements for vegetable remedies in the press.

As Thomsonianism declined, homeopathy rose to take its place. Founded by German physician Samuel Hahnemann at the end of the eighteenth century, homeopathy was based on two principles. The first, the law of similars, held that a disease could be cured by medicines that produce the symptoms of the disease in a healthy person. The second, the law of infinitesimals, asserted that medicine was effective in inverse proportion to the size of the dose; the smaller the dose, the higher the chances of cure. The second law, however absurd on the face of it, was probably the key to homeopathy's success. Homeopathic practitioners used many of the same medicines as regulars; but the homeopathist's doses were so small that in effect he was leaving the cure to nature and the placebo effect. If he did not cure, at least he did not kill, and his therapies were more palatable and less painful than those of regular medicine (or of the Thomsonians for that matter). Homeopathic physicians showed a strong interest in insanity and were often quite familiar with the leading treatises and theories on the subject. They applauded the trend toward milder therapies for the insane in asylums and had a beneficial influence in encouraging the move away from drastic medications.[56]

Homeopathy did not have as strong an organized following in South Carolina as botanic medicine. The state did not have a homeopathic institute, or apparently many homeopathic physicians, but homeopathy did have some influence. Regular physicians, although often hostile, treated homeopathy with more respect than Thomsonianism. Eli Geddings, a professor at the Medical College of South Carolina, reviewed several homeopathic books sympathetically in 1830. Moreover, although homeopathy was not a home-cure movement, some homeopathic physicians produced domestic manuals to guide those who lived far from the nearest practitioner. These manuals won some converts. Among them was planter James Henry Hammond, whose despair with the ineffectiveness of traditional medicine drove him to try homeopathy in the 1850s. Hammond hit exactly on the appeal of homeopathy: "When you hit right you make a speedy cure. If you miss, you do no harm."[57]

In addition to the medical sects, many people continued to place faith in the power of folk practitioners, some of whom had the reputation of having occult powers.[58] The practice of "using," which German immigrants brought to the state during the eighteenth century, retained some adherents in the central part of South Carolina at least into the early twentieth century. Practitioners of using would rub the affected part of the patient's body, blow their breath upon it, and repeat ancient charms and incantations. Among the remedies that has survived is the following one for epilepsy: "Take a new broom and sweep from three corners of a room. Throw the sweepings over the person who has the sickness, while you say these words: *In God's name, Falling Sickness, you must depart till I these seed do cut.* So do it three times." Like most forms of alternative medicine, using thrived on both faith and skepticism. One practitioner who defended using argued that it was just as effective as prayer, because the names of the Father, Son, and Holy Ghost were always used. If it did no good, she continued, at least it could do no harm, "and in this respect it differs from the drugs used by physicians."[59]

The ranks of the irregulars included numerous black herbal practitioners, root doctors, and conjurers, who provided an alternative medicine for blacks and, sometimes, for whites. Some of the black folk healers dealt exclusively in herbal remedies; others employed occult means, often referred to as conjure, hoodoo, or root. Blacks, like whites, were often skeptical of the abilities of regular physicians. Many plantation slaves understandably preferred the folk doctor's concoctions, even those containing boiled cockroaches or sheep's dung, to the painful and debilitating therapies of regular medicine. Some former slaves recalled that they placed little faith in white physicians and relied mostly on herbal medicines. Often the local folk doctor was also the plantation nurse, who practiced both white and black medicine. It was not uncommon for planters and other whites to consult black healers when sick and to learn black herbal lore from them. Many of the home remedies in planters' prescription books derived from black doctors.[60]

The popularity of folk practitioners among blacks did not derive solely from the negative image of white medicine. Root doctoring or conjure was appealing for cultural reasons, because it was connected with traditional African religion. Root doctors employed ritualism, which combined incantations and charms designed to add supernatural aid to the natural properties of the herbal remedy. Given the faith many people had in the powers of the conjurers and root doctors, they may have functioned effectively at times in combatting mental troubles whose origins were psychological or psychosomatic. But there was a negative side to the conjurer's work. According to those who believed in conjure, or hoodoo, the practitioners could cause as well as cure sickness through their charms and spells.[61]

Among the disorders the conjurers had a reputation for both inflicting and curing was insanity. A woman committed to South Carolina State Hospital in 1902 claimed that she was being pursued by devils who were trying to kill her. The physician who recorded her case commented that her disorder was "in all probability aggravated by a 'root doctor.'" Those who believed in conjure often held that a disease caused by conjuring could only be removed by conjuring. This belief is reflected in the words of a man admitted to the state hospital in 1906. According to his case history, he kept "saying he has been poisoned or conjured . . . says that medicine will do him no good."[62]

Belief in the power of root or conjure remained widespread long after emancipation. Many patients admitted to the state asylum around the turn of the century claimed that they had been conjured, hoodooed, or bewitched. The majority of these patients were black, but some were white.[63]

An example was a white farmer committed in the 1880s who believed that he had been bewitched after associating "with a certain old colored man."[64]

Those seeking to cure insanity at home had yet another alternative to regular medicine: self-medication with proprietary (patent) medicines or over-the-counter drugs. By the early nineteenth century, Americans had established a flourishing patent remedy industry. Throughout the century, newspapers and journals were full of advertisements for proprietary remedies that claimed to relieve or cure a variety of mental or nervous problems. In the 1840s, Moffatt's Vegetable Life Pills and Phoenix Bitters promised to cure "hysterical affections, hypocondriacism, restlessness, and many other varieties of the Neurotical class." In the 1870s, Hulmboldt's Extract Buchu guaranteed relief to "Nervous and Debilitated Sufferers" and warned that if left untreated, the symptoms of these conditions would lead to insanity, epilepsy, or imbecility. In the 1890s, Manetic Nervine combatted "nervous Prostration, Fits, Mental Depression, Softening of the Brain, causing Misery, Insanity, and Death."[65] Many other proprietary medicines claimed to combat nervous or mental disorders. Advertisements for vegetable remedies were particularly numerous. Their popularity reflected both the influence of the botanic doctors and a widespread aversion to the regular physicians' heavy use of calomel and other mineral remedies.[66] Most of the patent remedies were manufactured in the North, but some were locally produced. Mrs. E. A. Jenkins's "Celebrated Colleton Bitters" was billed as "the only Reliable Southern Medicine" for the cure of various digestive and nervous disorders.[67]

Proprietary medicines often contained powerful purgatives, opium, or large amounts of alcohol. But this did not stop their makers from exploiting the public's distrust and fear of regular medicine. Advertisements frequently stressed how much less painful and dangerous remedy X was compared to regular therapies. But the advertisers also spoke the well-understood language of traditional therapeutics. They sought to assure potential clients that their remedy would restore the internal balance by regulating the secretions. Advertisements for Dr. Benjamin Brandreth's Vegetable Universal Pills, which claimed to cure nervous diseases, referred to mercury as a poison and prominently proclaimed that "Calomel is not Used. . . . The Brandreth Pills are made ENTIRELY of Vegetable extracts, known by long experience to be perfectly innocent." But the puff paradoxically added that the power of the pills as a purgative was greater than that of any other medication. The apparent contradiction derived from popular ideas about medicine. Many people who were skeptical about the specific remedies of the regular physicians accepted the ancient wisdom of the humoralists about the need to cleanse the system. Brandreth's advertisements espoused a theory of disease and therapeutics that was simpler than the simplest system of the regulars and yet shared the same concern with regulating bodily fluids. Brandreth declared that all disease sprang from "impurity of the Blood," which inhibited the circulation and produced inflammation. His medicine was designed to "purify, and remove by its purgative powers all bad humors from the blood by the stomach and the bowels." [68]

Even if a remedy did not rely on any drug or medication, its promoters might describe its effects in the traditional terms of regulating and balancing the bodily fluids. Dr. Christie's Galvanic Belts, Bracelets, Necklace, and Magnetic Fluids claimed to cure a variety of nervous diseases and ills "caused by an impaired, weakened, or unhealthy condition of the Nervous System." Christie's advertisements appealed to the widespread interest in "the mysterious powers of GALVANISM and MAGNETISM" and exploited the understandable desire of many people to avoid traditional medications: "In Nervous Complaints, Drugs and Medicines increase the disease, for they weaken the vital energies and the already prostrated system; while under the strengthening, life-giving, vitalizing influence of Galvanism . . . the exhausted patient . . . is restored to former health, strength, elasticity, and vigor." For people tired of having their insides ravaged by violent medications, Dr. Christie offered welcome relief. His galvanic contraptions would "arrest and cure disease by outward application, in place of the usual mode of drugging and physicking the patient until exhausted Nature sinks hopelessly under the infliction." Best of all, they would painlessly accomplish the goal that drugs and medicines strove for in vain: "They strengthen the whole system, equalize the circulation of the blood, promote the secretions, and never do the slightest injury under any circumstances." [69]

Sellers of patent remedies also exploited traditional faith in folk medicine. An example from South Carolina is Ezxba W. Dedmond, a mill worker who capitalized on the widespread fear of pellagra in the early twentieth century. Pellagra, a niacin-deficiency disease that often produced psychotic symptoms in its advanced stages, sent hundreds of patients to the state hospital during these years. In 1911, four years after Dr. James Babcock had first diagnosed pellagra at the hospital, Dedmond began selling his remedy, "Ez-X-Ba River, the Stream of Life," for five dollars a bottle. Backed by some wealthy businessmen, Dedmond advertised his wares prominently in the state's newspapers and claimed to have cured himself and many others of pellagra. When Babcock and other physicians denounced him as a quack and called upon him to reveal the content of his nostrum, Dedmond struck back and questioned the competence of the regular medical men. It was "not a compliment to our present day doctors," he wrote, "that they cannot cure this awful disease . . . and they realize it." Like many folk practitioners, he stressed his humble background and associated himself with divine and occult powers:

When [the regular physicians] failed to even give relief, the God of Heaven sent a remedy. . . . Thus he called a boy who was raised at the plow handles. . . . It is galling to the smart men [to] let a poor uneducated man raised in the backwoods, and almost entirely without education, take their patients way from them. . . . I am my mother's 13th child, born on the 13th of the month, lost my dear old father and had to become a man at 13 years of age. Everything containing 13 with me is lucky.

In one advertisement, Dedmond claimed that he had cured "an insane woman" and included testimonials to that effect, including the following letter, allegedly from the woman's husband: "My wife was treated for Pellagra by my family physician, J. Lee Young. She grew worse until he said he had done all he could do. . . . She had been crazy about 7 weeks until she became a raving maniac. On Jan. 25 I sent for Mrs. Dedmond, she came, and said it was too late, but she would do the best she could, so we began the treatment and in 7 days my wife came to her mind and has steadily improved; we all thought she would die." [70]

The Public Health Service subsequently claimed that many of Dedmond's testimonials were false and that there was nothing of value in his remedy. Laboratory analysis showed that his medicine consisted of a dilute solution of iron, magnesium, aluminum, and calcium salts mixed with a mold growth. His cures, if cures there were, probably resulted from the tendency of pellagra's symptoms to retreat with seasonal improvements in diet. But regular physicians whose treatments were no more valid and perhaps more dangerous would have reaped the same benefits. [71]

Anyone could readily purchase patent remedies as well as the most powerful generic drugs by mail, from peddlers, merchants, or physicians. Antebellum planters often purchased medicine chests containing medications such as calomel, quinine, opiates, and various "powders" that they, their wives, or overseers used to treat their slaves and their families. Brandreth's advertisements assured planters that his pills would "INSURE HEALTH to the people of their estates." [72]

Throughout the century, many people concocted their own medications using recipes from the manuals or other sources. Planters sometimes kept recipe books in which they recorded prescriptions and the medications they had given to slaves.[73] The mother of a patient sent to the asylum in 1894 wrote that she had treated him for years with a homemade tonic that combined corn whiskey, quinine, and citrate of iron. She had also given him two courses of Dr. Pierce's medicine, two quart bottles of extract of nettle-root, and Koenig's Nerve Tonic. Only the tonics, she reported, seemed to do him any good. Another patient had received an unnamed prescription from the World's Dispensatory in Buffalo, New York.

Sufferers from nervous or mental conditions often dosed themselves with powerful medications. The commitment papers of one man stated that he had been treating himself with large doses of quinine and purgatives. In another case, a physician claimed that a woman had taken poisonous doses of bromides, laudanum, and sulfonal. The family of a Hampton County farm laborer gave her bromides, lavender, quinine, iodine, and a mustard plaster on the spine. The home remedies reported on the commitment papers of late-nineteenth-century patients included blistering, calomel, laudanum, opium, morphine, chloral, camphor, assafoetida, and whiskey. Some home therapies were decidedly bizarre. The friends of a man suffering from religious mania combatted his excitement by dashing water in his face, pricking him with pins, and pinching him. Families who could afford it sometimes tried to divert the patient's mind by the time-honored method of taking them on trips to the mountains, the seaside, or a mineral spring. In the 1850s, a Charleston man took his deranged wife to Virginia Springs, where she met some of her old friends and soon got well.[74] Ironically, despite the influence of the botanic physicians and the other medical sects, calomel remained perhaps the most popular home remedy throughout the nineteenth century. In 1845, Alfred Folger called calomel "the most important of our medicines."[75] In 1891, a South Carolina doctor wrote that calomel was the most commonly used domestic medicine in the state. It remained in many medicine cabinets as late as the 1930s.[76]

It is difficult to determine the impact that the various forms of irregular medicine had on the treatment of insanity. Their practitioners seldom left behind much evidence of their efforts. Yet we get an occasional glimpse of their presence in the comments of regular physicians on commitment papers, such as "No [treatment] Except by Quacks," or "*No Professional Treatment.*"[77] Although some of the patent remedies were positively dangerous, the folk healers and sectarians may have done less harm than orthodox physicians. It may be significant that asylum physicians were more critical of the attempts of their regular colleagues to cure insanity than of those of the irregulars.[78]

Community therapy for insanity in nineteenth-century South Carolina was indeed various and conflicting. The victims of mental disorders might be subjected to a bewildering array of treatments—regular and irregular, medical and magical—or to no treatment at all. In any given case, therapeutic choices might be determined by a host of social, economic, cultural, geographical, racial, and medical circumstances and attitudes. Many people could influence the kinds of treatment ultimately adopted, including the patient and the patient's family, friends, and owner (in the case of slaves), regular and irregular healers, nurses, and local officials.

Yet there was a certain consistency and continuity within this apparent therapeutic chaos. Physicians, both regular and irregular, might differ widely about theories of insanity and the best means to combat it. But in practice, they often tended to use similar remedies and sought to achieve much the same goals. As in other diseases, they generally agreed that treatment should be directed toward regulating bodily secretions and restoring the body's natural internal balance. The means by which healers sought to accomplish these aims changed, slowly, during the nineteenth century, as healers gradually abandoned bleeding and drastic purging. Old therapies persisted in modified forms, partly because that is what patients and their families expected. The lay public, whether or not they were skeptical about the regulars, shared many of their assumptions about mental disease and its treatment. This is reflected in the writings and advertisements of the medical sects and the patent remedy sellers, who emphasized the ability of their treatments to regulate secretions and restore proper bodily functions. Ironically, the irregulars capitalized on both the public's skepticism toward and acceptance of regular medicine to secure a significant role in the treatment of insanity.

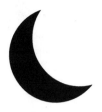

PART FOUR

The Postbellum Asylum

1861–1920

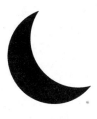

Ten

THE FEARFUL ORDEAL

THE ASYLUM DURING CIVIL WAR

AND RECONSTRUCTION

In 1877 Dr. Joshua Ensor summarized the experience of the South Carolina Lunatic Asylum during Reconstruction by claiming that "no other Asylum for the insane has ever passed through the fearful ordeal this one has during the past few years."[1] Ensor, who was then superintendent of the asylum, might have extended his remarks to include the years of war and chaos that preceded Reconstruction. The Civil War not only brought an end to the construction of the new asylum; the financial privations of the war and its aftermath brought about severe deterioration of the already inadequate existing plant. The Reconstruction government inherited an institution that was both decrepit and obsolescent by the standards of the time. The Republicans who ruled South Carolina during Reconstruction appointed an able superintendent in Ensor. But they were unable or unwilling to provide the resources necessary to overcome the years of neglect. The patients, particularly the black patients who first entered the asylum in significant numbers after 1865, suffered severely as a result of its financial problems during the years of war and Reconstruction. Hard pressed simply to keep the patients alive, the asylum's officers had little time to promote their recovery. The events of Reconstruction also politicized the care of the insane to a greater extent than ever before, as the asylum became the source of political patronage and political charges and countercharges.

Soon after the outbreak of the war, the always precarious financial situation of the asylum became desperate. As the regents had foreseen, the exigencies of war left the state with little revenue to devote to public charities. Even though the asylum was not dependent on state aid for ordinary operating expenses, the war created an emergency situation only the state government had the resources to deal with. The war, however, diverted much of the state's resources to military purposes and greatly weakened its overall economic position. By preventing the export of cotton and rice, the federal blockade deprived the state of hard currency and the imported manufactured goods it needed. Many of the state's citizens were caught between eroding incomes and rampant inflation.[2]

The asylum shared the misfortunes of the general populace. The officers had to pay increasingly high prices for food, medicine, clothing, and other essentials, while they found it increasingly difficult to collect payment for patients, never easy in the best of times. Those responsible for the paying patients often paid irregularly, if at all, and the number of pauper patients increased. The payments for pauper patients arrived more regularly, but the amounts paid for their care had always fallen below the actual cost of their care, and the gap widened considerably as the war caused prices to skyrocket. By the end of 1861 the asylum owed six thousand dollars and had no means of meeting its liabilities. The regents had already decided by then that the situation could only be solved by the end of hostilities: "We must share in the disturbed state of the country, and bowing to a destiny which we cannot resist, look forward with patience to a brighter and better future."[3]

Although they recognized the impossibility of removing a situation caused by events beyond their control, the asylum's officers tried to ameliorate it in several ways. One was to seek an increase in the rate paid for pauper patients, which had always been below the actual cost of their care.[4] In response to these appeals, and as the situation at the asylum worsened, the legislature raised the annual payment for paupers several times and made increasingly large appropriations for the asylum.[5] But inflation rendered such assistance inadequate before it was granted. Every year of the war the asylum ran out of funds several months before the legislature met to allocate appropriations. Each summer, the regents appealed to the governor for aid, but they were always rebuffed on the grounds that only the legislature had the power to grant the necessary relief. To meet these emergencies, the asylum's officers economized, borrowed, begged, and pledged their own resources and credit.[6] They sent out printed appeals soliciting contributions from the public, with some success. Parker discharged as many patients as he could, and the regents temporarily prohibited the admission of persons from other states. These measures helped reduce the patient census from 192 in November 1860 to 128 at the end of 1865.[7]

In spite of these efforts, the condition of the asylum deteriorated badly during the Civil War, especially during its later stages. The ordinary business of the asylum was complicated by the regents' inability to attend the regular monthly meetings.[8] Under these conditions, Parker had all he could do merely to keep the asylum operating. In July 1864, he confessed that the institution had retrogressed in every respect since the beginning of the war. The patients were constantly pleading for better diet and clothing, and the employees had become discontented and despondent. Dissatisfied with their board and unable to clothe themselves with their wages, several attendants had already left for more attractive jobs; the rest were only waiting an opportunity to do so. The superintendent could do little, for he had no money and only a day's supply of food. The regents met the immediate crisis by raising the attendants' wages and borrowing money, but conditions worsened in the following months. Mortality, which had averaged 8 percent of the patients under treatment in the decade 1853–62, increased to 13 percent between 1863 and 1865.[9]

Insult was added to injury. In 1862 the state established a nitre works close to the asylum, adding noxious odors to the trials of the patients and staff.[10] A greater indignity came in the waning months of war when the asylum served briefly as a prison for captured Union officers. Late in 1864, Confederate authorities brought more than one thousand of them to a site near Columbia. The location was soon found to be insecure and unhealthy, and more than three hundred escapes prompted vociferous complaints from the local citizenry. In response to these problems, Confederate military authorities decided to move the prisoners to a site fourteen miles north of Columbia. As an interim measure, the commissary general of the Confederate Prisons, General Winder, requested temporary use of the wing of the new asylum to house the prisoners until the new prison camp could be readied. The regents initially protested that they lacked legal authority to put the asylum to any other use than that for which it was established. But they agreed to allow the prisoners the use of several acres and some outbuildings.

The Union prisoners arrived at the asylum in mid-December 1864 and remained for about two months. Some were able to take refuge in existing buildings; the rest had to build their own quarters with wood and materials furnished by their Confederate captors. One of the POWs left the following description of the camp: "The yard in which we were confined contained about five acres, and was surrounded on three sides by a brick

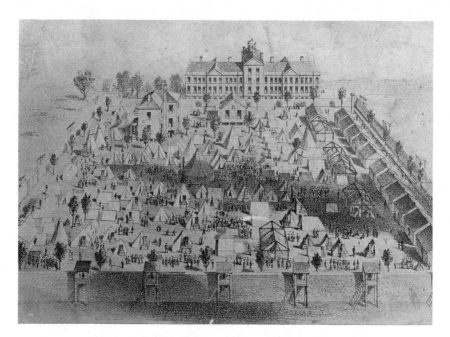

Asylum camp for captured Union officers, 1864–65.
(From A. O. Abbott, Prison Life in the South, 1864–1865, *1865;*
courtesy South Caroliniana Library, University of South Carolina)

wall ten feet in height, while on the fourth was a board fence, the same height. [This fence separated the prisoners from the old asylum, which was] pretty well populated, judging from the numerous doleful sounds emanating thence."[11] In mid-February 1865, the Confederate authorities removed most of the prisoners from the asylum grounds and sent them by rail to Charlotte. The hasty evacuation was prompted by the approach of General Sherman's Union army, which arrived in Columbia on February 17. The asylum's brief career as a POW camp does not seem to have greatly worsened its already straitened condition, although Parker complained that the Confederate guards had destroyed fences and consumed large amounts of wood without paying for it.[12]

The asylum's service to the Confederacy was not yet over. No sooner had the federal prisoners left than citizens of Columbia began to pour into the institution seeking refuge from the advancing enemy. The asylum was an obvious choice, because its main building was fireproof and its large yard was surrounded by a ten-foot brick wall. Moreover, its hospital status and the nature of its clientele encouraged citizens to believe that it would be spared from enemy attacks. The day before the Union army entered Columbia, Mary Leverette decided to send several members of her family to the asylum, "which we were fully sure would be respected." Parker took them in and even buried some of the family's silver.[13] Some citizens had long anticipated going to the asylum in the event of a Union attack on the capital. Several weeks before Sherman arrived, Mary Chesnut recorded in her diary that Frances Parker Waties, the superintendent's daughter, had decided to go there when the Yankees arrived: "Mrs. Waties . . . was calm and serene. She would take refuge in the insane asylum of which her father is the head. She knew no Yankees would venture there—and it was bomb-proof." Chesnut, less calm and serene, recalled that "Mr. [James Louis] Petigru said all South Carolina was an insane asylum. That will not save us now from fire and sword."[14]

Certainly, bedlam was about to descend on the state capital. On the night after Sherman's army occupied Columbia, much of the town was destroyed by fire.[15] The conflagration and the fear of drunken, looting Federal soldiers turned the trickle of refugees going to the asylum into a flood. One woman, Mrs. Campbell Bryce, decided to go there only after she discovered her house was on fire: "Someone rushed in and told us the roof of the house was on fire. We ran out. . . . [I]t was bitter cold, the streets filled with blue coats wild with delight at their success. I suddenly thought of the lunatic asylum, and suggested that as a shelter, saying, 'Surely they will not burn up the poor crazy people.'"[16] She proved correct. Except for a few threats of violence from drunken soldiers, Sherman's soldiers left the asylum alone. The end of the fire brought a further influx of refugees, as people who had lost their houses arrived at the institution in search of food and shelter. One woman reported that she and her family "wandered up to the Lunatic Asylum" at dawn, where they were given breakfast and housed for several days.[17]

In all, several hundred Columbians took refuge in the asylum. Many of them had escaped from their houses with nothing more than they could carry. Some were already refugees from the countryside who had fled the approaching army and lost most of their possessions. The scene at the asylum was one which Mrs. Bryce declared she would never forget: "The whole front of the enclosure was covered with people, their little effects tied up in sheets, and some few had boxes and small trunks." Another witness commented that the grounds of the institution "were covered with one moving, miserable mass of beings" whose dishevelled and haggard appearance made them difficult to distinguish from the regular residents: "Sometimes the permanent inmates of the asylum would elude their attendants and mingle with the new-comers, who in their hasty toilets made the night before, would present such grotesque figures as to look much more in need of the surveillance of the keepers than those for whom they were engaged."[18] Parker, already overwhelmed with the job of caring for the asylum's patients, welcomed the refugees and did what he could to provide food and shelter. His actions at this time of crisis won him the gratitude of many of the town's citizens. All of those who left accounts of the event commented on the kindness and attention of the superintendent and his family. Among those who came to the asylum to help at this time was Parker's former colleague, Dr. Trezevant.[19]

The asylum survived Sherman, but its condition worsened further in the following months. The strain of feeding the refugees, some of whom remained for weeks, reduced the already meager supplies of the institution. Moreover, the arrival of the Union army disrupted trade and rendered Confederate currency virtually worthless. At the beginning of April 1865, Parker told the regents that he had no more than three weeks supplies left and was pessimistic about his ability to continue to secure adequate provisions. For a time he managed to purchase enough food by buying at the City Depot and by sending agents into the countryside to buy direct from farmers. But these sources were now failing. Many people were refusing to take Confederate money, and it was seldom possible to secure wagons to transport food from the few country farms willing to sell or barter their produce. The regents appealed to Governor Magrath for aid without success, and by the beginning of May the asylum's provisions were exhausted. A few days later Parker informed the regents that he could no longer get supplies by any means and the patients faced starvation. He appealed to the regents to supply him with the only resource he believed could secure the necessary provisions: federal currency.

By the summer of 1865 Parker procured some federal money with which to purchase supplies, but the situation remained desperate for months. In July, the *Columbia Daily Phoenix* reported that the patients were without meat and were in grave danger of starvation and called upon the citizens to give or lend aid to the asylum. Among those who responded was Mrs. Campbell Bryce, grateful for the aid she had received on the night Columbia burned. By the end of 1865, these efforts had managed to exorcise the specter of starvation, but further shocks lay ahead.[20]

The end of the Civil War did not immediately bring about any major changes in the organization or staff of the asylum. Here, as elsewhere in the state and in much of the South, former Confederates continued to hold authority.[21] Parker and the regents remained in their positions. But they had to adjust to new realities. The outcome of the Civil War revolutionized the situation of the black insane, at least in theory. With emancipation, responsibility for the majority of insane blacks devolved from their masters to the state. The Union government of occupation insisted that insane freedmen be admitted to the state asylum on the same terms as whites. As soon as the war ended, the federal military authorities, the Freedmen's Bureau, and former slave owners began to send blacks to the asylum.[22]

Initially, some whites resisted this development. The Freedmen's Bureau censured the mayor of Columbia, Thomas Stark, in 1867 for refusing to sign orders for the admission of blacks into the asylum. Stark replied tartly that if the federal government wanted to treat the freedmen as its "Pet Lambs," it should pay for their care and not lay the burden on the white people of the state. The federal authorities forced Stark and those who agreed with him to give way, and blacks began to enter the asylum according to the same laws as whites. From only five in 1865, the number of black patients grew to seventy-five in 1871.[23]

The postwar asylum was not prepared to cope with an influx of patients, black or white. Physically, the institution had deteriorated considerably during the 1860s, and there was little prospect of immediate improvement. South Carolina had suffered staggering economic losses as a result of the war. Many of her citizens were impoverished by the accumulation of debt, loss of property, slaves, and the breakdown of traditional patterns of trade and agriculture.[24]

The economic crisis placed severe strain on the financial condition of the asylum. The number of paying patients, whose higher fees had previously subsidized the care of pauper patients, dropped from 88 in 1860 to 52 by 1868. At the same time the pauper patients (whose fees were paid— when they were paid—by the counties) increased from 106 to 152.[25] Many families who had previously paid for their relatives' care either removed them or transferred them to the pauper list. In either case the asylum lost revenues, and the situation was worsened by its inability to collect payment for many of the paying and pauper patients who remained. Unable to obtain sufficient revenues from either the patients' families or the counties, the asylum's officers turned to the state for help.[26]

But the postwar state government was unable or unwilling to solve the asylum's financial problems. The legislature began making annual grants for maintenance during the war and continued to make them afterward, but the amounts were insufficient to keep the institution out of debt. The officers kept the asylum running only by putting off badly needed repairs and improvements and by withholding employees' salaries. By the late 1860s it had deteriorated to the point where various observers declared its condition a scandal to the state.[27]

By then, South Carolina had embarked on the experiment of Radical Reconstruction. Protected by federal troops, Republicans took control of the state government with the support of the newly enfranchised black majority and a minority of whites. The state's traditional leaders watched in outraged disbelief as its constitution was rewritten and its government taken over by the Radical Republicans and their black allies. The asylum was soon affected by this revolution. Indeed, the Republican government's management of the institution became a prime target of their enemies, the Conservatives (Democrats).

The new state constitution of 1868 brought the asylum into the political maelstrom by giving the governor the power to appoint the superintendent and all "other necessary officers and employees," including the regents.[28] Previously, the regents had essentially controlled all appointments, including filling vacancies in their own ranks. Before the first Reconstruction governor, Robert K. Scott, was even inaugurated, members of his party were pressuring him to replace the asylum's officers with Republicans. Racial concerns played a central role in the conflict. One of the charges the Radicals brought against the existing officers was that they refused to provide black patients with the same facilities as whites. Scott initially resisted efforts to remove the asylum's officers, but at the end of 1869 he bowed to legislative pressure and replaced the existing regents with Republicans. Six of the new board were black and three white.[29] For several months more, Scott continued to oppose the removal of Parker, who had the support of both the old elite and the most influential asylum reformer of the day, Dorothea Dix. Dr. Clement A. Walker, superintendent of the Boston Lunatic Hospital, inspected the asylum in November 1868 and praised Parker's management. In the end, however, the demands of party proved more powerful, and during the summer of 1870 Scott agreed to remove Parker.[30]

The changes at the asylum enraged and alarmed many white South Carolinians. When the new regents were appointed, the *Columbia Daily Phoenix* accused the legislature of sacrificing the insane to the political spoils system and putting their care into the hands of "colored men, and others equally unfitted for their parts."[31] At bottom, the Conservatives' objections to the new regime were based on racial as much as on medical concerns. Many whites feared that the new board, with its black majority, would use its power to mix the races and put the white patients under the control and care of blacks. These apprehensions seemed realized when the new regents appointed blacks to the positions of assistant physician and steward.[32]

The ouster of Parker aroused similar concerns. Conservatives were convinced that the position of superintendent would inevitably be filled by a Republican party hack who would turn the asylum into another means of humiliating the white race and securing its subordination to Negro rule.[33] As early as March 1868, one of Parker's supporters wrote that the superintendent's removal was to be anticipated at some time, "but then with a Government and Legislature of South Carolina's we would have had the assurance that his place would have been filled by one who at least was a Gentleman, a qualification which I am loath . . . to grant to any Radical." From a government dominated by "Baboons and Pickpockets," it was not to be expected that anyone but a coarse, ignorant rascal would be appointed.[34]

The history of the South Carolina Lunatic Asylum during Reconstruction is significant, because Conservative politicians exploited events there as part of their attempt to discredit the Republican government. Historians eventually accepted the Conservatives' condemnations and wove them into what became the traditional historical view of Reconstruction in South Carolina: it was a dismal failure, an unrelieved morass of incompetence and corruption.[35] Historians who accepted this thesis often cited the asylum as a prime example of the effects of Radical misrule. The traditional view was well summed up by one of the biographers of Dorothea Dix: "[South Carolina] was under the control of a legislature packed almost solid with brutal plantation negroes. The influential leaders who swayed them were largely 'carpet bag' politicians from the North. . . . What would be the inevitable policy of such a legislature and such leaders toward a State Insane Asylum can readily be conceived. It would be to put in some ignorant, thievish black as steward, [and] some greedy, half educated white doctor as superintendent."[36]

Undoubtedly, the asylum suffered from corruption and maladministration during Reconstruction. Conditions were often desperate during these years, and some of those appointed to administer the asylum's affairs may well have been incompetent or corrupt. Yet the view presented by traditional historians is both exaggerated and misleading. For one thing, the asylum's problems during Reconstruction were partly the result of the ravages of the Civil War and the economically depressed state of South Carolina in the postwar years. Moreover, conditions at the asylum did not improve much after Reconstruction; in many respects, things got worse. Finally, the man the Republicans chose to run the asylum, Joshua Ensor, was acknowledged even by the Conservatives as honest and competent.

Ensor, who replaced superintendent Parker in 1870, was a Republican active in party affairs. But he was by no means a party hack. Born in Maryland in 1834, Ensor had received his medical training at the university of that state. During the war he had compiled a good record as a surgeon in the Union army. Although he does not seem to have had experience in the care of the insane prior to his South Carolina appointment, Ensor had been in charge of military hospitals. His selection as superintendent seems to have been a compromise between Scott and legislators who favored another candidate. Ensor quickly proved himself a man of ability, integrity and courage.[37]

Ensor frequently criticized the government that appointed him. At times, his strictures on the government's treatment of the insane were so harsh as to lend credence to the traditional interpretation of Reconstruction. Yet he remained a Republican even as he struggled against extremely adverse conditions to provide decent care for his patients. Looked at from the perspective of his record as superintendent, Reconstruction appears in a more positive light than in traditionalist accounts. His career could be seen as a confirmation of the claims of revisionist historians that Reconstruction, despite some moral lapses, produced both positive achievements and able leaders.[38] In a fundamental sense, however, the legacy of Reconstruction at the asylum was ambiguous. The Republican government deserves credit for appointing someone like Ensor as superintendent and keeping him there in spite of his attacks on its policies and personnel. Yet the government was also responsible for many of the problems he had to confront.

When Ensor assumed his duties at the asylum, he was appalled by its condition. The buildings were badly overcrowded and lacked essential facilities for the insane. The original building, erected in the 1820s, he declared "a shame upon the humanity of the age." Its rooms were "mere cells or chinks in the walls, dark and illy ventilated," and those on the ground floor were "so damp and unhealthy that it would be the grossest inhumanity to require the patients to occupy them." The only means of heating the old building was with fireplaces, which was inconvenient, dangerous, and expensive. The sanitary and bathing facilities were totally inadequate, there was no adequate means of classifying patients, no library, clinical ward, amusement hall, or chapel. Some of these facilities had existed at one time but had been abandoned or turned to some other purpose, such as accommodating the increasing numbers of patients. The patient population, which had dropped to 128 during the war, expanded to 245 by 1870. Despite Ensor's strenuous efforts to limit the numbers of patients, by 1877 there were more than three hundred. In addition to these problems and debt totaling twenty thousand dollars, the asylum buildings were badly in need of repair and new furniture was needed.[39]

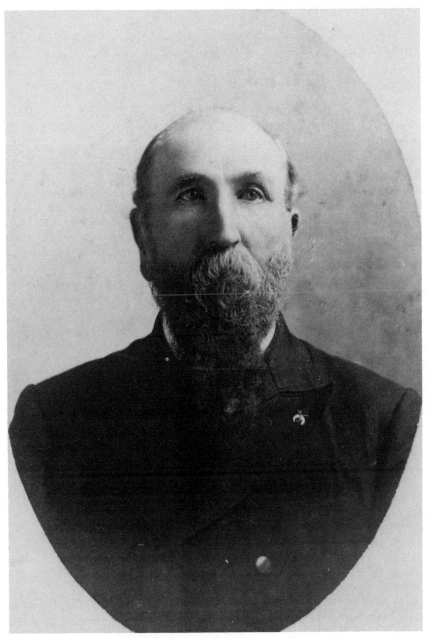

Joshua F. Ensor.
(Courtesy South Caroliniana Library, University of South Carolina)

Ensor did not blame his predecessor at the asylum for the conditions he encountered. Given the privations of the war and its aftermath, he conceded, Parker and the other officers had done as well as they could. The true source of the asylum's problems, Ensor argued, had been the general unenlightened conservatism of South Carolina's antebellum leaders.[40] The solution lay in the new Republican regime. It had introduced a new "spirit of enterprise" that would soon turn the institution into an "ornament" to South Carolina.[41]

If Ensor believed his own rhetoric, he was quickly disappointed. The Republican government, although willing to spend money on a variety of dubious projects and financial schemes, was less willing or able to provide adequate support for the asylum. During his tenure the institution was almost always critically short of funds. Sometimes this was because of an inadequate appropriation by the legislature, but more often it was because the appropriation was never fully allocated or was allocated months after it was due. As a result, Ensor found himself forced to support the asylum on credit received from merchants and banks, and at times had to pledge his own salary and personal credit as collateral.

At the session of 1870, the legislature failed to provide the support Ensor considered necessary to solve the asylum's financial problems. After it ended, Ensor informed Governor Scott that the condition of the institution was critical and appealed for emergency aid. Because of the officers' inability to collect the arrears of the counties for pauper patients, the asylum's debts had continued to mount. Loans from local merchants had allowed the asylum to continue operation, but its credit with these men had reached its limits. Many of the employees had not been paid for more than a year and some for as much as two years. Apologizing to Scott for his gloomy message, Ensor nevertheless vowed to conduct the asylum "upon principles of a broad and liberal humanity."[42]

Scott did not extend the aid Ensor requested, and during 1871 the financial position of the asylum worsened. At the 1870 session the legislature, at Ensor's request, had passed an act to transfer responsibility for pauper patients from the counties to the state. But this act initially did little to help the asylum. The general assembly appropriated half the sum Ensor considered adequate for the patients' support. The asylum's indebtedness increased. The situation was exacerbated by the failure of the state treasurer, Niles G. Parker, to pay the institution's appropriations on time. Once again the asylum had to rely on "the charitable indulgence" of Columbia's merchants and "the personal credit of the superintendent." If proper provision were not soon made for the maintenance of the institution, Ensor warned, it would have to close its doors and send the patients home.[43]

By the end of 1871 Ensor was becoming disillusioned with the government from which he had held such high expectations. The financial embarrassment of the asylum coincided with a generous use of public funds for less worthy objects, and the superintendent was not reticent in noting the connection.[44] Ensor's remarks about the state's legislators, which he sometimes recorded in the press, became increasingly bitter and sarcastic. In a letter to the *Columbia Daily Union*, he accused those opposed to a higher appropriation for the asylum of barbarism and inhumanity.[45]

The ostensible reason for the legislators' opposition to higher appropriations for the asylum by 1871 was the need for retrenchment. The government's extravagance over the previous several years had outraged many citizens and led to the organization of the Taxpayer's Convention in May 1871. Governor Scott, although conceding the needs of the asylum in his annual message at the end of 1871, cautioned the general assembly "against making more liberal appropriations than the income of the State at present justifies."[46] Ensor showed no patience with this argument. South Carolina's insane, he claimed, were already supported more cheaply than those of other states and would continue to be even if the legislature granted all that he had requested. Retrenchment was overdue, but to accomplish it by neglecting the needs of the insane showed "littleness of soul" on the part of legislators who had been "wonderfully lavish with the public money for other less worthy purposes."[47]

The conditions that sparked these harsh words remained much the same throughout Ensor's tenure at the asylum. The asylum's financial problems after 1871, however, were caused less by low appropriations than by the state treasurer's failure to disburse the money on schedule. Between 1870 and 1875 disbursements were often nearly a year behind schedule. During that time the asylum had to survive most of each year on credit, which greatly increased its costs and aggravated its already dire financial condition.[48] Credit was expensive and difficult to procure in the depressed economy of postwar South Carolina. At times Ensor was reduced to virtual begging on the streets of Columbia and Charleston in attempts to secure credit or loans. Often he had to offer his own salary as collateral.[49] On at least two occasions he traveled to Philadelphia to seek assistance because state merchants were unable to extend further credit. At one point he had spent seven thousand dollars of his own money to feed the patients.[50]

Keeping the asylum operating under these conditions often required extreme measures of retrenchment. In addition to holding back employees' pay, the staff was cut back to the point where at times there were no subordinate officers between the superintendent and the attendants. For months or years Ensor performed the duties of the secretary-treasurer, steward, and assistant physician in addition to his own. In order to relieve overcrowding and cut down on the number of patients he had to feed and clothe, Ensor returned many chronic pauper patients to their counties and discouraged probate judges from sending new patients unless they were acute and dangerous.[51]

Despite the asylum's financial difficulties, Ensor insisted on implementing numerous improvements he considered essential to bring it up to the standards of similar institutions elsewhere.[52] According to his own figures, the asylum spent about twenty-five thousand dollars between 1870 and 1874 on central heating, indoor plumbing, underground sewers, furniture, carpeting, and new dining and bathing facilities. Pianos for the parlors and games and books for the patients' amusement were purchased.[53]

The asylum's problems ultimately had important political repercussions. That Ensor aired his grievances in the press as well as in his annual reports was a decided embarrassment to the Republican regime. Ultimately, it aided the conservatives in their bid to overthrow the Reconstruction government.[54] Conservative papers gave much publicity to the asylum's plight, for it seemed to provide manifest evidence of the government's ineptitude and corruption. The *Charleston Daily News*, for example, subtitled one article on the asylum "A Sad and Shameful Picture of the Results of Extravagance and Maladministration."[55] The *Columbia Daily Phoenix* declared that the previous government had handed the asylum to the Radicals "intact" (conveniently forgetting its accumulated debts and run-down condition at the end of the war). Yet the Republican government had allowed the institution to descend to a level where its superintendent had to take to the "streets in the quest for food." The government, the paper claimed, could not adequately support the asylum because it had squandered the state's revenues to pay largely fraudulent legislative expenses. The *Phoenix* expressed incredulity that men who had "so grossly and criminally defrauded" a charitable institution could consider themselves entitled to reelection.[56]

Given Ensor's sharp and public criticism of the Republican government's policies toward the asylum, it may seem surprising that he was not removed. There was, indeed, at least one attempt to discredit him and force his resignation. In the spring of 1873, rumors circulated that the cause of the asylum's financial problems was the officers' extravagant and illegal use of state appropriations. At one point the board of regents asked Governor Franklin Moses to appoint a committee to examine the asylum's accounts.[57] Ensor defended himself vigorously in the press and in his reports. He conceded that the expenses of the asylum had been higher than normal. But this, he claimed, was the inevitable result of two unusual circumstances. The first was that he had inherited an institution that had deteriorated so badly that extensive repairs and improvements could no longer be postponed. The second arose from long delays in securing appropriations, which had forced the asylum to borrow at high rates of interest. The payment of these loans consumed a substantial part of the asylum's annual income.[58] Ensor also charged that the attack on his management of the asylum was simply an attempt by corrupt politicians to deflect attention from their own malfeasance: "It has been insinuated if not openly charged, that the expenses of this institution are unnecessarily large, and even fraud and peculation have been hinted at by some whose own craven natures are so corrupt that they can't see anything but dishonesty in others, and they are always nosing around with an eye of suspicion to see if other people are not stealing as well as they."[59]

The attempt to discredit Ensor failed completely. Individuals and newspapers of both parties leaped to the superintendent's defense. The Democratic *Charleston News and Courier* denounced what it claimed was a "treacherous and secret effort to injure [Ensor's] fair fame."[60] The *Aiken Tribune*, a Republican paper, attributed the attack on Ensor to "a spirit of retaliation created by [his] refusal to lend himself and his influence to the successful perpetration of schemes led by a set of heartless plunderers, intent upon robbing the grand and noble charity, in common with other institutions of the state."[61] One of Ensor's strongest defenders was Dr. Maximilian Laborde, a professor at South Carolina College who had served on the board of regents of the asylum for almost thirty years before the Radicals removed him in 1870. In a letter to the press, Laborde noted that he continued to visit the asylum occasionally and found it to be well managed. Dr. Ensor, Laborde concluded, deserved the trust of the state's citizens. He was not only a worthy successor to superintendent Parker but also in every respect "the right man in the right place."[62]

Ensor's disgust with the corruptionists led him to join a Republican reform movement that was emerging by 1872. He supported the election of the reformer F. L. Cardozo as state treasurer in 1872.[63] Later, in 1874, he served as campaign manager for the successful reform candidate for governor, Daniel H. Chamberlain, who had previously served for a time as one of the asylum's regents. Together, Cardozo and Chamberlain managed to eliminate much of the corruption in the Reconstruction regime.[64]

Ensor expected that the asylum would benefit from the advent of more honest and less wasteful leadership, and to some extent he was correct. In April 1875 he informed the regents that the asylum's financial condition was the best it had been for many years. For the first time in a decade, the asylum was able to begin a new year without owing back salaries and wages to the employees.[65] Yet he had to endure many of the same financial woes under the reformers as he had under the corruptionists. He continued to have difficulty in getting state appropriations paid on time. The source of the problem was no longer government extravagance but economic depression. As a result of the Panic of 1873, state revenues declined in the last years of the Republican regime. At the same time, reformers such as Cardozo and Chamberlain remained determined to bring government spending into line with revenues and expected all state institutions to share in the burden of retrenchment. This goal brought them into conflict with Ensor, whose first concern was the condition of his institution. Soon after Cardozo became treasurer at the end of 1872 he issued sixty thousand dollars in appropriations for the asylum. But before long the treasury was empty, and he refused to issue more funds. By May 1873, Ensor and Cardozo were openly clashing over the issuance of appropriations, with the treasurer claiming that the asylum had been overpaid and Ensor vehemently denying it.[66]

Ensor came into conflict with Chamberlain soon after the governor was elected. The new governor was determined to reduce government expenditures not only as a measure of reform but also as a means of attracting Democratic support for the Republican reformers.[67] In his message to the legislature in January 1875 Chamberlain praised the condition of the asylum and conceded that it deserved liberal support. But he refused to recommend the appropriation Ensor and the regents had requested because it would require him to break a recent law that made it a felony for any public official to spend in excess of revenues. This was sufficiently bad news for Ensor, but he was infuriated by another part of the governor's speech. In referring to the accumulated debt of the asylum, Chamberlain implied that the superintendent himself was partly to blame for the situation.[68]

Ensor was disappointed and stung by Chamberlain's speech. He complained bitterly to the regents that on the amount of money the governor was willing to give the asylum it could only be kept open by running it like a county poorhouse. As far as the debt was concerned, the governor's accusation was hypocritical. Chamberlain, Ensor charged, was well aware of "the compulsory nature" of the asylum's indebtedness, for he had approved much of it himself while a member of the asylum's board of regents. Ensor believed that Chamberlain was making him a scapegoat for the past excesses of the Republican regime.[69]

Chamberlain subsequently tried to placate Ensor. In his annual message to the legislature in 1875 the governor admitted that the asylum's debts were the result of inadequate and irregularly paid appropriations. He made a strong appeal to the legislature to provide greater support for the asylum. The legislature responded with an appropriation of sixty-five thousand dollars. But a few weeks later Chamberlain announced that state spending would have to be slashed in order to balance the budget and recommended a series of drastic cuts in the funding of public institutions, including the asylum.[70]

In spite of his conflicts with Chamberlain and the asylum's continuing financial difficulties, Ensor supported the governor's reelection in 1876. In October, Ensor attended the annual convention of the asylum superintendents and told them that the situation of the insane in South Carolina was improving under the Chamberlain regime: "We have at last gotten an honest and able Governor who takes an earnest interest in all that concerns the welfare of our State, and as we are almost certain to reelect him for another term, I begin to feel hopeful." [71]

The outcome of the 1876 governor's race was much different from what Ensor had predicted. After a violent and disputed election, Chamberlain and the Democratic candidate, Wade Hampton, each formed rival governments. Chamberlain was forced from office in April 1877 when President Hayes ordered the removal of federal troops from South Carolina, assuring the victory of the Democrats. Hampton had by this time virtually seized control of the state anyway, for he had been able to prevent the Chamberlain government from collecting enough revenue to sustain the operation of its institutions.[72]

By January 1877 the financial situation of the asylum had become critical. Ensor told the regents on January 4 that he had no money or food and that the merchants who had been supplying credit were threatening to shut it off. For a week the patients had been on half rations, and for two weeks no laundry had been done, because he had been forced to release many of the employees, including the washerwomen. A few days later Ensor appealed to Hampton for emergency aid and received it. As he later explained, it was the only rational thing to do: "To have relied upon the Chamberlain government under the circumstances that then surrounded us would have been ample evidence of our own insanity." [73] By his act, however, the superintendent had given the Democratic government its first recognition of legitimacy by a state official. The fact contained an irony one of Hampton's supporters could not overlook: "It was one of the many absurd pranks of fate in the 1876 revolution that Hampton's first and strongest claims on the governorship went to him through the lunatic asylum and the penitentiary—and he backed by the best and clearest brains and highest character of the country."[74]

Although he remained a Republican, Ensor seemed willing to continue in office under the Democrats (or Redeemers, as they were calling themselves at the time). Given his experiences under the Reconstruction government, he may have believed that the Democrats could not do much worse. Moreover, he had won the respect if not the friendship of some Democrats. He welcomed the new government in terms reminiscent of his first favorable comments on the Republican regime. A "new era" had "dawned upon the fortunes of the State," he proclaimed in his annual report, and a "higher plane of politics has been inaugurated." He praised the Democrats for having saved the asylum's patients from starvation and from "a reign of profligacy and corruption unparalleled in the experience of man."[75] Such language seems like a fawning attempt to curry favor with the Redeemers, but Ensor was not the fawning type. He may have been simply expressing the disillusionment with Reconstruction that many Republicans felt by the time it came to its inglorious end.[76]

There was, in any event, little chance that the Democrats would retain Ensor as superintendent. Having finally seized power from the hated Reconstruction regime, they were determined to remove its appointees from positions of power and replace them with loyal Democrats and former Confederates. In June 1877 Hampton replaced the Republican regents with men of his own party. In November the new board requested the governor to remove Ensor in favor of a Redeemer, Dr. Peter Griffin. Ensor submitted his resignation a few weeks later.[77]

The decision to remove Ensor seems to have been purely political. No one brought any charges against him. A legislative commission appointed by the Hampton regime in 1877 to investigate the state's charitable and penal institutions not only absolved Ensor of any wrongdoing but also commended his faithful and efficient administration of the asylum.[78] That several conservative historians of Reconstruction later praised Ensor indicates that he had won the respect of some of the Redeemer leaders.[79] Democratic admiration for Ensor, however, was not due simply to his honest and capable administration of the asylum. Some Democrats viewed him as the man who prevented the Radicals from carrying out a "nefarious" plan to institute racial equality and race mixing at the asylum. Conservatives credited Ensor for having forced the removal in 1871 of Dr. Harris, the black assistant physician, because he was obnoxious to the white patients.[80]

Ensor did request Harris's removal, although on what grounds is not clear. In any case, the regents, a majority of whom were black, granted the request. Ensor undoubtedly shared, or came to share, the antipathy of most contemporary whites to integration, although he did not make any public statement on the subject until near the end of his tenure. In his last annual report (1877), he noted that experience had convinced him that black and white patients ought not to be mixed together because of the "mutual antagonism of the races." On the other hand, he complained bitterly on numerous occasions about the inadequate facilities the asylum provided for the black patients. After the Civil War, the legislature had authorized the construction of two wooden pavilions for black patients. More wooden buildings were added as black admissions increased. Ensor referred to these structures as "miserable cattle stalls" unfit for the treatment of the insane and claimed that their substandard condition was responsible for the deaths of numerous black patients. "Is it any wonder," he wrote, "that nearly every one of them that sickens dies?" The asylum's facilities for black patients, he charged, were "a cruel imposition upon humanity, a reproach to the Republican party, and a disgrace to the state."[81]

Whatever his racial attitudes, the Redeemers had little incentive to keep Ensor at the asylum. To do so would not only have been an affront to Democratic stalwarts but would have conspicuously contradicted the Redeemers' claim to have saved South Carolina from a thoroughly corrupt and incompetent regime. Ensor may have been an asset to the Democrats during Reconstruction, because he had repeatedly exposed the problems of the asylum in the public prints, but he was now a liability and had to be sacrificed to the Redeemer campaign to condemn Reconstruction in toto.[82] Ensor was acutely aware of this, and expressed a fear that his resignation would be interpreted as a confession of guilt. He was particularly concerned about his reputation, he claimed, because he had no intention of leaving the state: "I have earned a reputation here for honesty under the most adverse circumstances that almost ever encompassed a Public Officer . . . and I do not propose now, at this critical moment, to fritter that boon away, among the people with whom I expect to live and die, sharing their fortunes and misfortunes, to gratify the caprice of anybody."[83]

To the Democrats, Ensor's removal was politically necessary for another reason. The Redeemers' program, like that of Governor Chamberlain before them, included a pledge of retrenchment in state spending. The asylum, as one of the most expensive of state institutions, was going to have to bear some of the pains of fiscal conservatism. Indeed, during the following decades per capita expenditure on South Carolina's insane was to be driven ever lower. Ensor had shown himself adept at economizing when he had no choice, but he had never accepted financial limits graciously. His reports were peppered with references to the "niggardly" and "illiberal" provision the Reconstruction government had made for the insane.[84]

Despite his welcome to the new regime, Ensor quickly made it clear that he was unwilling to acquiesce in a program of retrenchment. His first monthly report to the new Democratic regents consisted largely of a list of needed improvements and complaints about the "scanty appropriation" the Democratic legislature had given the asylum, along with statistics showing the superior facilities and more generous support North Carolina and Georgia provided their insane. In his annual report a few months later, he set forth a plan for the improvement of the asylum, which he admitted would require large annual appropriations. But, he added, "if the State of South Carolina intends to make the provisions for the care and treatment of the insane that are being made in every other part of the world, and which an enlightened humanity demands, we may as well make up our minds at once that we will be obliged to spend annually a considerable sum of money for this noble charity."[85] This was not what the new rulers of South Carolina wanted to hear.

After leaving the asylum, Ensor remained in South Carolina until his death in 1907. He continued to be a member of the Republican Party and held several federal jobs, including postmaster of Columbia and chief raiding deputy for the Bureau of Internal Revenue. In this latter post he even won the admiration of the men he was employed to prosecute. According to A. B. Williams, Ensor was the "idol of the moonshiners because he never was afraid of them and never broke his word or was harsh or unfair. He could go into the most dangerous places, arrest the most dangerous men, alone and without show of weapons and never was even fired at."[86]

Ensor's career at the South Carolina asylum should caution us against any simplistic interpretation of the effects of Reconstruction on southern institutions. That the Reconstruction government often treated the asylum shabbily is undeniable. Yet it was the Reconstruction government that placed Ensor in the post of superintendent and kept him there despite his public and often acerbic criticism of Republican officials. That Ensor was an honest and able administrator, and that he fought valiantly against extremely difficult conditions, seems undeniable. It is more difficult to judge his ability as a physician. Recovery rates during his tenure averaged 31 percent upon admissions, a somewhat lower proportion than his predecessors claimed. The decline may have been due as much to more rigorous conceptions of what constituted a recovery as to any failing of Ensor. In any case, recovery rates continued to fall under his immediate successors, Peter Griffin and James W. Babcock.[87]

Ensor's reports show that he was conversant with contemporary ideas about the kind of facilities needed for the care of the insane. But neither the reports nor the asylum's case records tell us much about his efforts to treat patients. What evidence there is indicates that Ensor's views of insanity and its treatment were similar to those of most American alienists of his time. He considered insanity to be a physical disease that required the care of a physician. But that did not make him an advocate of vigorous medical therapy. Medicine, he declared firmly, had "a very narrow sphere in the treatment of insanity." Like most contemporary alienists, he condemned the copious bloodletting and drastic purging that had been common in the early nineteenth century. The decline of such depletive measures left little in the medical armory besides tonics designed to build up patients' strength and sedatives to calm their excitement or anxieties. Thus, it is not surprising that the few references to medical treatment in Ensor's case reports are to the use of tonics and sedatives such as potassium bromide.[88]

Medical treatment, however, was only one part of the nineteenth-century asylum's therapeutic armory. Moral treatment comprised the other part, and it was to this, Ensor declared, that he looked "for the largest measure of success." In common with other asylum superintendents, he promoted moral treatment through the provision of such things as concerts, lectures, dances, games, musical instruments, reading matter, and agricultural and other employment. Providing proper facilities for moral treatment was expensive, however, and it was Ensor's insistence on doing so that led to many of his conflicts with the state government. The lack of such facilities, he charged, contributed to low recovery and high mortality rates. As he wrote of the black patients in 1872, "These people are placed in the asylum to be cured of insanity, and with proper facilities for their treatment, fifty per cent of them may be cured. But with the present imperfect accommodations, we cannot hope to cure any of them."[89]

Despite his advocacy of moral treatment, Ensor apparently came to share the growing pessimism of superintendents about the prognosis of insanity. By the 1870s asylum physicians were turning away from the therapeutic optimism of the antebellum period. They were coming to believe that a large proportion of the insane suffered from organic and hereditary disorders that would not yield readily to any known therapeutic measures.

Many superintendents had already concluded that the asylum's main function was to provide humane custodial care rather than to cure large numbers of patients.[90] That Ensor may have accepted this outlook is indicated by the relative absence of discussion in his reports about therapeutics and the large number of patients he diagnosed as incurable.[91] On the other hand, Ensor showed repeatedly that he was determined to provide high quality care for his patients and not let the asylum deteriorate to "the level of a county poor house."[92] In this respect if no other, he was indeed the right man in the right place.

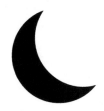

Eleven

I AM NOT AN OFFICE SEEKER

THE POLITICS OF INSANITY

By the end of Reconstruction, the question of who held the post of superintendent of the state asylum in South Carolina had become a matter of considerable political importance. The number of patients in the South Carolina Lunatic Asylum increased rapidly during the last part of the nineteenth century, from about three hundred in 1877 to almost eleven hundred by 1901. This growth created internal problems that are the subject of the following chapters. But it also contributed to the growing politicization of the asylum. In the late nineteenth century, appropriations for the asylum became one of the largest items in the state budget and thus a major concern of taxpayers and politicians.[1]

The burden of caring for a rapidly increasing number of mental patients was borne by an economy severely weakened by the effects of war and agricultural depression. South Carolina began to industrialize between 1880 and World War I, and the Piedmont became dotted with textile mills. But well into the twentieth century, the state remained overwhelmingly agricultural and more dependent than ever on the cultivation of cotton. During the postbellum decades, many of the state's farming families suffered severe distress from falling cotton prices and the peonage of the sharecropping and crop-lien systems. Along with the reaction against the relative free spending of the early Reconstruction years, economic hardship produced demands from voters that state spending be kept as low as possible.[2]

Under these circumstances, the asylum became a target of politicians seeking to cut state expenditures. To keep spending down, the Democratic politicians who dominated the state after 1877 needed a superintendent sympathetic to their aims. During Reconstruction, Ensor had shown the ability of an articulate and independent-minded superintendent to embarrass the state government with charges of niggardly treatment of the insane. His successor, Peter Griffin, proved more willing to acquiesce in politicians' attempts to reduce spending on the asylum; Griffin's successor, James Babcock, was perhaps even more cooperative.[3]

Griffin, like Ensor, owed his position largely to political considerations. As a South Carolina native, a Confederate veteran, and a Redeemer, Griffin had excellent qualifications for high state office in the wake of Reconstruction. "Like all true Southern men, he did his whole duty in the late war,"[4] the *Charleston News and Courier* noted approvingly of his appointment as superintendent of the state lunatic asylum in December 1877. Griffin demonstrated his political loyalties soon after he became superintendent when he urged the regents to give the asylum coachman an increase in wages because he was the only asylum employee who had voted Democratic in the 1876 election.[5]

Yet Griffin, like Ensor, was no mere political hack. Although most of his career had been spent as a country doctor in his native Society Hill, his medical education was superior to that of many contemporary American physicians. He took an M.D. at the University of Pennsylvania in 1855 and followed with two more years of study in the hospitals of Paris, then the world's leading medical center.[6] Griffin lacked experience in treating the insane, but he was assisted during the first few years by the former superintendent, Dr. Parker. Ensor persuaded Parker to return the asylum as assistant physician in November 1876, and he remained until his death in 1882. When Ensor resigned, Parker might have seemed a logical choice as his replacement. As the man the Radicals had turned out after thirty years of faithful service, Parker had experience and sentiment on his side. A Charlestonian pleaded that the veteran superintendent, "who so long and ably held the fort, be reinstated at once into the position which he graced in the days of Auld Lang Syne."[7] But Parker was now nearly seventy-five, and he may have compromised himself somewhat by accepting employment under the Reconstruction regime. He was also not a Confederate veteran, a qualification many Redeemers considered essential for holding important state offices.[8]

Griffin succeeded in reducing the per capita costs of the asylum. But its total costs rose substantially with the rapid increase of the patient population, and charges of extravagant management became common. The critics

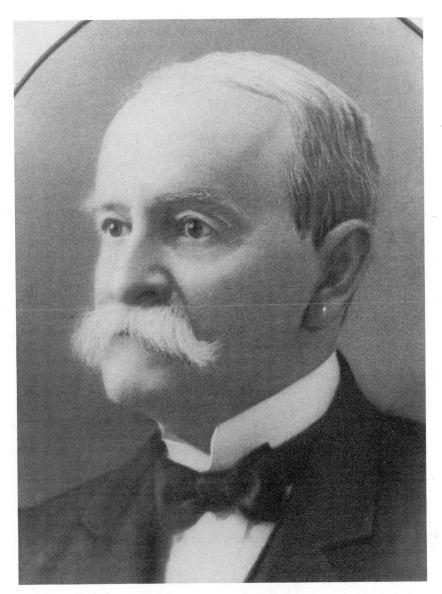

Peter E. Griffin.
(Courtesy South Carolina Department of Mental Health)

were mainly people disgruntled with the leadership of the ruling elite of the Democratic Party. The disaffected group, predominately farmers, charged that the party's leaders, the Conservatives or so-called Bourbons, favored the rich planters, lawyers, merchants, and industrialists over the middling and poorer farmers, and Charleston and Columbia over the rest of the state.

Buffeted by agricultural depression and convinced that state taxation was unnecessarily high, many white farmers and their allies demanded a series of reforms to make the state government more efficient and economical. They also sought to make the Democratic Party and the state more democratic—for whites—while eliminating the black vote. By the later 1880s these "reformers," coalesced around Benjamin Tillman's Farmers' Movement, became a powerful force within the Democratic Party. In 1890 they succeeded in electing Tillman as governor.[9]

The election of "Pitchfork Ben" Tillman ushered in South Carolina's third political revolution within twenty years. As with Reconstruction and Redemption, the triumph of Tillmanism brought changes in the personnel of state institutions, including the asylum. For several years Tillmanites had been attacking the management of the asylum as extravagant and wasteful. After the 1890 election, Tillmanite legislators quickly proposed bills to reduce the superintendent's salary and the per diem and number of the regents. The inaugural speech of the new governor dwelt on extravagance at the asylum. Tillman charged that the asylum's low per capita cost compared to similar institutions in other states was misleading, because the other asylums were predominantly white institutions. The South Carolina Lunatic Asylum had a large proportion of black patients, the cost of whose care was well below the per capita amount, which meant that "the white patients are costing much more per-capita than is shown in [the Annual] Reports." Tillman charged that the state was supporting too many patients who could afford to pay for their care or who ought to be cared for elsewhere. Of these, he demanded, "the Asylum should be purged as soon as possible." He also made clear that he was determined that patients dependent on the bounty of the state should be cared for as economically as possible. Humanity and public safety demanded that society should provide for the insane. Pauper patients should be supplied with kind care, skillful medical treatment, and adequate food and clothing. But South Carolina's impoverished taxpayers should "not be expected to support pauper lunatics in better style than they themselves are able to afford."[10]

Tillman soon decided that his plans for the asylum required the removal of Griffin as superintendent. As the object of Tillmanite charges of extravagance, the superintendent was a logical candidate for replacement. Moreover, the fact that he had been an appointee and a supporter of the Conservative regime made him suspect in the eyes of the new governor. Finally, although Tillman's campaign had accused the Conservatives of monopolizing state offices, his own followers expected to be rewarded with political appointments. As one Tillmanite office seeker put it: "The malignant faction which maligned you through all the campaign will continue the war till it is annihilated. Concession will do no good. . . . [I]f the enemy is dislodged from every office which the Governor can reach, the people of the State may still hope for a future. The case demands *heroic* treatment."[11]

A few days after Tillman's inauguration, the legislature appointed a committee to investigate conditions at the asylum. The pretext for the inquiry was the murder of a patient by another patient during the previous year. The asylum investigation that followed in March 1891 was conducted in secret. The committee examined more than one hundred witnesses, including the officers and many employees of the institution. The committee issued a report in early April that contained its conclusions but no testimony. The committee decided not to release the testimony as a whole, although they provided a synopsis of portions of it to the newspapers three weeks later.[12]

The committee investigated both the general management of the asylum and various aspects of patient care and treatment. The report concluded that the patients' food was of a lower quality than "might be expected considering the liberal appropriations made by the Legislature," that the asylum farm was poorly managed, and that the regents had failed to inspect the institution as thoroughly or as frequently as their rules required. The committee acquitted the attendants of various charges of cruelty and neglect but found its officers guilty of "gross negligence" and "lack of judgment" in allowing dangerous patients to move about without restraint.[13]

It is difficult to judge the validity of the committee's conclusions, as only a small part of the testimony was published. The committee appears to have drawn up the report hastily; the charges were generally vague and unsupported by references to specific testimony, and the conclusions were not presented in an orderly and convincing manner. Undoubtedly, the committee was looking for evidence to justify personnel changes at the asylum as well as Tillmanite charges of extravagance. One of the committee's members and a Tillman ally, Senator T. J. Strait, wrote the governor while the inquiry was in progress that they "could not find anything wrong with the books" but that he (Strait) still felt "that things were not just what they ought to be." The committee had learned from "a reliable source" that a reputedly dangerous patient who had threatened several people possessed a pistol and a knife as well as various sharp tools. The patient, named Milne, was employed at the asylum as a cabinet maker and painter, and he allegedly also held a key that allowed him access to any department of the institution. Strait obviously saw this information as something Tillman might use to discredit Griffin: "I feel [it] my duty . . . to give you an inkling of what is transpiring and if you think it best or of importance to you can correspond with Dr. Timmerman [another Tillmanite] who can give you more information. . . . We have given out nothing to any one, but feel you out [*sic*] to know." [14]

Tillman subsequently made the revelations about Milne the centerpiece of his case against Griffin. Before the committee reported, the *Columbia Daily Register* published a story claiming that Milne had attacked and beaten an attendant named McDowell, who was one of Strait's sources. According to McDowell, Milne had threatened him repeatedly and accused him and another attendant of "reporting him to the investigating committee for carrying a pistol." Although what actually happened is unclear, the story revealed to the public the existence of Milne's pistol, tools, and key. Another attendant reported to the paper that he had informed Griffin of Milne's threats on several occasions. The superintendent had replied that he did not consider the patient dangerous and that he needed the tools to do his work around the asylum. Confronted by the press, Griffin refused to comment on the matter. [15]

Based on the press synopsis of the testimony, it appears that Milne had a pistol at one time but surrendered it at Griffin's request. As to the key, Milne testified that he had received it from Griffin, but the superintendent denied it and suggested that Milne may have found a lost key. Although the evidence was inconclusive, the Tillmanites made as much of it as they could. The *Charleston News and Courier*, admittedly a Conservative newspaper with no love for Tillman, charged that a "very disproportionate part of the investigation" was concerned with Milne. The paper also contended that much of the testimony was contradictory; the evidence of the attendants was especially suspect. [16]

Griffin and the regents labeled the investigation an inquisition in which they had been "put on trial" without being informed of the charges or allowed to defend themselves. They complained that they were not given any opportunity to cross-examine or rebut the testimony of witnesses or to be present during any testimony but their own. Griffin asserted that he had not seen any of the testimony until almost three weeks after the report appeared, and then only those portions that were unfavorable to him. Most of the witnesses giving unfavorable testimony, the regents claimed, were discharged or disgruntled employees.

The regents denied most of the allegations against them. They conceded that they did not always visit every ward during their inspections of the asylum. But this was because it had become too large for them to view thoroughly in one day, and because it was "manifestly improper for strangers to intrude too often" in the wards that contained violent patients for fear of exciting them and retarding their recovery. Moreover, they claimed, one of the regents inspected the entire asylum once or twice a month. As to allegations that the food and general care of the patients was poor, the regents recalled that Tillman himself had recently charged that the "pauper lunatics fared better than the poor toiling farmer who was taxed for their support." Griffin refused even to discuss most of the charges against him, except those regarding his alleged failure to restrain dangerous patients. He wrote to the newspapers, defending his handling of patients as examples of enlightened and humane methods of managing the insane. Like all "scientific and progressive" superintendents, he claimed, he was an advocate of nonrestraint who believed in giving his patients as much freedom of movement as possible. The alternative (which he essentially accused his detractors of advocating) was to "undo the humane progress of sixty years" and return to the "brutal method . . . used to lash the convict to his cell." On the basis of one homicide and one assault, he protested, the investigating committee had erroneously implied that patient violence had become common at the asylum. The only sure way to prevent a homicide like that that had recently occurred, the superintendent pointed out, would be to place all potentially dangerous patients under constant mechanical restraint. The homicide had occurred because an attendant had permitted the offending patient to leave his ward in violation of orders. As for Milne, he was "a man of unusual intelligence, skilled in painting and other artistic work." He had been employed for some time around the asylum for both the economic and therapeutic value of his labor.

Griffin insisted that he did not consider Milne dangerous. Many patients made similar threats and never harmed anyone. The superintendent conceded that he may have erred concerning Milne but vowed that it was an isolated mistake and not indicative of general laxity. Besides, he added, the day-to-day supervision of the patients was carried out by the assistant physicians and attendants. His duties were largely administrative.[17]

For several weeks following the investigation, the superintendent and the governor traded charges and counter-charges in the press. Tillman demanded that Griffin answer the accusations against him fully and offered to let him cross-examine witnesses. Griffin insisted that he would remain silent unless the investigating committee was reconvened, retracted its charges, and conducted a proper inquiry in public. Tillman refused, returning repeatedly to the case of Milne and linking it to one of his favorite political trump cards: the defense of southern womanhood. The key Milne possessed, the governor claimed, gave him access to the female wards.

Although there was no evidence that Milne had ever done anything beyond assaulting an attendant, Tillman emphasized the dire possibilities in
the situation: "The mind revolts at and the imagination is sickened by the
thought of what could have happened." Griffin remained obdurate in the
face of the governor's assault; Tillman finally asked for the superintendent's
resignation, then dismissed him when he received no reply.[18]

With Griffin gone, Tillman turned to the regents. During the exchange
between Tillman and Griffin, the regents had published a letter defending
the superintendent. Tillman referred to it in one of his replies to Griffin, noting that the regents' "flattering endorsement of your conduct . . .
may prove a boomerang to themselves." The *Charleston News and Courier*
interpreted the threat as a sign that the governor would also remove the regents.[19] That did not turn out to be necessary. The legislature passed an act
reducing the number of regents from nine to five and giving the governor
the power to choose the members of the new board. When Tillman asked
the existing regents to draw lots to see who would leave the board, they
resigned in protest.[20]

Tillman's treatment of Griffin and the regents, like so many of his actions as governor, was highly controversial. The *Columbia Daily Register*, a
paper generally sympathetic to Tillman, claimed that the investigation was
thorough and fair. But anti-Tillman papers such as the *Columbia State* and
the *Charleston News and Courier* condemned it as incomplete and one-
sided and questioned the necessity and the constitutionality of Griffin's
removal. Even one of Tillman's supporters remarked that Griffin had been
"put out in a shabby manner."[21] The *News and Courier* conceded that the
investigation might ultimately benefit the state by instituting a more economical regime at the asylum but described Tillman's methods as savage.
The test of the governor's sincerity in trying to reform the asylum, the newspaper implied, would be the selection of Griffin's replacement: the new
superintendent should be chosen "solely for his competency as a physician
and his experience in dealing with the insane," not for any "partisan or
political services."[22]

Tillman's Conservative enemies claimed that he had planned all along
to get rid of Griffin and replace him with a political crony. The governor
consistently denied any such intention. In one of his letters to Griffin he
referred to the fact that "your friends and some newspapers charge that you
were being persecuted, and that the investigation of the asylum was instituted for the purpose of making room for one of my political adherents. . . .
I have not found a man to my liking. It is the most important office in the

State, and I would be the last man to allow political motives to influence my choice."[23]

Tillman's denial was genuine—in part. There is no firm evidence that he purposely set out to oust Griffin in favor of a Tillmanite. He had not chosen Griffin's successor at the time he dismissed the superintendent. But political motives played a part in the choice he ultimately made. Tillman's followers clearly expected him to reward supporters with asylum jobs. Rumors that Tillman intended to replace Griffin with one of his Edgefield cronies were given credence soon after the inauguration, when the governor appointed an Edgefield relative, J. W. Bunch, to succeed the asylum's recently deceased secretary-treasurer.[24] As soon as Tillman was elected, he began to receive applications and nominations for the jobs of superintendent and assistant physician. All the correspondents were confident that changes in the staff of the institution were imminent. One applicant wrote that he had learned that the governor intended to appoint a new superintendent shortly after the inauguration. He assured Tillman that he was a thoroughgoing "reformer" and that he had "been looking forward . . . to this position as resident physician of the Lunatic Asylum" for some time.[25] Tillman does not seem to have taken any of these applicants seriously. Indeed, he was genuinely angered at their impertinence in applying for a position that he had not even declared open.[26]

Tillman probably did not know precisely what he intended to do with the asylum when he became governor. He had promised before his election that he would make it run more efficiently and cheaply, but he never spelled out a specific program. After he became governor, the need to carry out his promise became an economic as well as a political necessity. He had also pledged to increase state revenues by raising the royalty on phosphate mining in South Carolina waters from one to two dollars a ton. His efforts to obtain this goal, however, led the Coosaw Mining Company to secure an injunction to stop mining operations for a year, and the state lost more than sixty thousand dollars in annual revenues. The loss of the royalty was a political embarrassment to the new governor and forced him to make a commensurate cut in spending on state institutions. One of Tillman's supporters suggested that they should get "the Asylum and the Penitentiary if possible to counterbalance the loss of Phosphate royalty."[27]

To carry out retrenchment at the asylum, Tillman needed a superintendent who would cooperate with him. He conducted the search carefully; both publicly and privately he insisted he wanted the "best man" for the job and not someone whose chief qualification was personal friendship or political loyalty.[28] Yet he could not totally abandon political considerations. He wanted a physician of administrative and business ability who was also sympathetic to the aims of the reform movement.[29] Tillman took two months to find a successor for Griffin. One of the candidates for the job of superintendent was the first assistant physician, Dr. James M. Thompson. Indeed, Thompson applied for the job more than a month before Griffin's removal. Tillman does not seem to have seriously considered Thompson or anyone who applied for the job. James Woods Babcock, the man Tillman chose, was told by one of his supporters not to apply himself but to let his friends put his name forward.[30]

Babcock's medical credentials were impressive and quickly grabbed Tillman's attention. Only thirty-five in 1891, he was a graduate of Phillips Exeter Academy, Harvard University, and Harvard Medical School. He was also—unlike any previous superintendent of the South Carolina Asylum— a specialist in mental diseases. After he received his M.D. in 1886, he served as assistant physician at Massachusetts's most prestigious private asylum, McLean Hospital. Prior to that, he had interned at the Insane Department of the Massachusetts State Almshouse at Tewkesbury. He had also spent some time studying mental diseases in Europe.[31] Politically, Babcock was perhaps an ideal candidate from Tillman's perspective. He was a native of Chester, South Carolina, but he had been out of the state for some years and had taken no part in the recent political struggles. Yet his family were Tillmanites sympathetic to the Farmers' Movement. His father was a former Confederate army surgeon who shared Tillman's political and racial views. Sidney Babcock had sent his son north to be educated in the 1870s, James explained some years later, because the Reconstruction government had opened South Carolina's schools to blacks.[32]

Babcock's supporters assured Tillman that he was the perfect candidate for the asylum job, but the governor was not immediately convinced. Tillman was impressed by Babcock's medical credentials but was more concerned about his other qualities. In a revealing letter to one of Babcock's backers, the governor argued that the superintendent's post required "executive ability, firmness, tact, and business sense . . . rather than skill as a physician."[33] Babcock's promoters assured the governor that the young doctor was "a practical and systematic business man," but Tillman was not so sure. Neither was Babcock; when first informed that he was a candidate for the job, he exhibited a lack of confidence in his fitness and an understandable reluctance to enter the rough and tumble of South Carolina political life. As he told his brother Brooks, "The asylum problem in

South Carolina—as I understand it—is a grave one, and should be trusted only to the most experienced humanitarians. I do not think I am capable of assuming such responsibilities. Besides this, I am *not* an office seeker."[34] Dr. Edward Cowles, the superintendent of McLean Hospital, told Tillman of Babcock's doubts; Cowles himself did not think that Babcock was prepared for the job of administering a large state asylum.[35] Babcock's father was dubious about his son's fitness for the post, too, but for another reason. Brooks wrote to James that "Father does not seem to think much of your accepting the job. . . . He thinks you would worry yourself to death over the miserable niggers."[36]

In the end, Tillman offered the superintendency to Babcock, but only after another candidate declined it. Tillman confessed that he had "some misgivings" about appointing Babcock, but he later came to brag about his Harvard physician. The two men, whose birthdays were coincidentally on the same day, soon became close friends. Babcock became Tillman's personal physician and on his death wrote the inscription for his tomb.[37]

Babcock possessed attractive personal qualities. By most accounts, he was a gentle and self-effacing man. At McLean he had won the admiration of colleagues, trustees, and patients alike. One of the trustees at McLean recalled that Babcock had "one characteristic he had never seen equaled . . . that of knowing all about the patients" and seeming "to be acquainted with them individually."[38] After a visit from Babcock in 1897, Dr. T. O. Powell, superintendent of the Georgia State Hospital, wrote to a mutual friend that the South Carolina doctor was "certainly a lovable character. My family all fell in love with him." Another friend of Babcock described him as a man "of gentle and rare personality . . . governed by unfailing modesty and a cheerful readiness for self-extinction." Whether this was a personality fitted for the rigors of running a large public institution dependent on politicians not known for gentleness or modesty may well be doubted. Nor was Babcock's task eased by the fact that he was a painfully sensitive man "easily misunderstood by those who knew him but slightly."[39]

Babcock's shy and gentle nature often led him to avoid conflict. He tended to work around problems rather than attack them directly, especially if the direct course meant fighting with politicians, the regents, or some of his subordinates. This became evident soon after he became superintendent. His first report to the regents praised the institution's "excellent condition," except the wards for black patients, which were "out of repair and insecure." Otherwise, the asylum was up-to-date and admirably conducted:

It is rare to find a building devoted to the care of the insane better adapted to its purpose than is the New Asylum. Its wards were planned and built on a liberal scale. The corridors and sitting rooms are unusually wide, well-lighted and cheerful! The patients' rooms are commodious, clean, well-ventilated, and comfortably furnished. The diet is liberal. The nursing service compares favorably with similar service elsewhere. . . . The people of South Carolina should take pride in this institution as a retreat for afflicted white men and women.[40]

Babcock's private correspondence shows that his real opinion of the asylum was much less positive. His years spent in the progressive and modern atmosphere of McLean left him unprepared for the shabbier and more conservative environment of the South Carolina institution. Soon after he arrived he wrote to Katherine Guion, a McLean nurse he had hired to help him establish a nurses' training school. He warned her that she might experience some "surprises and disappointments" upon her arrival. The South Carolina Lunatic Asylum, he told her, differed greatly from McLean and other northern hospitals they were familiar with, and there would be "many obstacles to overcome both within and without the Asylum."[41]

As Babcock settled in and got to know the institution better, his letters to Guion became even more gloomy: "I feel it my duty to prepare you, so far as possible, for some very *un*hospital like customs and surroundings." The main problem, he believed, was the conservatism of the asylum staff and their resentment of the new regime. She should expect, he told her, to endure "an unusual amount of hospital bickerings and jealousies. . . . We have to contend not only with ordinary conservatism, but also with the jealousies and prejudices of people who have been at the helm for fifteen years. It could not reasonably be expected of them to give up ways that they think best for methods altogether novel, not to say revolutionary."[42]

Despite his disappointment with conditions at the asylum, Babcock told Guion that he did not regret having come. But within a year, the situation had become so unpleasant that he tendered his resignation and began to look for another job. The main source of his dissatisfaction was his inability to shape the asylum staff to his liking, and replace the "conservatives" with more "loyal people" of his own choosing.[43]

From the outset of his tenure at the asylum, Babcock's freedom of action in personnel matters was limited and complicated by political events and realities. Because of the way Tillman had dismissed Griffin, many of the older staff resented Babcock and feared for their own positions. The first assistant physician, Dr. Thompson, had unsuccessfully applied for Babcock's job. Mrs. Carter, the matron, was Thompson's mother-in-law. According to Babcock, she was at the center of a group who fought against his innovations. Although Tillman undoubtedly wanted to help the new superintendent in staff matters, the furor over Griffin's removal discouraged major personnel changes, as they were likely to arouse charges of political manipulation in the anti-Tillmanite press. This happened in 1892 when one of the assistant physicians, L. G. Corbett, resigned for reasons that apparently had nothing to do with politics. In selecting new staff, Babcock was also constrained by political considerations. For example, he had to choose South Carolinians for jobs at the asylum, and he had to accept some employees who were political appointees or relatives of the regents.[44]

Babcock's attempts to make personnel changes periodically brought him into conflict with the regents, because they had the power to appoint and dismiss all the subordinate officers. Although he won a partial victory in 1892 and retracted his resignation, conflicts with and over his subordinates continued. In 1897 he nearly resigned again to take the job of superintendent at the new Lakeside Hospital in Cleveland. One of the most attractive aspects of the Lakeside post, Babcock confided to a fellow superintendent, was that he would be the undisputed executive head, with all other officers subordinate to him.[45]

Babcock decided to seek the Cleveland job after one of the nurses, a Miss Koon, accused him before the legislative committee on the asylum of mismanagement, extravagance, favoritism, misuse of state property, and neglect of duty. He protested that Koon attacked him because she was opposed to his innovations at the institution. The regents and the legislative committee conducted an investigation that exonerated Babcock and commended his management of the asylum. In the following weeks he was able to secure the removal of several "insubordinate" nurses.[46]

Despite his victory, he decided that he could no longer tolerate the situation in Columbia and resolved to leave when the trustees of Lakeside Hospital offered him the superintendent's position. Only the opposition of Ben Tillman and a sense of duty to his state seems to have changed his mind. Tillman, now a U.S. senator, virtually ordered Babcock not to go: "I will never consent for you to accept any of these offers unless things get in much worse shape in the state than they are. You can not have many enemies here—certainly none who can bother you much." In South Carolina, Tillman claimed, he had the protection of the state's most powerful politician, Tillman himself. In another state, that would not be the case: "You might be subjected to the same animosities and jealousies . . . in a less limited degree . . . and there you would have nothing but your medical knowledge and skill to back you up."[47] A month later, Babcock told a fellow superintendent that he was on the verge of accepting the Lakeside job, but his "feeling of allegiance to the State was born in me and it comes harder than I realized to think of giving up my work here."[48] He decided to remain in South Carolina.[49]

Staff problems continued to plague Babcock. Combined with inadequate appropriations, they made it impossible for him to achieve his goal of modernizing the South Carolina Lunatic Asylum and making it one of the best in the nation. A more aggressive man might have overcome some of these obstacles, but Babcock's distaste for personal and political conflicts often led him to avoid them if at all possible. The result was that he failed to insist on the removal of officers he found it difficult to work with or had little confidence in, such as Dr. Thompson.[50] Babcock threatened to resign on at least two more occasions but never carried out his threat. Eventually, he abandoned efforts to mold the staff to his standards and left the assistant physicians to run their departments with minimal supervision. He rarely called staff meetings or visited the wards. The supervisor of the white men's department remarked in 1909 that "Dr. Babcock's management was all right for several years after he came here. . . . [But] in recent years he has appeared indifferent."[51] The superintendent increasingly busied himself with outside consultations and other work, such as overseeing the construction of buildings, that should have been done by others. He also spent much time on scholarly pursuits, reading and writing on the history of insanity and the care of the insane. Although some of his research, notably that on tuberculosis and pellagra, was directly relevant to conditions at the state hospital, none of it brought much benefit to its patients.[52] As we shall see, the asylum environment deteriorated during his tenure and reached a critical point by the first decade of the twentieth century. By then, the effects of politicization and rigid economizing had created scandalous conditions at the institution.

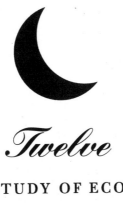

Twelve

THE STUDY OF ECONOMY

MANAGING THE POSTBELLUM ASYLUM

The South Carolina Lunatic Asylum changed markedly after the Civil War. During the antebellum period, the asylum's officers viewed their mission as largely therapeutic. The small patient population was overwhelmingly white, and many of them paid for their care. By the 1880s, it was becoming clear that the asylum had added a new function. Without officially abandoning its therapeutic mission, it became a receptacle for large numbers of "mental defectives" of both races, who were accepted regardless of curability or ability to pay. In common with other public mental hospitals, it settled down to become a basically custodial welfare institution. The patient population expanded rapidly, placing new demands on the institution and its staff. The superintendents had to adjust to the uncomfortable role of custodians and to become adept at managing a massive state-supported institution. Administrative and financial concerns took up more and more of their time. To add to their difficulties, they operated under severe economic and political constraints that required them to support their patients as cheaply as possible.[1]

An 1891 addition to the asylum's by-laws succinctly summarizes the new priorities of the institution: "The same principles of economy, order, and efficiency which regulate a well-managed private enterprise should prevail in a charitable institution supported by the taxes of the people; and a disposition towards extravagance and wastefulness in any form will disqualify any person from employment here."[2]

The asylum's officers did not accept these constraints entirely without protest. They frequently pointed out that the appropriations for the institution were inadequate. Soon after Peter Griffin became superintendent in 1878, he told the regents that the appropriation for the asylum needed to be at least one-fourth higher than it was. A few years later he informed the general assembly that he could not reduce the per capita cost of maintenance further without lowering the asylum to the level of a jail or a poorhouse. Griffin's successor, James Babcock, frequently pointed out that the per capita costs of the South Carolina Lunatic Asylum were lower than those of virtually every other hospital in the country and lower than a proper standard of care would demand.[3] Yet the pleas of Griffin and Babcock for more adequate funding lacked the intensity, persistence, and righteous anger of Ensor's. Moreover, unlike Ensor, they did not appeal to the press and public. Whatever their personal misgivings, Griffin and Babcock generally cooperated with the politicians' desire to retrench. They devoted themselves, in Griffin's words, to "the study of economy."[4]

In one respect, the financial situation of the asylum improved after the end of Reconstruction. The Democratic regime generally issued appropriations on time and assumed the debts that had accumulated during the administrations of Parker and Ensor. Freed from the necessity of borrowing at high rates of interest, the asylum was usually able, through strict economizing, to keep within its appropriations.[5] But the appropriations were exceedingly meager. The number of patients increased much faster than the amounts the legislature appropriated for their maintenance. Between 1875 and 1905, the average daily census of patients quadrupled from 312 to 1,210. Meanwhile, the appropriation for the maintenance of the patients only doubled, from $70,000 to $140,000. Annual expenditure per patient fell from $210 to $102. During this period, according to Babcock, prices of food and supplies increased by about 25 percent. Other state asylums faced similar problems. But, as its officers regularly pointed out, per capita expenditures for maintenance at the South Carolina Lunatic Asylum were well below the national average and frequently among the lowest of American public mental institutions. The average annual expenditure per patient for fifty-three state hospitals in the early 1890s was $179. In South Carolina between 1891 and 1895, it was $127, slightly below the southern average of $129.[6]

No matter how much the asylum's officers pared down expenses, however, politicians continually accused them of extravagance. Griffin fumed that every election brought forth such charges, made by people who "will not read our statistics, never visit the asylum, and really know nothing of the necessary costs of such institutions."[7] In 1886 a special legislative committee investigated the asylum's expenditures, but could not find any room for further retrenchment.[8] Nevertheless, the charge that the asylum was wastefully managed was one of the main planks in the successful gubernatorial campaign of Ben Tillman in 1890. As we have seen, Tillman discharged Griffin partly on grounds of mismanagement and replaced him with Babcock.

Griffin's experience weighed heavily upon Babcock, a shy man who hated the rough and tumble of politics. In effect, he capitulated to the forces of retrenchment. In 1909 Babcock told a legislative investigation that the attacks on Griffin had made him "unusually economical" in managing the institution: "When I came here the previous administration had been assailed on the ground of extravagance. . . . [M]y administration started with the idea that the money that was supplied for this institution must be made to go as far as possible. . . . This money that is sent to the asylum comes from the people, from so many taxpayers, and it is by the special providence of God that you get a penny . . . but above all things, don't go to the Legislature and say you haven't got a plenty of it."[9]

At first, Babcock protested vigorously against conditions at the asylum. In 1892 he complained bitterly that overcrowding made it necessary to use some "dark rooms" as bedrooms for violent patients: "From a humanitarian or even a hygienic standpoint they are such dungeons as one would never confine healthy criminals in lest they might be made insane thereby. Shall we longer then place the sick entrusted to our care in such receptacles?"[10] But already he was concluding that it was fruitless to appeal to the legislature for a remedy. The same year he told the regents that the asylum needed more land, but that experience had taught him that it was useless to go to the legislature for a special appropriation. Instead, he suggested that the asylum purchase land piecemeal by setting aside a part of the regular maintenance fund each year—in other words, by reducing the funds available for patient care and treatment. Year after year Babcock reported that the asylum had one of the lowest per capita costs in the nation but took little action to change things, beyond pointing out some of the institution's needs in his reports to the regents.[11] Rather than fight the general assembly for desperately needed appropriations, he settled for trying to make the most of whatever it would give him. A member of the 1909 investigating committee asked him if he had kept the legislature informed of his needs. He replied, "There the reports are. I would like to say that

I am not robust, and I do not consider that it comes within the line of my duty to go down to the State House and pull the honorable members of the General Assembly out of their seats to listen to the needs of the asylum."[12]

Many taxpayers and legislators were unsympathetic to the needs of the asylum, because they were convinced that its charity was frequently abused. As proof, they pointed to the fact that most patients admitted since the Civil War were paupers or beneficiaries; paying admissions had dwindled to insignificance. During the antebellum period, the number of pauper patients had only slightly exceeded the number of paying patients. As late as 1865, there were 60 paying and 68 pauper patients in the asylum. By 1881, beneficiaries outnumbered paying patients almost twenty to one (464 to 26). The trend continued and outraged taxpayers and politicians. Governor Tillman remarked only half-facetiously in 1890 that the proportion of pauper patients was so high that "we are forced to ask whether only the poor people go crazy."[13]

It was not only the poor who went crazy, of course. As was true in public asylums elsewhere, many beneficiary patients in South Carolina were not paupers in the sense of being totally destitute. Many had occupations, land, or other property. Moreover, insanity, like any serious illness, creates poverty and dependence by eliminating the ability of the victim or other family members to earn income. But the proportion of beneficiary patients in South Carolina increased so rapidly in the late nineteenth century partly because its citizens were poorer than before. Many families who had once been able to pay for the care of their insane relatives at home, in boarding-houses, or in asylums could no longer afford to do so. "There is no doubt," Griffin wrote in 1878, "that the poverty of our people forces now to the Asylum many harmless and inoffensive patients who have heretofore been cared for at home."[14]

Emancipation also greatly increased the potential number of beneficiary patients by fully opening the asylum to blacks. African Americans constituted a majority of the state's population, and nearly all were too poor to pay for asylum care. The number of black patients in the asylum increased from five in 1865 to more than four hundred at the end of 1901.[15]

Finally, a major change in social policy contributed to the sharp increase in beneficiary patients. In 1871 the state assumed financial responsibility for the care of pauper patients in the asylum. This freed the institution from the problem of trying to collect payment from the counties. But it also made it easier for local officials such as the county commissioners to send an insane person to the asylum. Many families, too, were less reluctant to accept assistance from the state than from local poor-law authorities.

That the pejorative term "pauper lunatic" was abandoned in favor of "state patient" or "beneficiary" during the 1870s was both a sign of changing attitudes toward accepting public assistance and an additional inducement to such acceptance. Babcock stressed the importance of the new terminology from the point of the asylum physician. The law, he maintained, justly discriminated between the lunatic and the pauper. The lunatic was a victim of disease and was "therefore a patient deserving skilled medical attention." The pauper, on the other hand, was frequently a "victim of a vice" who "should be forced to labor and thus contribute towards his support." To its credit the state refrained from applying "the offensive word pauper to the needy insane" and instead viewed them as " 'beneficiaries' of her bounty."[16]

To many taxpayers and politicians, however, the sharp increase of beneficiary patients indicated abuse of the state's benevolence. The asylum's officers sometimes agreed. Griffin, for example, argued that the dramatic increase in the proportion of beneficiary patients happened because "many families have shifted upon the State a burden which they are able, but unwilling, to bear."[17] Governor Johnson Hagood echoed these charges in his message to the legislature in 1881 and demanded that "the pauper alone should receive the bounty of the State; those who are able to pay in whole or in part . . . should be required to do so."[18] In 1890, Governor Tillman explained his view of how the asylum's charity was being abused:

> The law provides that the lunatics who have property shall be supported out of the income therefrom. I have known instances in which this has been disregarded, and not only the income but the estate itself has been used by the relatives while the State was called on to support the lunatics. It is probable that many of the patients in the Asylum belong in this category, and the County Commissioners, whose duty it is to prevent it, have either been imposed upon or winked at the wrong to please some friend and curry favor with an influential voter. The law provides for punishment, it is true, but what is everybody's business is nobody's business. Few people know anything about such a law. The Asylum is at a distance; the patient enters and is soon forgotten. The neighbors talk a while and there's an end.[19]

Tillman implied that such abuses were common, but the evidence is inconclusive. No doubt some patients committed as beneficiaries could have contributed substantially toward the costs of their maintenance, but many could pay little or nothing. In impoverished postbellum South Carolina, few families had enough resources to pay for extended care and treatment. Moreover, insanity not only increased expenses, it also often reduced available income, because the patient or another family member was unable to work. The following letters and affidavits, which accompanied applications for beneficiary status, provide examples of what must have been common predicaments:

> I have had [my son] in the insane department of the Hospital in Charleston, S.C. for treatment but after staying a short while he escaped. I am not able to defray the expense of keeping him in the Insane Asylum. I am entirely out of employment and unable to do manual labor and have no income with the exception of $100 rent for my wife's place, and have a wife, mother, and five children dependent on me for support.
>
> J. D. Lange . . . upon oath says that he knows J. H., colored, and is fully acquainted with his financial condition. Deponent says that the said J. H. is almost entirely without means of any description; that he owns no real estate, and only a scanty supply of the most ordinary clothing, which constitutes the extent of his personal property. That his parents are both dead, and while they were living they owned only such effects as ordinary colored laborers used.[20]

Tillman and others believed that the best way to slow the increase in beneficiaries was to make the counties financially responsible, in whole or part, for the care of pauper patients. If each county were required to pay some of the costs of patients it sent to the asylum, Tillman contended, the numbers of patients and the cost to the taxpayers would be considerably reduced. Faced with the scrutiny of the local press and the county grand jury, he claimed, the commissioners would be sure to make everyone pay who ought to pay, "and instead of bundling off every idiot and harmless imbecile to Columbia, there would be careful calculation as to whether they should not go to the County Poor House." Moreover, families who were willing enough to send a harmless patient to the asylum to get rid of him might balk, out of pride, at putting him in the poorhouse. They would have no other option but to care for him themselves.[21]

Tillman's solutions assumed that the actions of local authorities and the patients' families were responsible for the alleged abuses of state charity. In the main, this was probably true, but the asylum's officers themselves contributed to the trend. Superintendents sometimes recommended that patients be moved from the pay to the beneficiary list as a means of easing the financial burden on their families. For example, Babcock wrote the friend of a family with two patients in the asylum that he had "suggested to Mrs. O. . . . that she allow her daughter to become a beneficiary patient. This will not make the slightest difference in her surroundings or treatment. As to Mr. O., I suggested the payment of a nominal sum — say $10 — that would allow me to keep him at the pay patient's table. . . . The afflicted family deserves our most considerate treatment and fullest sympathy."[22]

Babcock and Griffin generally supported a return to some system of county support, but the asylum's regents generally opposed it. They pointed out that the legislature had adopted state support in the first place because of the asylum's difficulties in collecting payment from the counties. Instead of abolishing state support, the legislature tried to reduce the number of beneficiary patients by tightening up commitment procedures. In 1881 and 1882, the general assembly passed acts that required the county commissioners to determine the financial status of patients before committing them and to investigate and report on the financial status of patients already in the asylum.[23] These measures did little to stem the tide of beneficiaries. Despite the provision of fines for noncompliance, many commissioners failed to carry out the required investigations or produced reports that were too vague to be of any use in determining a patient's ability to pay. Trying to get the required information, Griffin concluded, was a frustrating and often hopeless task that resulted in only a few patients being transferred to the pay list. Moreover, requiring the county commissioners to provide financial information on patients aggravated the perennial problem of getting acute cases to the asylum quickly. In most counties, the commissioners met only once a month; this meant that patients sometimes remained in the county jail or under severe restraint for weeks after their commitment hearing.[24] In 1894, the legislature tried to solve these problems by making the probate judges responsible for reporting on patients' financial condition.[25] This change, too, was unavailing. By 1900, less than 3 percent of the patients were paying anything toward the cost of their maintenance at the state hospital.[26]

The rapid influx of beneficiary patients combined with low appropriations overwhelmed the asylum's facilities. Severe overcrowding became a chronic problem. In 1875 Ensor reported that patients in the female department were crowded together "like sheep on the floors, in the corridors, and in rooms that are only large enough for one, or two at most."[27] The reports of Griffin and Babcock endlessly repeated the same theme. In 1878, Griffin reported that it was no longer possible "with present accommodations to admit patients without crowding our wards to an extent dangerous to health and fatal to the chances of cure."[28] In 1902 Babcock noted that "the overcrowded condition of our wards has so often been dealt with" in his reports that he feared it had "become a tiresome story."[29]

The problem of overcrowding was common to most public asylums in the United States and Europe in the late nineteenth century, and the explanation was much the same everywhere: over time, chronic, incurable patients tended to accumulate in institutions. In South Carolina, as in some other states, the law aggravated the tendency by requiring the asylum to receive epileptics and idiots.[30] From the 1860s superintendents complained that the asylum was clogged with chronic patients whose presence excluded the acute insane. Griffin lamented that many persons sent to the asylum were "simply idiots, imbeciles, dotards, or harmless epileptics."[31] Babcock made similar complaints every year. Local officials, he argued, sent many patients to the asylum who properly belonged in a general hospital, a poorhouse, or at home. Between 1891 and 1911, according to Babcock's statistics, more than 18 percent of the admissions to the state hospital consisted of imbeciles, idiots, epileptics, and inebriates. In 1897, he reported that one of the most important changes in the patient population was the increasing number of older patients. Between 1875 and 1895 the percentage of resident patients over fifty increased from 11.7 to 27.6.[32]

These developments reflected a change in the asylum's function in the late nineteenth century. The South Carolina Lunatic Asylum, like similar institutions elsewhere, increasingly served the purposes of a welfare institution for various classes of "defectives" whose common denominator was poverty.[33] In South Carolina, this tendency was aggravated by the lack of general hospitals and institutions for the feeble-minded and inebriates, the absence or decrepit condition of the county poorhouses, and the preferences of the patients' friends and county officials to place them in the asylum rather than in a poorhouse. Outside of Charleston, as the regents pointed out, the state asylum was virtually the only hospital in the state. It was not surprising that it received many patients who "were not fit subjects for an insane hospital," including "the undesirable elements of all communities—imbeciles, incorrigibles, waifs, the blind, and many aged persons . . . who justly belong to county almshouses."[34]

During the late nineteenth and early twentieth centuries, some American states and European countries experimented with alternative methods of caring for chronic patients. One option was to establish separate institutions for the chronically insane. The English county of Middlesex built two large institutions for the chronically insane near London in the 1860s. About the same time, New York state established the Willard Asylum for the Chronic Insane, and Massachusetts created a separate section of its almshouse at Tewkesbury to care for chronically insane immigrant paupers. Other solutions were influenced by the "Gheel system" of Belgium, where since the Middle Ages the insane had been boarded in private houses in and around the village of Gheel. The Gheel model inspired various schemes of supervised boarding out, decentralized "colonies" for the different classes of insane, and "segregate" hospitals that combined a central hospital building with smaller, less expensive buildings scattered around the grounds. Massachusetts adopted boarding out in 1885, placing the chronically insane in private homes, a method that Scotland had implemented with some success in the 1860s. The Whittingham Asylum in England, built in the 1860s, and the Illinois state hospital at Kankakee (1880) were examples of the segregate or "cottage" hospital, sometimes called the Kankakee system. Wisconsin took decentralization further by requiring the creation of small county asylums for the chronic insane in conjunction with the poorhouses. The Wisconsin system, as this method became known, was under the supervision of the State Board of Charities.[35]

Some states also established separate institutions or colonies for the feeble-minded, epileptics, or inebriates in the late nineteenth century. Several, including New York, Pennsylvania, Massachusetts, Ohio, and Kentucky, founded training schools for idiots before 1860, and after the Civil War, other states followed their example. In the 1890s, Ohio and New York established separate institutions for epileptics, as did a few other states in the next few decades. New York created the first state inebriate asylum in 1864; by 1900, more than fifty public and private inebriate institutions had been opened in the United States.[36]

The officers of the South Carolina Lunatic Asylum were aware of these alternative care plans and advocated most of them at one time or another. Parker proposed the creation of an idiot asylum in South Carolina as early as 1869. Ensor and Griffin both suggested using the original building at the state lunatic asylum as a residence for the chronically insane. After attending the 1883 National Conference of Charities and Corrections, Griffin advocated that South Carolina adopt the Kankakee system.[37] From the later 1890s, Babcock repeatedly recommended that the state establish separate institutions or colonies for epileptics, the feeble-minded, and inebriates. In 1903 Governor McSweeney urged that South Carolina adopt the Wisconsin system and require the counties to provide suitable accommodations for the reception of harmless chronic patients. But the state did not embrace any of these alternatives until after World War I.[38]

Faced with a constantly expanding crowd of patients, the officers of the South Carolina Lunatic Asylum frequently appealed to the legislature for additional accommodation. But they were never able to secure enough money from the state to keep pace with the demand for space. Obsessed with the need to keep taxes down, legislators seldom provided adequate funds for maintenance, let alone new construction. An example is the completion of the "new asylum" building begun in the later 1850s. One wing of this Kirkbride-style building was erected before construction was suspended by the Civil War. Work was resumed in 1870, but progress was glacial.[39] Construction was suspended several times because of delays in getting the appropriations paid on schedule. By 1875 the south (male) wing was finished, but despite Ensor's continued appeals, nothing more had been done by the time he resigned in December 1877.[40]

Construction resumed under Ensor's successor Griffin but was hampered by the paltry sums the legislature provided. As a result, the building was completed in several stages over a period of seven years and only by financing much of the cost out of the appropriations for the patients' maintenance. In 1878 Griffin asked for an appropriation of fifty thousand dollars a year for two or three years to complete the building. The legislature allocated five thousand dollars for one year, a sum, he told the regents, that was "more of an embarrassment than a benefit."[41] The legislature also directed the asylum's officers to save money on materials by using brick and granite provided by convict labor from the new state penitentiary in Columbia. Legislative cheeseparing at the penitentiary, however, largely negated this plan. State appropriations were so inadequate that penitentiary officials had to hire out most of the prisoners to pay the costs of their maintenance. The asylum could get brick and granite from the penitentiary only by paying for it, although at one-half the market cost. In 1879 Griffin again asked the general assembly for fifty thousand dollars a year until the new building was completed; legislators gave him ten thousand. With this money, plus some funds that he had saved from the appropriations of the previous two years, the regents decided to resume construction.[42] The north wing was completed in 1882. Work then commenced on the center, or administrative, building, which Samuel Sloan of Philadelphia designed. With the help of patient labor and a more generous appropriation, the building was finally finished in 1885, nearly thirty years after it had been begun.[43]

The completion of the new asylum, Griffin proudly announced, gave South Carolina a structure equal to the best in the country. But many patients still inhabited the original building, which Trezevant, Parker, and Ensor had condemned years before as obsolete. Moreover, the completion of the new building left many black patients housed in wooden buildings. Yet Griffin assured the legislature that it was "not probable that the State would ever be called on to erect another Asylum as expensive as the one just finished." When more accommodation was needed, it could be met by erecting "separate buildings of plainer construction" for the black patients.[44]

Securing even plain buildings for the black patients, however, proved more difficult than finishing the new asylum. Since the 1860s, they had been housed in "temporary" wooden structures, despite the obvious danger of fire and inadequate sanitation and amenities. When the new asylum was completed in 1885, the black women patients were transferred to the old asylum, but the black men remained in wooden buildings until 1898. Griffin and Babcock repeatedly reminded the regents and the legislature of the need for permanent brick buildings for the black patients, but to little effect. Soon after he became superintendent, Babcock protested that the legislature did not seem to understand "the true gravity of the [blacks'] situation here." Providing facilities for their care, he argued, was the most important question facing the people of South Carolina.[45]

Few of the state's leaders felt Babcock's sense of urgency. In the case of the black patients, the legislature's desires to economize coexisted comfortably with the racial views and policies of the white Democratic politicians who controlled the state after 1876. During the last part of the nineteenth century, South Carolina's political leaders gradually moved to eliminate all vestiges of racial equality and to erect a regime based on segregation and white supremacy. The markedly inferior accommodations allotted to the black insane did not arouse much concern among those in the white establishment. As a legislative committee of 1910 noted matter of factly, white patients required a superior quality of accommodations and care than blacks "by reason of [the whites'] higher standard of living."[46]

The problem of getting permanent facilities for the black insane was complicated by divisions over long-term policy toward their care. For several decades, South Carolina's leaders could not decide what to do with the state's insane blacks. One group, disturbed by the proximity of the races as well as the difficulties of managing a multiracial institution, wanted to establish a separate institution for blacks. Griffin and Babcock generally preferred this solution, which was adopted by North Carolina, Virginia, and Alabama. Another group favored retaining a single institution for both races on grounds of economy and ease of administration. The asylum's regents generally supported this policy. Both sides were fully committed to segregation of the races, but proponents of a second asylum believed that segregation could not be efficiently or fully maintained within one institution. Indeed, black and white patients often shared the same buildings, although they were kept on separate wards. The presence of both races within one institution also complicated attempts to classify patients according to type and severity of disorder.[47]

In 1887, a legislative committee recommended that the state investigate the creation of a separate asylum for blacks. But the proposal did not come before the senate until the last day of the session, and its opponents successfully moved to postpone consideration of the report. Two years later, the legislature passed a joint resolution requiring the board of regents to advertise around the state for donations of land or money to be used for the purpose of establishing an asylum for blacks. The regents received several offers of land, but they continued to oppose a separate asylum, and the proposal went no further.[48] The legislature did not begin to resolve the policy issue until 1910, when it authorized the purchase of a tract of land several miles from Columbia for the purpose of erecting a second state hospital. Development of this location, known as State Park, was seriously hampered by insufficient appropriations, disagreement over its purposes, and the opposition of Governor Coleman Blease (1910–14). In 1913, Blease denounced the State Park project as a scheme designed to enrich his political opponents at the expense of the taxpayer. An exhuberant racist, Blease did not oppose the separation of the races. He merely objected, he claimed, to spending white taxpayers' money to provide a new hospital for blacks. At one point, he proposed to sell the State Park land and convert the state penitentiary into an asylum for blacks. He was already engaged in a controversial move to empty the penitentiary by pardoning some convicts and sending others to the county chain gangs. As he explained to a legislative inquiry on the state hospital in 1914: "My idea is to take these insane colored people, spend a few dollars and put [the Penitentiary] in shape and put the colored people in there. . . . Take State Park—and I say sell it. . . . I would like for you to get half of the amount paid for it; [that] sandy land out there . . . you could not raise anything but an umbrella on it."[49] Despite Blease's opposition, the project continued and the transfer of black patients to State Park began in 1914. But development was slow, and black patients remained at the old state hospital until the 1930s.[50]

The failure to develop a second institution for the black insane before World War I forced the asylum authorities to provide permanent accommodation at the Columbia location. In 1893, the legislature gave the regents permission to begin construction of a brick structure for the black men patients. But the hospital received no appropriation for the building until 1897, when the legislature allocated a mere $7,500. To save money, Babcock acted as architect, and one of the hospital's black employees, Page Ellington, served as engineer and contractor. Black patients excavated the foundation; convicts made some of the brick, and an old brick wall provided the rest. Lack of money stopped construction with the structure nearly completed. In 1898, the legislature provided an additional $13,500 to complete and furnish the building, which was named for Parker. The total cost to the state of the Parker building, designed for two hundred patients, was only $21,000.[51]

The inability of the asylum's officers to secure sufficient accommodation forced them to seek ways to limit the size and nature of the patient population. In common with asylum authorities elsewhere, they sought to discharge chronic and incurable patients and to limit admissions to acute cases. Superintendent Parker had suggested the removal of some chronic pauper patients from the asylum as early as the 1850s. These "harmless and quiet" patients, he argued, "might receive benefit from domestic or agricultural employment in the society of their friends, and thus make room for admission of others continually applied for." Some states, he pointed out, had enacted laws that compelled the counties to remove such patients whenever the asylum authorities decided that they were not likely to receive further benefit from confinement.[52] In 1871, Ensor convinced the legislature to enact such a law, and during the next few years he discharged some patients to the counties whenever the asylum became too crowded.[53]

Griffin also periodically sent patients back to the counties. Between 1883 and 1885, the regents approved the return of more than 100 patients, 62 in March 1885 alone. One problem in making such removals was that the county commissioners sometimes failed to arrange the removal of patients. In 1884, the legislature made it a misdemeanor for a county commissioner to fail to remove a patient from the asylum within thirty days of receiving a request to do so from the superintendent.[54] But the law proved difficult to enforce. Griffin's efforts resulted in a small decrease in the number of patients, from 628 at the end of 1884 to 605 at the end of the following year. But the numbers soon began to climb again. Babcock occasionally carried out similar removals during the 1890s, but they, too, brought only temporary relief.[55]

The superintendents, like many of their colleagues in other states, viewed such removals as an expediency, not a reform. Ensor called the removals a "disgraceful and humiliating necessity" and ended them when he decided that the drawbacks outweighed the advantages. Only a very few patients, he told the regents, were suitable for removal, and often those had no friends or family to care for them. The alternative of sending such patients to the poorhouse, he argued, was a bitter one: "What heart does not revolt at the idea of subjecting our poor, unfortunate insane fellow-beings to the miseries of a county poorhouse?"[56] Most poorhouses were themselves overcrowded and lacked suitable accommodations and staff to care for the insane. Ensor described the poorhouse of Richland County in Columbia as typical: "A few dilapidated log cabins in an old field, that no respectable farmer would shelter his stock in."[57]

Griffin and Babcock also questioned the wisdom or feasibility of returning chronic patients to the poorhouses. According to Griffin, only Charleston County provided facilities suitable for the reception of the chronically insane. Several counties did not have a poorhouse at all, although the law required them to maintain one.[58] To make the counties provide suitable facilities and supervision for the insane would cost more than to extend the asylum, and the history of poorhouse care indicated that it would be likely to lead to considerable neglect and abuse.[59] Babcock agreed. He occasionally conceded that the poorhouses might be used to relieve overcrowding in the asylum, but only if the state forced the counties to markedly upgrade their facilities. "The present condition of the poorhouses," he wrote in 1895, "does not warrant the belief that they are proper receptacles for the helpless insane." In a modern, civilized society, the transfer of insane patients from asylums to poorhouses could not be justified except as a temporary expedient in times of excessive overcrowding.[60]

The superintendents opposed removal of patients to the poorhouses for another reason: many families thought it a greater disgrace to have a relative in a poorhouse than in an asylum. The advent of state care for nearly all the patients and the use of the term "beneficiary" in place of "pauper lunatic" had taken some of the stigma out of being in the asylum. As Griffin put it, "In the popular estimation it is more respectable to be in the Asylum than in the Poor House."[61]

Babcock virtually refused to discharge white women to the poorhouses, arguing that it "should never be the policy of the Asylum to place white women in the county poor house. The friends of the patient should be urged to take them home." To discharge white women patients to poorhouses, he predicted, would produce public outrage: "I scarcely believe that the officers of the Asylum would be sustained if they should resort to such a course in regard to the white female patients."[62]

Sending chronic patients back to the counties was often an exercise in futility. There was nothing to stop the commissioners from returning a patient or some other chronic under another commitment order. As an exasperated Griffin explained:

To show how difficult it is to exclude this class from the Asylum, I may mention that from the very Poor House to which three imbeciles had been sent was committed to the Asylum two days later a colored woman over eighty years old, whose insanity was simply dotage. Yesterday we had returned to us from the Poor House of another County a young negro man who was removed only 24 days ago. During his eight years residence in the Asylum he showed no vicious tendencies, and was regarded as a good-natured imbecile, who was willing and able to assist in many simple industries. As the commitment papers of both these persons were in legal form, we were obliged to admit them.[63]

In returning chronic patients to the asylum, local officials were not necessarily being obtuse or obstreperous. Sometimes they did not know what else to do. One magistrate sent a patient back to the hospital with the following explanation: "J. M., who was allowed to come home from your hospital about ten days ago, proved to be a dangerous man. A few nights ago, he knocked down his wife and had a knife in his hands, and told her I had authorized him to kill her. He was only prevented from doing some injury by his children. This afternoon, he attacked a white man with an axe and did hurt him to some extent. This man wants him arrested and punished. So I thought best to send him back to you for safe keeping."[64]

The superintendents themselves admitted the problem: no matter how much care was taken in selecting a patient for removal, it often happened that one who was well behaved and industrious in the asylum quickly became dangerous, suicidal, or a public nuisance when outside of it. One man wrote Griffin asking him to readmit a patient because "we cannot manage him at home. He will get up at night and ramble all night and disturb the neighborhood and there is danger of his being badly injured. . . . Please take him back again. . . . *[W]rite me at once* and I will send him on the first train."[65] A father petitioned for the recommitment of his son when the boy suddenly became violent: "He began to throw rocks at the other members of the family, destroyed some crockery and bit one of the children in the arm badly. He tried to kill me this morning with an axe. I can't control him or do any thing with him. I am afraid he will kill some of the family if he is left at home."[66]

The superintendents' attempts to send patients back to their communities were often inhibited by the reluctance of their families or the local authorities to receive them at all. In the early 1880s, Griffin established a system of probation, by which patients could be released for a three-month trial period upon the application of friends. At any time during that period, they could be returned on the original commitment order. At the end of the period, they were discharged or returned, or the period of probation was extended. The probation system made the asylum less crowded than it might have been, but the impact of probation was limited in that it required someone to take responsibility for the patient. Some patients had no family or friends able to care for them. Relatives or community members often feared that the patient would become dangerous or uncontrollable outside the asylum. Sometimes the family or the local officials simply did not want to be burdened with the care or the expense of the patient. A physician advised Babcock not to return an elderly woman to her family because her son and daughter-in-law both worked in a cotton mill and there was no one at home to watch her. She had previously attacked their small child with a stick.[67]

Even if a relative or friend was willing to accept a patient, local officials or physicians might oppose his release. A probate judge asked Babcock not to release a patient whose wife had petitioned for his release, unless he was "a great deal better than when I sent him down. . . . For months he made life a burden to all us county officials."[68] Another probate judge advised Babcock not to discharge a woman because if released she would soon "be thrown on the public or the charitable people of the community."[69]

Families, physicians, or local officials sometimes protested even the possibility that a patient might be discharged in the future. One physician wrote Griffin, cautioning him not to release a patient who had attacked two citizens with a knife: "In the name of all our ladies and children for God's sake don't let him come back here soon."[70] In another case, a patient's acquaintance wrote to an asylum employee and asked him to warn the asylum physicians of the dangers of letting the patient out: "I am requested by Mrs. V. to write to you in regard to Jim. She is afraid he will be able to fool the Doctors and get off and come home and do harm, as he did sweare death to several persons, and at last accused his wife and son of all the trouble. Charlie, you know Jim from old, you know he is keen, sharp and cunning."[71]

The difficulty of discharging patients was increased by the actions and attitudes of the asylum authorities themselves. Fear of releasing a potentially dangerous patient was only part of the problem. Until the early 1900s, the rules required that the regents personally examine the patients prior to dismissal. But the regents normally met only once a month, and sometimes they did not examine all or any of the patients the physicians recommended for discharge. Months might pass between the physician's recommendation and the actual time of release. Dr. Sarah Allan, who served as assistant physician in charge of the white women patients from 1895 to 1906, recorded in her diary the frustration she and her patients felt at these delays:

January 11 [1900]. . . . Board met today. We're trying to get off Mrs. H. B. and Miss L., but Board did not see patients.

February 8. Patients were much disappointed today because the regents did not see them. Mrs. M. was the only one fortunate enough to be sent home.

March 8. Crowd of disappointed patients again as regents did not see them.

April ——. Patients were disappointed at not meeting the Board yesterday.

May 10. Board refused again to see patients today, but [the patients] seem to be getting accustomed to this. Mrs. T., Misses D. and S. should be discharged.[72]

The second method by which the superintendents sought to control its patient population was through the commitment process. They demanded the power to discriminate among admissions and exclude patients they considered unlikely to benefit from asylum care. Those responsible for the commitment of patients, they argued, were largely to blame for the accumulation of chronic cases in the asylum. As Babcock put it in 1891, "There certainly must be a lack of appreciation of the purposes of the Asylum, as well as a disregard for the rights of individuals when two little sisters aged 7 and 9 years, respectively, are sent here at the same time as insane, when suffering from Chorea or St. Vitus's dance; or when the father of a sixteen year old boy, who had been idiotic from his fourth year, was allowed to think that his son's mind could be restored by treatment here."[73]

Griffin blamed carelessness on the part of certifying physicians for most of these improper commitments. As he noted, no one could be committed without the certificates of two physicians. Yet many medical certificates showed signs of hasty examination and an unwillingness to consider alternatives to commitment: "How often might [the physicians] say to the Commissioners: this vagrant negro is a natural imbecile; put him to work on your Poor House farm: this woman, 80 years old, is simply in her dotage; it will be more humane to let her die at home, and even cheaper to assist the family in her care, than to send her to the Asylum; or this man is crazed from drink; get him a physician and a nurse and in a few days he will be as well as usual."[74]

Commitment papers provide some support for the superintendents' charges. The physicians' certificates were sometimes so vague or general as to be of little value. Under the section "Facts indicating Insanity," physicians reported things such as "We find her insane," "Given by her father, brother, and several other neighbors," "General behavior," "He wants to be a Vagabond," "His mode of life, habits, and conversation."[75] A few certifying physicians were barely literate. The physicians in one case stated that "we say him have an Epileptic fit also his behavior towards runing at larg and disturbing the people. We therefore recommend his being confined in an Asylumm."[76] Certifying physicians occasionally cited secondhand evidence to justify a patient's commitment, as in the following example: "His talk and actions are rational, but information from his relatives and his being in the Milledgeville [Georgia] Asylum makes the case an asylum one. His appearance is calm and peaceful."[77]

Physicians sometimes confessed uncertainty about the propriety of commitment but signed the papers anyway. One doctor wrote the following about a patient he had certified: "I think he is dangerous — I have never seen him when he was so violent he could not be managed. I think he is a proper subject for admission to the Asylum but I cannot give any recommendation as to his admission. . . . I know that his family and himself are very poor people — I don't think them able to take care of him at home — I think his disease is chronic meningitis of old persons."[78]

Ensor, Griffin, and Babcock advocated a change in the commitment law that would allow the asylum to discriminate among admissions and give preference to recent, acute, and dangerous cases and exclude idiots, imbeciles, and harmless chronics. Before Babcock achieved this change in 1894, the superintendents appealed to county commissioners, probate judges, and physicians to be more selective in sending patients to the asylum. In a speech to the South Carolina Medical Association in 1879, Griffin urged physicians to exercise greater care in examining alleged lunatics and deciding whether or not they were fit subjects for the asylum. The following year, he sent a circular to the probate judges asking them to concede "by courtesy, what we cannot exact by law, namely the principle of discrimination."[79]

Griffin's complaints convinced the legislature to change the commitment procedure in 1884. The new law required physicians to state that the person they were recommending for commitment was "incurable at home" and "violent or dangerous." The act also limited the admission of idiots, epileptics, inebriates, and drug patients to those considered dangerous; made physicians liable to fine if they certified someone who was "simply idiotic, epileptic, physically infirm, or mentally imbecile"; provided fines for probate judges and county commissioners who committed someone without a medical certificate conforming to these new requirements; and required the families or counties of inebriate and drug patients to pay for their maintenance.[80]

The act brought about a drop in admissions in 1885, when there were seventy-seven fewer than in the previous year. But the decrease was only temporary. In 1894, Babcock convinced the legislature to pass an act giving the superintendent the power to refuse patients and spelling out more carefully the order of preference for admission. The 1894 act also took away the power of committal from the county commissioners and put it exclusively in the hands of the probate judges.[81]

These changes also had little effect on admissions. According to Babcock, the county commissioners continued to wield considerable influence over the committal of patients through their recommendations to the probate judges. Some of the correspondence regarding commitments bears this out. For example, Babcock sent back the commitment papers of an old woman with the statement that the hospital was overcrowded and urged she be sent to the poorhouse. The county supervisor wrote to the probate judge that they could not take her at the poorhouse, "so you will just have to take her on to Columbia." The patient was sent to the hospital and admitted a few days later.[82]

Babcock charged that the local officials and physicians tended to interpret the admission criteria too broadly, in an attempt "to relieve [the patients'] families and friends of unpleasant burdens."[83] Certainly, the commitment papers of many patients stressed the family's inability to provide care at home and the disruption or economic difficulties the patient was causing, as in the following examples:

> Her presence creates constant fear and alarm in her vicinity [so] that her natural guardians are worn out with care from constant watching and fear of bodily harm.
>
> N. H. [an idiot from birth] is now eighteen years old, is physically strong and is under the care of afflicted and aged grandparents with no other members of the family except two uncles both of whom are idiots. The grandparents are very poor and unable to support the said N. H. who is . . . very violent and refractory when excited.[84]

Yet the superintendents' charge that local officials were responsible for crowding the hospital with improper commitments was not completely fair. The absence of any suitable alternative to the state asylum led some probate judges and physicians to send patients there out of a sense of desperation. One judge wrote apologetically to Babcock that he was committing an eight-year-old boy, apparently an epileptic, rather than keep him in the county jail: "Under the law I have no power to send this Lunatic either to the poor house, or back to his Father and Mother, who say that they can do nothing for him. The County Superintendent says he cannot take him. I see no other way out of this difficulty but to commit to your care this boy and have issued a commitment to the Sheriff to take him to you."[85]

The superintendents almost always admitted such patients, however much they protested their commitment. Ensor sometimes turned away patients when the asylum was overcrowded, even when they were "brought to our doors in manacles."[86] But Griffin and especially Babcock were more reluctant to refuse admission to those who arrived with the proper commitment papers. Before 1894, they could argue that they had no choice. As Griffin put it, "It is often charged that the asylum is maintaining many persons who are not fit subjects of its charity. It is true, but it is not our fault. No one is admitted except in conformity to the law."[87]

After 1894, the superintendent could legally refuse admission to patients he considered unlikely to benefit by asylum care. But Babcock seldom used the power, because he conceived it his duty to accept whatever patients the local officials sent him. He told the investigating committee of 1909 that "it would be a great blessing if we did not have to receive [improper patients], but until you provide some other receptacle for them for the protection of innocent women and children, we have got to receive them here. . . . I am personally responsible for receiving these patients. . . . [M]y idea is to administer the institution with the broadest charity."[88]

Babcock often urged probate judges not to commit a patient. But if a judge persisted, the superintendent almost always admitted the patient. Babcock pleaded with one probate judge not to send an eighty-year-old woman who was at the county poorhouse and to make efforts to care for her there: "We are very crowded here and if we admit her we have to refuse a curable patient. At her age we can do nothing in the way of cure and the change to this institution may hasten her death. Please refer the case to the physicians and I will abide by their decision." The judge sent the patient, and the superintendent admitted him.[89] Babcock wrote another probate judge that he would accept a patient, although he was a harmless chronic, because he had accepted similar cases in the past. The superintendent's letter revealed clearly his personal responsibility for accepting such admissions: "I have agreed to admit other equally harmless cases here because the county officers and physicians did not consider them proper subjects for the County Poor House. . . . Having today agreed against the advice of

Governor Ansel and the Board of Regents to receive such cases, I cannot make an exception of yours." [90]

Babcock was particularly reluctant to refuse admission to white women patients. He felt a sense of special responsibility to protect southern white womanhood at its most vulnerable. In 1893 he told the regents that, although the wards for white women were badly overcrowded, it was "inadvisable" to refuse to admit more "as long as we can possibly crowd another patient in." The alternative, to send them to the county jails, was unthinkable, because they were the "very class of patients that should be best provided for." [91] In the following years he admitted on several occasions that he had not used the discretionary powers the law gave him. In 1896, for example, he reported that had received every application for admission "except three or four for small children of four and six years." [92] In 1909 he told the legislative investigation, with some exaggeration, that he had "not turned away three patients since I have been here. We take them and do the best we can, if we have to crowd them until they cut one another's throats." [93]

The superintendents' efforts to control the asylum's population met with little success. The consequences were tragic. Combined with the inadequate appropriations the asylum received, overcrowding produced an abominable situation for its patients, from both a medical and a hygienic standpoint. The patients may not have cut one another's throats, but they often died of one another's diseases. In 1903, Governor McSweeney remarked that he feared that the asylum's "lack of means has seriously handicapped the officers in their efforts to develop and maintain the institution up to the high standards to which they have aspired." [94] Just how far short of attaining these standards the asylum had fallen became abundantly clear a few years later.

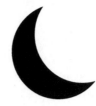

Thirteen

THE HORRORS OF THIS PLACE

LIFE IN THE POSTBELLUM ASYLUM

Thomas Doar was a patient in the South Carolina State Hospital (formerly the South Carolina Lunatic Asylum) during the early years of this century. He wrote many letters to his sister Annie. Often, as in the following letter of August 1908, he complained about conditions in the hospital:

> It is utterly impossible for me [to] form any idea of things in the noise and tumult of a Crazy house where you have to be on the watch all the time to keep from being trampled under foot and mashed to pieces. . . . I have tried to . . . describe to you what the horrors of this place is, but you seem to willing to beleave what others tell you, that I am doing well in here. . . . It would be oh! like new life to be out of this dirty filthy place. . . . I am jammed into a little Cell which is really not big enough for one person . . . with another patient, and am locked up like some wild Animal every night. . . . Often the person in the room with you is sick, and to be locked into a close Cell in this *not Enervating* climate with fumes of all descriptions is enough to make you fade out of existence.[1]

Doar's family and friends were inclined to dismiss his complaints as delusions.[2] But we should not. By the turn of the century, conditions at the South Carolina State Hospital approached the horrific. Retrenchment weighed heavily on everyone associated with the hospital in the late nineteenth and early twentieth centuries, but the burdens fell most heavily on its patients. The hospital's rules, as revised in 1891, stated that "the South Carolina Lunatic Asylum was established and is maintained for the benefit of the insane alone. The health, comfort, and humane custody of these unfortunate patients must therefore receive the highest consideration."[3] In their quest to keep down expenditures, however, the hospital's administration sacrificed the patients' health, comfort, and even their lives.

In 1895, the South Carolina Lunatic Asylum became the South Carolina State Hospital for the Insane. Babcock proposed the change to emphasize that the institution was a hospital, not a prison or an almshouse.[4] Ironically, by the time its name changed, the asylum's function had become essentially custodial. The percentage of patients the hospital discharged as recovered fell from about 30 percent in the 1870s to less than 17 percent of those admitted between 1902 and 1911.[5] Although the decline may have reflected the adoption of more rigorous criteria for what constituted a recovery, there is little doubt that the hospital's primary emphasis had shifted from cure to care. It was not an unusual development. By the 1870s, asylums throughout the Western world were becoming clogged with chronic patients, and most of those concerned with the care of the insane were discarding the therapeutic optimism of the early nineteenth century. But the retreat to custodialism at the South Carolina State Hospital was more thoroughgoing than in many other mental institutions. In 1904, a special report of the United States Bureau of the Census revealed that the South Carolina State Hospital's recovery rate was about 5 percent below the national and South Atlantic averages.[6]

One sign of the emergence of a custodial regime was the gradual decline of moral treatment. During the late nineteenth century, asylum physicians everywhere were losing faith in the therapeutic effectiveness of moral treatment as they confronted the accumulation of large numbers of chronic cases in their institutions. Increasingly, experts on insanity stressed that it was a disease of primarily somatic origins, and that psychological therapies could do little to influence it. "Any other conclusion," the *American Journal of Insanity* claimed in 1865, was "an absurdity."[7]

The move away from moral treatment was gradual. Asylum superintendents in South Carolina and elsewhere did not suddenly abandon the antebellum emphasis on the physical and mental benefits of occupation and amusement. They continued to preach the value of work and recreation as a means to divert the patients' minds and to promote order within the institution. Superintendents valued occupation and amusement not only for its therapeutic benefits but also as a benign means of keeping patients calm and manageable. More activity meant fewer disturbances and less use of drugs and mechanical restraint.[8]

But however much the superintendents may have wanted to keep their patients occupied and amused, their ability to do so declined considerably in the late nineteenth century. The hospital population grew much faster than the staff and the facilities. Hampered by overcrowding and poorly de-signed buildings, the physicians found it increasingly difficult to classify and separate patients according to their mental or physical condition. They mixed violent and suicidal cases, epileptics, idiots, the criminally insane, and the feeble-minded and senile of all ages through the wards, making any systematic program of moral therapy nearly impossible. At the same time, relentless pressure for retrenchment left little money available for activi-ties many taxpayers seem to have viewed as frills. The hospital authorities, facing constant charges of extravagance, were determined neither to be nor appear to be wasteful. In 1878, after a Columbia newspaper reported on a Christmas dance at the asylum, the executive regent reported that the danc-ing "was not done with his knowledge nor was his consent asked." Such "scenes of revelry," he added, were "not in keeping with his idea of the proper management of such an institution."[9]

Occasional dances continued during the following decades, but many other traditional diversions, such as bowling, billiards, and rides and walks through the city, gradually disappeared. By the early years of the new century, patients were providing much of their own entertainment. Many patients made their own checker sets. In 1908, the white men patients started a baseball team, but the games soon came to an end due to lack of support from the administration. A former patient complained that the hospital did not encourage occupation or recreation, and that "there were no diversions except by the patient's initiative."[10]

The emphasis on the need for amusement and occupation also gradu-ally disappeared from the institution's annual reports. After the early 1890s, Babcock ceased to write about the subject, probably because there was little to report; he was increasingly overwhelmed by the sheer problems of keep-ing the ever-increasing mass of patients fed, housed, and clothed. In 1909 he admitted that the hospital provided little amusement for the patients and blamed the situation on the rapid growth of its population combined with the emphasis on economy: "In the good old days when there were two hundred and fifty patients in the institution it was possible to have the patients go driving and to give them all those little pleasures of life, but with this overwhelming population, how are we going to have patients go to drive without going up against the question of favoritism? To give those patients proper buggies and carriages . . . would cost enormously."[11]

By the beginning of the twentieth century, the South Carolina State Hospital was doing less to occupy its patients than most other American institutions for the insane. The legislative investigation of 1909 claimed that the proportion of the hospital's patients who participated in occupation and amusement was well below the average for American hospitals. The scope of occupational and recreational activities available was also much smaller at the South Carolina State Hospital; its staff made no systematic attempt to match patients with suitable employment. Most of the hospital's patients spent their lives sitting in their rooms or wandering about the corridors and yards.[12]

Although some patients did have employment, its nature and purpose changed during the later nineteenth century. It became more economic than therapeutic, and race increasingly influenced the allocation of tasks. During the antebellum period the rationale for getting patients to work was primarily therapeutic. In the 1850s, for example, Trezevant wrote that he didn't care how long the patients took to lay out a garden, because his aim was to occupy them. After the Civil War, asylum authorities increasingly tried to cut costs by having patients do much of the institution's cleaning, repair, and general maintenance. Patients worked at mending shoes, making clothing, sewing, cleaning, laundering, painting, and farming. In 1893, Babcock wrote that the patients' work substantially reduced the hospital's expenses. Former patients testified in 1909 that they did "most of the inside work" and that they kept busy "washing [other] patients, scouring out the spittoons, everything that was needed on the ward."[13] During the 1880s and 1890s, patients also provided labor for hospital construction. They made bricks, dug foundations, and helped erect buildings.[14]

As in the antebellum period, occupation and recreation was rigidly differentiated along gender lines. Women patients continued as before to engage primarily in indoor work and passive, sedentary recreations; men patients tended to work outdoors and be involved in more vigorous activities. Griffin reported in 1878 that "some of the more delicate ladies are driven out every pleasant day, [while] many of the men take frequent walks in the suburbs. . . . In the female department, though a few of the colored find employment about the kitchens, the chief occupation is sewing. . . . On the male side as many as will are employed in the farm and garden and in work about the grounds." Like his antebellum predecessors, he complained that it was much easier to find work for the women patients than for the men. The women could find plenty to do around the wards, the kitchen, the laundry, and the sewing room. Finding work for the men was more difficult, because the asylum did not have enough land to occupy more than a small percentage in outdoor activities.[15]

Employment was also differentiated along racial lines. As the number of black patients grew in the late nineteenth century, they came to dominate certain types of work. Black women patients began to specialize in cleaning, laundry, and kitchen work, whereas black men took over most of the menial work outdoors. The increased use of black patient labor complicated the problem of providing occupation for the white men patients. The hospital established a workshop in the early 1890s, where white males made mats, rugs, and picture frames and did horn and scroll work. But few of them could be prevailed upon to do this or any sort of work. Babcock attributed the difficulty to the presence of black patients: "If we did not have the negroes here, we would get very much more work out of the white men, and work is a means of leading to the restoration of health . . . but with white men the work is unpopular because we hire the negro man to do the hauling out of the slops, the shoveling of coal, and things like that."[16]

The use of black patient labor around the hospital increased considerably from the 1880s, and its justification was primarily economic. In 1909, Babcock claimed that he had saved the state a great deal of money on new buildings because he had used "negro male patients for hod-carriers, excavations and things like that."[17] Black patients also did most of the work in the laundry, kitchen, dining rooms, and dairy. Babcock decided to employ black men patients to do the milking because the hired black workers frequently went on strike. The hospital's treasurer argued that it would be impossible to run the asylum economically without the labor of the black patients, because "it is impossible to get any work of any consequence out of white people, and the negroes do quite a lot of the drudgery."[18]

Race substantially influenced the hospital's provision of both occupation and amusement. The investigating committee of 1909 estimated that 40 percent of the black patients were employed, but only 24 percent of the white women and 16 percent of the white men. When it came to amusement, however, the positions of the two races was reversed. The hospital gave the white patients cards, a weekly dance, the use of a gramophone, and occasional other entertainments. For the black patients, the investigation reported, the hospital provided "no amusement whatever."[19]

According to the hospital's officers, all work was voluntary. Much of it probably was. Some patients helped with cleaning and caring for other patients because they wanted to keep occupied, to be helpful, or merely to ameliorate their unpleasant surroundings. One former patient recalled that he and his fellow patients "did a heap of work" on the ward trying to keep it clean and free of bedbugs.[20] Many patients worked in return for privileges and presents. Like superintendents elsewhere, Babcock encouraged patients to work by giving them extra food, tobacco, and clothing. The substandard diet and amenities the hospital provided probably increased the number of such "volunteer" workers. Tom Doar wrote home that he had been working on the infirmary ward because he was "allowed to eat what is provided for the sick patients, which is better prepared than what we have in the mess room." The patients learned, he claimed, that it was "a privilege to be allowed to work, and of course I get a few advantages in the way of a glass of milk occasionally and a little better fare than what the crowd gets." But he did not consider the work voluntary. He complained that he was forced to work "in order to get something that is fit to eat," and that the more he did, the more he was asked to do. After a few months at the hospital, he told his sister that he wouldn't mind getting a job as an attendant after his discharge, because he was "working as hard as any of them." [21]

The superintendents and other officers claimed that they never used coercion to get patients to work; it was against the rules. But in the case of black patients at least, this rule was sometimes bent. During the investigation of 1909, a legislator asked Babcock if the hospital had ever forced patients to work:

A: No sir. Nobody in this institution has ever been forced to work. If they work it is of their own volition, and that entirely.

Q: Is that a set rule . . . for blacks and whites?

A: Yes sir. . . . The only departure from that is occasionally colored women would circulate among the other colored women and say they should not work. Whenever I have known of that in my department, I have had those women who were stirring up strife locked up.[22]

The decline of moral treatment at the South Carolina State Hospital in the late nineteenth century was not matched by an increase in medical therapy for insanity. The hospital's physicians used a lot of medicine, but primarily to combat the patients' abundant physical maladies. Many patients arrived suffering from one or more diseases, some of them, as the physicians frequently complained, on the verge of death. The overcrowded and unsanitary conditions of the institution bred more illness, and altercations among patients, falls, and other accidents produced many cuts, bruises, and occasional broken bones. The physicians were constantly confronted with malarial and other fevers, tuberculosis, influenza, pneumonia, worms, ulcers, tumors, infections, abscesses, boils, hernias, venereal diseases, and a host of bowel, stomach, menstrual, skin, eye, ear, nose, and throat disorders. They also had to deal with occasional invasions of smallpox, typhoid, and other epidemic diseases. After 1907, they diagnosed and treated large numbers of pellagra cases.

Some idea of the challenge they faced can be garnered from the experience of the hospital's first woman physician, Sarah Allan, hired in 1895. Allan kept a diary between January and May 1900. During this period her "doctoring" was confined to the treatment of physical illnesses, as the following selections illustrate:

> January 1, 1900. Smallpox scare in town again. Vaccinated four nurses. . . . Early in the a.m. Mrs. J. was pushed down by another patient and left hip dislocated or fractured. . . .
>
> January 8. L. C. vomited two round worms this a.m. . . .
>
> January 11. Mrs. G.'s eye to be removed Saturday. . . .
>
> January 14. L. T. bit off the end of Miss W.'s left thumb today, just below nail. Could not find the piece. . . .
>
> January 27. As Dr. B. did not take charge of the Negroes, I had to amputate the big toe of A. R. . . .
>
> February 13. Poor Mrs. M. after much misery to herself and others died today of general tuberculosis. . . . M. W. also died of tuberculosis. . . .
>
> February 15. Colored woman came with a bad burn on the abdomen with flat iron, big slough. . . .
>
> March 6. A good many [patients] have malaria aches. . . .
>
> March 17. Had a series of tooth pullings this morning, about six patients were relieved of some of their teeth. . . .
>
> April 3. . . . Miss D. cut Miss A. on head with knife at table, one stitch needed.[23]

It is difficult to determine precisely how the hospital's physicians viewed and used medical therapy for insanity itself. They recorded almost nothing about their psychiatric theory, principles, or practice. Nor do the patients' case histories of this period provide much information about treatment.[24]

The available evidence indicates that the physicians employed much the same medicines as their colleagues in other contemporary mental institutions. The emphasis, as in the later antebellum period, was on supportive and calmative treatment. The most commonly used medications were tonics and stimulants—such as iron, quinine, and alcohol—and various sedatives and hypnotics, particularly potassium bromide and chloral hydrate.

During the 1890s and early 1900s, patients often received drugs such as strychnine, sulphonal, and potassium iodide. The physicians occasionally prescribed old standbys such as calomel, opium, morphine, and digitalis. They gave alcohol—mainly whiskey—to inebriates and morphine for drug cases, gradually reducing the amounts. Some of the physicians began to use the antisyphilitic drugs salvarsan and neosalvarsan shortly after Paul Ehrlich developed them in 1910 and 1912.[25] Until 1910, however, the hospital had no facilities for hydrotherapy, which many other American hospitals for the insane had been using for some time. Babcock claimed that the hospital could not afford to buy the equipment or hire nurses with training in hydrotherapy.[26]

During the investigations of 1909 and 1914, most of the hospital's physicians professed little faith in the efficacy of medical treatment for insanity. Experience played a part in this development, but so did changing theories about the nature and causation of insanity. Late-nineteenth-century psychiatrists tended to reject the antebellum view that mental disorders were largely environmental in origin and functional in nature. Increasingly, they came to see insanity as an organic disorder in which heredity, along with syphilis and alcohol abuse, played a major role. The physicians at the South Carolina State Hospital gradually came to accept these views, and with them, a more pessimistic outlook about the chances of curing insanity through any existing medical therapy.[27]

Babcock testified that he considered medicine less important in the treatment of the insane than outdoor activity, occupation, and amusement (which he confessed the hospital was unable to adequately provide). The primary value of drugs in cases of insanity, he claimed, was to relieve insomnia. Most of the assistant physicians held similar views, to judge by their testimony before the legislative investigations of 1909 and 1914. For example, Dr. Thompson stated that the hospital's patients did not receive any systematic treatment for insanity, because there was no effective treatment; the hospital, he declared, was a mere custodian. Dr. Eleonora B. Saunders, the hospital's second woman physician who replaced Dr. Allan in 1907, was somewhat more optimistic. She argued that insanity itself could not be cured by medicine, but that drugs, if properly used, could help both mind and body. Saunders was energetic and well informed about the most recent trends in medicine. She studied hookworm, pellagra, and other diseases and promoted the use of new therapies and laboratory techniques, including salvarsan, hydrotherapy, and electric massage. In 1913 she became the first physician at the state hospital to use the Wassermann reaction, a test for syphilis that August Wassermann and his colleagues developed in 1906.[28]

Babcock supported Saunders's efforts, but the other assistant physicians were more pessimistic, if not fatalistic, about their work and resented her enthusiasm for new therapies and techniques. In their testimony before the 1914 investigation, they admitted that they did not follow Saunders's lead in introducing the Wassermann reaction into their departments. Doctors H. H. Griffin and W. E. Fulmer testified that the test was not essential in diagnosing syphilis; they claimed that they could diagnose the disease without it. Fulmer asserted that syphilis had been diagnosed "ever since the world has been here" but confessed that he did not know how many of his patients had the disease.[29] Fulmer did not seem to think that it mattered much what the physician did: "You can make a diagnosis of one kind with an intention and expectation of [curing them], but you fail to cure them. They get well themselves." He even seemed to be uncertain as to whether or not insanity was a disease:

Q: As I understand you are there to keep them and not to cure them?
A: I cure them when they get sick, if possible.
Q: Well, they are sick when they come there?
A: Well, they come there for insanity, not sickness.
Q: Ain't that a form of sickness?
A: Well, it is a brain affection, as I consider it. . . .
Q: You would not have brain trouble unless you had some disease?
A: Well, of course, that is the source of the majority of it. I am no authority on insanity whatever.[30]

How patients viewed the treatment they received at the hospital is difficult to know. Few of them recorded their impressions, and those who did, invariably, were white males. One former patient who testified at the investigation of 1909 stated that he was given no medical treatment during two stays in the hospital. The only treatment he got, he said, was restraint and baseball, and he had initiated the baseball. When a legislator asked him if he had observed any systematic efforts toward treatment of the patients, he replied that he had never seen any: "The inebriates and the dope fiends had a sort of drug treatment, and medicines were given to other patients—certain medical prescriptions, but I never saw myself any specific treatment." The hospital, he concluded, "surrounded me with unhealthy conditions, and left me to struggle and get well the best way I could in spite of them."[31]

This patient's emphasis on restraint as a treatment accurately reflected the nature of the hospital around the turn of the century. Seclusion and mechanical restraint flourished during these years. Methods of restraint in use at the hospital around 1900 included various types of leather mit-

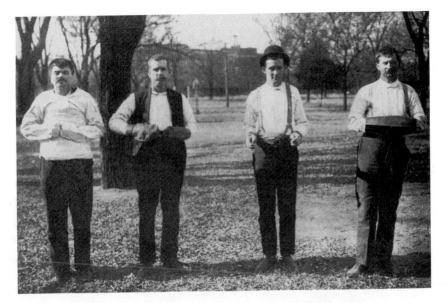

Restraints used at South Carolina State Hospital, 1909.
(From Report of the Legislative Committee on the State Hospital, *1910;*
courtesy South Caroliniana Library, University of South Carolina)

tens, muffs, belts and wristlets, bed straps, restraint sheets, straitjackets or camisoles, and canvas sleeves. The case histories of the period indicate a routine use of restraint. Many records contain statements such as "restraints are kept on him night and day," "generally in restraint," "requires constant restraint," and "keep him restrained all the time."[32]

During Babcock's tenure, the hospital probably used mechanical restraint more than at any time since the 1830s and more than many contemporary mental institutions. The authorities of many American state hospitals were trying to reduce the use of mechanical restraints during the later nineteenth century. Babcock's heavy reliance on restraint may have been connected with the fate of his predecessor. Griffin's critics had accused him of being lax about controlling dangerous patients. Although the South Carolina State Hospital, unlike most other contemporary state hospitals, kept no statistical records of restraint, the impression of widespread use of mechanical restraint is verified by other sources. According to the investigating committee of 1909, the average proportion of patients under restraint at any time in American hospitals for the insane was 1 percent; the committee estimated the proportion at the South Carolina State Hospital was 7 percent overall and 10 percent in the white men's department.[33]

Routine use of mechanical restraint at the hospital was partly a consequence of a high ratio of patients to attendants and physicians. Over-whelmed by the mass of patients and free from close supervision by the physicians, it is not surprising that attendants sometimes used restraint to make their job easier. Tom Doar wrote home that when he complained about things going missing from his room, the attendants told him "you can have your room locked and be locked in it yourself if you dare to com-plain too much."[34] The supervisor of the white men's department testified that the lack of discipline at the hospital was such that attendants frequently put patients in restraints without notifying the physicians or himself, as re-quired by the rules. Some attendants may not have been aware of the need to report the application of mechanical restraint; a former attendant stated that he had never received a copy of the hospital's rules.

But the liberal application of mechanical restraint was not merely due to laxness. It was also the result of conscious policy by the physicians. The assistant physician for the black men told the investigating committee of 1909 that the heavy use of mechanical restraint in his department was necessary because his patients were so violent that it was impossible to control them in any other way.[35] Babcock used the same argument. Large numbers of women patients were restrained, he stated, because "women are rather violent." He also defended the use of mechanical restraint as "a good therapeutic measure." Like other superintendents who defended me-chanical restraint, he asserted that its use was preferable to manual restraint by attendants or heavy reliance on chemical restraint. Moreover, many hos-pitals that had supposedly abolished mechanical restraint still used it: "I have visited asylums in which it was advertised that restraint was not used and seen a camesole in use."[36]

The patients' dietary condition also deteriorated during the late nine-teenth century. The officers constantly sought ways to cut down on the ex-penditures for food. A month after he became superintendent, Peter Griffin suggested that the institution could save money by providing black patients a less expensive diet. A cheaper diet, he argued, would be "more in accord with [the black patients'] habits and tastes" than the existing one, which all patients received. The regents doubted the feasibility of further cuts in rations but gave the superintendent and steward power to change the diet as they thought fit.[37] A few years later the regents themselves ordered that grits should be substituted for rice wherever possible and that beneficiary patients should receive fewer "luxuries."[38] Milk was a luxury. After a visit to the North in 1890, Griffin told the regents that one of the things that most impressed him about the asylums he had visited was their liberal provision of milk. He reported that New York's Bellevue Hospital, with a patient population only about one-third larger than that of the South Carolina Lunatic Asylum, consumed almost ten times as much milk.[39]

Shortly before Babcock took over as superintendent, his brother wrote him that he had heard that "the food furnished [at the asylum] was very poor." Babcock came to the same conclusion. One of his first monthly reports referred to the asylum's food service as the weakest aspect of its management. But he was unable to improve the quality of the dietary; if anything, it got worse.[40] The 1909 investigation declared the food service to be extremely poor. Frederick Wines, a national expert on welfare institutions, inspected the hospital for the investigating committee and reported that the food was unappealing and insufficient in amount. The regular menu was starchy and monotonous, with a heavy concentration on hominy, corn bread, and bacon.

Both Wines and the investigating committee described the main kitchen as poorly designed and equipped and extremely unsanitary. Flies had easy entrance through the unscreened windows. The head cook was said to be incompetent and his department totally undisciplined. The previous cook had died of tuberculosis shortly after leaving the hospital. The kitchen for the black women patients was located in an old brick building without a floor and was unscreened despite its proximity to the stable and a dirty urinal swarming with flies. The men's dining rooms were dirty, and the patients were served unappetizing and poorly prepared food on greasy tin plates. The women's dining rooms (especially those for white women) were generally cleaner and more attractive, but all suffered from overcrowding and inadequate staff and equipment. The hospital dairy was poorly equipped and filthy.[41]

A few patients recorded their impressions of the hospital food service in the early twentieth century, seldom with fondness. A former patient in the white men's department described the basic diet in 1909. Breakfast regularly consisted of hominy with ham, biscuits, and coffee; eggs were served occasionally. For dinner, the patients generally got mushy rice, ham, or bacon with cornbread; potatoes and other vegetables were plentiful in season. Supper was usually bread and molasses with coffee. He was served ground beef two days a week. The rice, grits, and coffee he found to be "pretty poor." The beef was "unpalatable," but the milk was "usually very good." This patient's diet was superior to that of many other patients. He ate in the so-called pay room, which served the higher class of white patients, paying or beneficiary. The patients in the mess hall or main dining room, he believed, never had fried meat or milk. Whereas patients in the pay room had their meals served on china, mess hall patients' meals were served on "tin plates which were very greasy, and usually it was all put together in one plate. The patients in the mess hall complained very bitterly. . . . They say [the food] was very poor, and it was served in such a way that all the appetite they had was destroyed." On one occasion, he had seen corn full of weevils being ground for hominy. The eggs, he said, were often dirty, and many patients would not eat them.[42]

Another former patient with serious bowel trouble agreed that the food was "pretty tough" and that he and the other patients could not eat some of it. The rice was like "glue," the eggs were dirty, and the milk had "black, dirty settlement at the bottom." He said he had watched the milking, which was done by black men patients: "During the time they were milking they were chewing and spitting [tobacco] across the bucket. . . . I saw a cow that had her foot in filth raise it and set it in the bucket, and I was looking for him to wash it out, and he just milked right on into the bucket."[43] A former patient who had also been confined in the New York State Hospital at Poughkeepsie recalled that its diet was far superior to that at the South Carolina State Hospital.[44]

Patients with some money could supplement the hospital fare by purchasing food from outside vendors, a situation that aroused envy. Tom Doar wrote home that the paying patients were "better cared for than the non-pay ones. Some of them send out for orders each week for delicacies to eat." He got enough to eat but complained that the preparation "is very rough, and the food is far inferior to what we are accustomed to." Worse than the poor quality of the food was the lack of time the staff gave the patients to eat: "we have to bolt everything, which is all the harder on [the stomach]."[45]

Patient complaints about the food usually made little impression on the administration. Such grumbling was "to be expected," according to one regent, who claimed to have found the diet "clean, wholesome, and substantial."[46] Yet some of the officers and employees admitted that the food was monotonous and often prepared and served in unappetizing and unsanitary ways. In 1909 Dr. Thompson agreed that the food in his department (white men) was not particularly wholesome or appealing to a sane person. He conceded that the white men's mess hall and the main kitchen were dirty, and that the patient helpers did not clean the dishes properly. The assistant physician in charge of the black men's department, H. H. Griffin, claimed that his patients' food was "better than they are accustomed to," but he would not "care to live on it himself."[47] In 1912, one of the regents declared that much of the bread was neither palatable nor wholesome. The dough was not properly mixed, and the result was that much of the bread

TABLE 3. *Percentage of Deaths of Patients under Treatment at the South Carolina State Hospital, at Five-Year Intervals, 1890–1910*

Year	All	Blacks	Whites
1890	14	21	9
1895	13	17	9
1900	16	23	10
1905	13	17	9
1910	14	21	8

Source: *Annual Report*, 1889–90, 1894–95, 1900, 1905, 1910.
Note: Averages are rounded to the nearest number.

was indigestible: "A well and strong man at hard labor might afford to eat the bread . . . but sick people cannot do it." He recommended that the hospital buy a dough mixer and hire a professional baker. Two years later, the regents were still discussing the purchase of a dough mixer.[48]

The most horrific consequence of the hospital's frugal and inefficient management was exhibited in high mortality rates, especially for black patients. Between 1890 and 1913, nearly 14 percent of the patients under treatment died. Black patients were about twice as likely to die as white patients.[49] These mortality rates were apparently much worse than those of similar institutions in the nation and region. In 1904 a special report of the United States Bureau of the Census revealed that the mortality rate at the South Carolina State Hospital for that year was more than double the national average and almost double the average for the South Atlantic states. The black death rate was double the regional average and more than double the national average for blacks in mental institutions.[50]

The high mortality at the South Carolina State Hospital was not due entirely to substandard conditions. The severe poverty that afflicted much of the state's population undoubtedly contributed to it. Many patients arrived at the hospital suffering from severe physical diseases in addition to, or that may have produced, their mental symptoms. Nor can the comparatively higher black mortality be blamed solely on the hospital environment. Blacks in the general population had much higher mortality and morbidity rates than whites. Blacks also had a lower resistance than whites to one of the biggest killers of the hospital's patients, tuberculosis. Because of their greater poverty and lower access to health care, blacks may also have been more likely to arrive at the hospital near death than whites.[51]

Yet the hospital's manifest deficiencies undoubtedly increased its mortality rates. A dietary heavy in grits and bacon may have contributed to deaths from nutritional disorders such as pellagra, a niacin deficiency disease Babcock first diagnosed at the hospital in 1907. The physicians attributed more than eleven hundred deaths to pellagra between 1908 and 1914. Overcrowding hastened the spread of infectious diseases. By 1909, the hospital housed fifteen hundred patients in buildings designed for one thousand. Most of the buildings were badly maintained, poorly designed, or obsolete. Many patients slept in corridors or in basement rooms that were poorly ventilated and devoid of natural light. These rooms were "more suggestive of dungeons than of living and sleeping apartments for the afflicted," charged the chairman of the State Board of Health.[52]

The facilities provided for the hospital's black patients were particularly bad. All the superintendents between the 1870s and the 1920s blamed the institution's high black mortality rates largely on inferior accommodations. The old asylum building erected in the 1820s, crammed with black women patients, had a mortality rate of more than 34 percent of the average number of inmates in 1908 and more than 28 percent during the previous five years. In 1909, about sixty patients in this building were living in damp ground floor rooms that Trezevant had condemned as unhealthy more than half a century earlier. The previous year, two patients had died from smoke inhalation in one of these rooms, which was next to the antiquated furnaces. Almost twenty years before Babcock had complained that the patients in this building were "surrounded by such hygienic evils as insufficient ventilation, defective plumbing, want of sunlight, and overcrowding."[53] More ideal conditions for the spread of tuberculosis, typhoid, and other infectious diseases could hardly have existed. In the Parker building, which housed black men, conditions were no better. The death rate in the Parker building averaged 27 percent between 1903 and 1908. This building was infested with vermin, and many patients slept on straw. Designed for about 200 patients, it housed 330 at the beginning of 1909. The investigating committee estimated that almost 500 black patients had died unnecessarily between 1903 and 1908 because of conditions in these two buildings.[54]

Tuberculosis was the leading cause of patient deaths during these years. Between 1900 and 1908, the physicians ascribed one patient death in three to tuberculosis. Much of this mortality was preventable, but the hospital's authorities did little to prevent it. Their inaction was not a matter of ignorance. In 1895, Babcock wrote an article for the *American Journal of Insanity* on the prevention and care of tuberculosis in hospitals for the insane. He argued that the disease was communicable and that its spread in institutions could be prevented by various hygienic measures and isolation of confirmed cases. "If my facts are true," he concluded, "then a high death rate from tuberculosis means bad hospital hygiene; and a very high mortality, criminal negligence."[55]

For several years thereafter, he pleaded for the creation of isolation wards or separate pavilions for the tuberculous patients as the only measure likely to greatly reduce the mortality rate. But he was unable to secure the necessary money and took no effective action to solve the problem. The investigating committee of 1909 expressed amazement that he had not undertaken any of the preventive measures he recommended in his article. The superintendent, the committee pointed out, was among the first to insist on the contagiousness of the disease, "yet in our Hospital no steps are taken to prevent contagion. Patients suffering from this disease are on most of the wards, mingling freely with other patients, drinking out of the same vessels and sometimes sleeping in the same rooms. . . . The State is now maintaining in its Hospital a breeding-place for this disease."[56]

The hospital's high rate of mortality was aggravated by other deficiencies. Among them were the high ratio of patients to staff and the low quality of attendants. Under Griffin and Babcock, the hospital never had enough physicians and attendants, and the situation became worse over time. Although the number of assistant physicians increased, the number of patients increased much faster. The ratio of patients to physicians (including the superintendent) rose from 105:1 in 1878 to 376:1 in 1909. In comparison, in 1894 the nine state hospitals of New York had an average patient-physician ratio of 171:1; in 1923, American mental hospitals averaged 234:1.

The reality was often worse than the official physician-patient ratios implied. Between about 1903 and 1910, Babcock had charge of the black women patients as well as the general administration of the institution. After Dr. Sarah Allan resigned from her position as physician to the white women patients in 1906, he handled seven hundred women patients of both races for several months. An assistant physician hired in 1906 to care for black men patients spent only one to four hours a day at the hospital; the same was true of the assistant physician the hospital appointed in 1910 to relieve Babcock of the care of the black women patients. The report of the legislative investigation in 1914 concluded that the care of the black patients was effectively "left to ignorant nurses."[57]

Forced to deal with so many patients, the physicians found it increasingly difficult to provide the patients with personal attention. Dr. Allan's diary from 1900 provides some sense of what the rapid growth of the patient population meant from the physicians' perspective:

January 16. . . . Number up to 1016 and we find hard work accommodating them. . . . Number of women patients present today, 570.

January 19. . . . As Dr. B[abcock] is away for a few days, I had all the women to see today.

January 23. I have the darkies again owing to numerous calls to the Superintendent. . . .

February 21. . . . Darkies come in rapidly and not hopeful cases either. . . . The house is so crowded that bed patients have to room with others . . .

February 22. Very glad to give up C[olored] to Dr. B[abcock].[58]

As the number of patients per physician increased, their contact with the physicians declined considerably from the antebellum period. This was happening in other state hospitals, but it was hard for both staff and patients to accept. In 1897, a nurse complained that Babcock visited the wards so seldom that there were "many patients whom he does not know."[59] Other staff members and patients made similar charges in the following years. Dr. Thompson complained in 1909 that Babcock was out of touch with conditions in the wards because he seldom visited them or consulted with his assistants. The only part of the hospital Babcock spent much time in according to Thompson was the white women's wards. The superintendent acknowledged the charge with pride: "I honestly admit that I have paid more attention to the white women here than to any other department, but at the same time I do not mean to apologize for it. . . . I think they were entitled to the best we had."[60]

Some patients were content with the attention they received from the physicians. One wrote to Babcock after his discharge that he would "never forget you and your assistants, but more especially you and your kindness. . . . If you had been my own son you could not have been more considerate of me in a sad and trying experience."[61]

But other patients complained about the lack of attention from the physicians. Tom Doar wrote to his sister that the doctors were kind and "polite and attentive, but it is not often that you see them. . . . I seldom ever have the opportunity of speaking with Dr. Thompson and never see Dr. Babcock at all." In another letter, Doar described a rare visit by Babcock: "Dr. Thompson has not been on the ward today. I hear he is sick, and I think it must be so for Dr. Babcock came through the male wards today, something I never knew him to do before. I spoke to him and asked him if he knew me, telling him my name. He asked me how I was getting along, and seemed to know that I had been to the Hospital in Rhode Island. . . . All this he said to me in passing me in the hallway, hardly stopping at all, and out he went, so I am as much in the dark as ever." From the patient's perspective, the physicians' ward tours resembled the levees of royal dignitaries, with the patients playing the role of humble supplicants. When the physicians appeared on the wards, Doar claimed, he had to compete with the other patients wanting to speak to them. On one occasion, he told his sister that he would try to speak to Thompson at the first opportunity, but that he did not want "to impose on a man who is beset on all sides as soon as he enters the ward." One day when Babcock made an appearance, Doar "begged him for a few words. He told me to make it short."[62] A former patient told the investigating committee in 1909 that he saw "very little" of Babcock while in the hospital on two different occasions: "I saw him once when Dr. Thompson was away. I saw him just as he went through a side door. . . . My first stay I saw him three times and my second stay I saw him twice."[63]

The medical staff was also unable to cope with the increasing volume of paperwork regarding patients. The hospital's clerical establishment did not grow or change with the size of the institution. The investigation of 1909 found the clerical department totally inadequate for a large, modern hospital. Babcock did not have his own office or his own secretary and did not keep regular office hours. The three assistant physicians shared an office and a secretary in the main hospital building, but they had no filing cabinets or any system for dealing with correspondence and records. Relatives of patients, and patients themselves, frequently complained that their letters asking for information went unanswered. In his early years, Babcock seems to have been able to answer correspondence about the patients. But he was unable to keep this up. On several occasions Governor Martin Ansel ordered Babcock to reply to correspondents trying to find out about the condition of relatives or friends in the hospital.[64]

Due to the lack of clerical staff and facilities, the keeping of case and other patient records became increasingly perfunctory. The staff physicians, according to the 1909 investigation, did not generally make complete physical or mental examinations of newly admitted patients, nor did they keep records of such examinations as they made. The hospital kept no regular clinical records, only the commitment papers and brief case histories, which rarely contained much information about the progress or outcome of the case. Often the case histories merely repeated information in the commitment papers. By 1914, the situation in the white wards had improved, but the physicians in charge of the black patients still made no specific examinations. The physician of the black women's department, Dr. Fulmer, admitted in 1914 that he did not routinely diagnose or examine new cases on admission. He merely recorded the diagnosis on the commitment papers and looked the patients over: "I think any one who looks at them can tell whether they are a healthy woman or depressed or anemic person."[65]

As in other large mental institutions of the time, the physicians' limited contact with patients enhanced the importance of the attendants and nurses. But the number of the attendants did not keep pace with the growing patient population, either. It is difficult to ascertain the ratio of attendants to patients for particular times, because the officers did not usually include this information in the annual reports. Nevertheless, the general trend at the hospital between 1880 and 1910 was toward a higher ratio of patients to attendants.

The hospital's regulations, as well as expert opinion, stipulated that the ratio of attendants to patients should be 1:10. But Babcock reported in 1893 that this proportion had seldom been maintained. In 1877, the ratio was 1:10.6; by 1909 it had risen to 1:18 in the departments for white women, white men, and black women. In the black men's department it was an astonishing 1:36; on one ward there were only two attendants for 111 patients. Around the turn of the century, the proportion of attendants to patients in American mental institutions averaged about 1:12; in the South, it averaged 1:15. Such averages can be misleading, however, because they only record the situation at one point in time. Various circumstances could lead to sudden reductions in attendants' numbers. Governor Tillman pressed for staff reductions soon after he took office in 1891. Dr. Thompson, who was then acting superintendent, responded by discharging several attendants and other employees. Attendants sometimes suddenly resigned or were discharged for breaking the rules; they could not always be replaced quickly. The number of attendants could also be substantially reduced at times because of sickness. Dr. Allan's diary refers constantly to sick nurses. During the first half of 1900, she seldom had a full complement of nurses for the women's wards because of illness, resignations, and leaves.[66] The hospital's officers often complained about the difficulty of procuring and retaining sufficient numbers of qualified attendants.

The attendant corps changed radically in some respects during the later nineteenth century. The increasing number of black patients led to the hiring of black attendants to care for patients of their race. Simultaneously, South Carolina natives of both races gradually took over all the attendants' positions, ending the dominance of Irish immigrants. In 1860, three-fourths of the attendants were of Irish birth. In 1900, all of them were born in the United States, and all but one of them in South Carolina. The decline in the number of Irish did not reflect an improvement in the status, conditions, or remuneration of the position of attendant. Few immigrants were attracted to economically declining South Carolina in the decades following the Civil War. At the same time, the state's chronically depressed economy made native whites more willing than they were in the antebellum era to apply for asylum work. Politically, too, it became difficult to hire any but South Carolinians for state jobs.[67]

Yet many attendants did not stay at the state hospital long. Although the position of attendant was more secure than many other jobs, its long hours, unpleasant duties, and relatively low wages reduced its attractiveness. Attendants often had to spend much of their time cleaning up the patients and the wards. They had to endure taunts, insults, abuse, and occasional violence from patients. Dr. Allan recorded that one violent patient had put the nurses "in a state of terror lest she get out and attack one [of them] alone for the keys." Another entry described the attempt of an epileptic patient to escape: "Day before yesterday Mrs. S. jumped the fence, ran away, attacked the nurses who followed and then fell into convulsions just as they restrained her. . . . After this very violent, kicking, etc. They finally got her in and in her room; for 24 hours she was alternately crying and kicking."[68] When a legislator asked one former attendant in 1909 how he liked the work, he replied, "I can not say that I liked it. I have always had it to do." He recalled having to clean out the rooms of some of the "filthy" patients several times a day. According to Dr. Saunders, most attendants viewed the hospital as "a mere stepping stone, because asylum work is not altogether pleasant work. . . . [A]fter staying here a week or . . . a month, they get something better."[69]

Many attendants strongly resented the hospital's attempts to enforce strict control over their personal lives. The rules, as in most contemporary hospitals, required the attendants to devote virtually all their time to the needs of their patients, even to sleep on their wards. Attendants were not allowed to leave the institution without the approval of the superintendent.[70] The lack of free time away from the asylum, along with the tendency of attendants to become involved in employment and business outside the asylum, led to the development of what Babcock described in 1892 as the "substitute system." This was a practice of allowing attendants time off if they could procure a substitute to perform their duties. Babcock did not approve of the system, and he initially modified it by insisting that he have the right to name the substitute; then he asked the regents to abolish the practice and prohibit the attendants from outside work. As compensation, he recommended that they receive two weeks paid vacation every year after a stipulated period in the service. In 1912, the regents granted all nurses two weeks' vacation after one year's service.[71]

Comparatively low wages reduced the attractiveness of work as an asylum attendant. During the late nineteenth century, the regents tried to keep attendants' wages as low as possible. In 1877 the base salary for men attendants was $300 per year; for women, $200. The following year the regents reduced the attendants' wages on the grounds of the general depression of the economy. The base wages of women attendants fell from $16.50 to $12.50 per month; of white men attendants, from $25.00 to $18.50. Black men attendants suffered the steepest cut: from $25.00 to $12.50. The salaries of the physicians and administrative officers remained the same. In 1909 the wages for white men attendants ranged between $25.00 and $31.00 per month. The pay for black male attendants was $17.50 to $21.50 a month—at a time when, as one assistant physician put it, they could get a dollar a day shoveling dirt on the streets.[72]

The superintendents supported differential pay scales for black and white attendants. Griffin opposed the reduction of wages for white (but not black) attendants in 1878 and generally supported white attendants' attempts to secure wage increases. He claimed that the only way to retain quality white male attendants was to keep wages competitive; otherwise they would leave for less arduous jobs with the police force or the railroads. He could get acceptable black attendants at low wages, he claimed, because they had fewer opportunities for alternative employment than whites.[73]

But Griffin's approval of racial differentials in pay was more than a matter of economic calculation. It was also an attack on the relative racial equality among asylum employees that existed under the Reconstruction regime. In his view, it was essential to maintain a distinction between attendants based on race as well as on gender. For example, in 1878, the wages of white and black women attendants were set at the same rate: $12.50 per month. When the white female attendants petitioned a few months later for an increase to $15.00 per month, Griffin supported the increase, "provided that no change be made in the compensation of the colored attendants, which I think is already sufficient." The regents agreed.[74]

Despite the differential between black and white attendants, wages for both groups were low compared to similar occupations elsewhere. Shortly before Babcock became superintendent, his brother wrote to him in astonishment at "the remarkably low wages for which the Asylum employees work. How can [the asylum] expect to get competent persons for so little?"[75] The answer, as Babcock often repeated in the following years, was that the institution could never get, or keep, enough competent attendants. Even the best attendants seldom had much knowledge about the care of the insane or even much education at all. None had any formal preparation for their positions until after 1892, when Babcock established a training school for nurses at the hospital. Many were illiterate or semiliterate. The investigation of 1909 revealed that attendants who could not read the labels on medications sometimes gave medicine to the patients. One patient testified that he sometimes wrote out the monthly ward reports for attendants who could barely write. Dr. Allan frequently complained to her diary about the student nurses' poor academic preparation. "It takes strength to teach them," she concluded wearily after one class.[76]

As in the antebellum period, drunkenness among attendants was a chronic problem, and dismissals for alcohol-related offenses remained fairly common. The superintendents also discharged attendants for insubordination, obscenity, inefficiency, unauthorized use of restraint, abusing patients, and various violations of the asylum's rules. Sometimes the problem was not the attendant but a relative. In 1877 one of the regents reported a nurse in the female department for neglecting her duty to care for her husband. "If left to herself," he related, "she is a good and efficient person, but she is almost daily beset by a good for nothing drunken husband who occupies entirely too much of her time." The regent noted that he would have discharged her but had been unable to procure a suitable replacement.[77]

Because it was difficult to replace attendants quickly, the hospital authorities were reluctant to discharge even the incompetent or abusive. The investigation in 1909 revealed that several attendants who had abused patients remained at the hospital for months or more. In one case, a nurse was discharged twice for abusing patients. When a legislator asked Dr. Thompson why the hospital retained such attendants, he replied that they were so short of help that they could not afford to let them go. The supervisor on the white male wards complained during the same investigation that the lack of suitable replacements forced him to keep undisciplined and incompetent nurses on his wards.[78]

Securing a sufficient supply of suitable attendants and nurses was a problem all nineteenth-century hospitals faced. After the 1870s many hospitals sought to improve the quality and quantity of their staff through the establishment of in-house training schools. Hospitals in Boston, New York, and Philadelphia established the first training schools in 1873; Charleston's City Hospital followed suit in 1881. In 1882 Boston's McLean Hospital created the first training school at a mental hospital; by 1895 training schools existed at more than thirty other hospitals for the insane in the United States. The training schools were designed to teach nurses through a more formal course of study than traditional on-the-job learning. The promoters of such schools anticipated that most of the pupils would not remain at the hospital after graduation but become private-duty nurses. The great advantage to the hospital was that the trainees provided a source of inexpensive and, the hospitals hoped, easily disciplined labor.[79]

Babcock, who had spent several years at McLean Hospital as assistant physician, started a training school for nurses soon after he came to the South Carolina Lunatic Asylum. In establishing the school, Babcock was strongly influenced by his experience at McLean. He quoted McLean's superintendent, Dr. Edward Cowles, in support of his view of the school's role and organization. Babcock envisioned the school as having a dual purpose: to train attendants for the asylum and "to fit young women, as in general hospitals, to undertake nursing in all its branches. Nurses who enter the School will be regarded as coming here to fit themselves for an honorable calling, as well as to assist in caring for the sick and afflicted in this Asylum."[80]

A training school had other advantages, according to Babcock. It could aid the work of the medical staff, introduce the more efficient methods of general hospitals, and banish the idea that the asylum was a prison. To help him establish and run the school, Babcock hired Katherine Guion, a nurse from North Carolina who had trained at McLean Hospital, the Government Hospital for the Insane in Washington, D.C., and Massachusetts General Hospital. Babcock saw mental nursing as a branch of general nursing and wanted a comprehensive, two-year curriculum that would provide instruction in that field as well as in elementary anatomy, physiology, and hygiene. Such a foundation, he argued, was essential to prepare students to learn mental nursing and to fit them for other nursing jobs outside the asylum. The instruction was to include daily training in ward duties, reading assignments, and weekly lectures by members of the asylum staff.[81]

Babcock told the regents that the staff showed considerable interest in the training school. But this seems to have been the bravado of the young enthusiast determined to convince his reluctant and conservative superiors of the feasibility of his plan. Many of the staff, as he well knew, were opposed to or unattracted by the idea of a training school. Babcock told Guion shortly before she arrived that she would have to overcome many obstacles to make the school a success. The personnel, he warned her, were neither well informed about nor receptive to new methods in psychiatry:

"To be frank, the idea of a training school for nurses . . . probably does not meet with the entire approval of those now in the service."[82]

Babcock's more pessimistic assessment was closer to the mark. He initially proposed a school that would train all attendants, with separate classes for each sex and race, but he was apparently unable to convince the regents and the staff to support this ambitious plan. A few months later he announced that the school would enroll all the currently employed women attendants first, then require all newly hired attendants to enroll as probationers. In practice, this turned out to mean white attendants. He noted in 1893 that the black men attendants were being "given a modified course of instruction." But sixteen years later, the physician in charge of the black men's wards stated that the black attendants did not receive any formal training: "You see as a rule they are very ignorant. We have some over there that cannot write."[83]

The decision to begin with women only was also soon changed, perhaps because too few women enrolled. In 1892, Babcock reported that the school had opened, with fourteen women and ten men enrolled in the first two classes. He claimed to be pleased with the beginning and with the improved "care and attention intelligently given the patients." But many attendants did not enroll or dropped out before completing the course, and the requirement that new attendants enroll was quickly abandoned. In 1893, at Babcock's suggestion, the regents agreed to determine merit pay for attendants in part by completion of the training school curriculum. This incentive may have increased enrollment for a time. Between 1893 and 1900, the school graduated about six nurses a year, but during the next ten years (1901–10) the average was about four. Virtually all were women. Men stopped enrolling in the school after the second year. Babcock explained that men were reluctant to enter the training school because they could obtain higher wages elsewhere and often took attendants' jobs "as a temporary makeshift" until they could get something better. Some men were reluctant to take the nursing course because they feared to fail it. One told the supervisor of the white men's department that he didn't want to take the classes because he could not write and could barely read. If the officers forced him to take it, he vowed to quit. In 1909 only two white men graduates of the training school worked at the hospital, as opposed to twelve white women graduates. Both men were supervisors.[84]

It is difficult to measure the impact of the training school on the quality of attendants. Any improvement was limited mainly to the white women nurses who cared primarily for white women patients. In the other departments, the quality of nursing was little affected; if anything, it got worse, because the ratio of attendants to patients declined. Vastly outnumbered, poorly trained, and often inadequately supervised, the attendants could hardly have provided a high quality of patient care. One catches a glimpse of the situation in Dr. Allan's diary entry for February 18, 1900: "Intensely cold this a.m. and old Rosa M. found in bed stiff and almost pulseless. . . . Tried administering restoratives and heat. There was a little response, but I do not think she will rally. . . . Urine froze on floors. . . . [I] fear these old darkies were neglected by Miss S. Minerva."[85]

The investigation of 1909 revealed numerous examples of neglect and mistreatment of patients by attendants. As was often the case in asylum investigations elsewhere, witnesses (both attendants and patients) accused some attendants of assaults on the patients, misuse of mechanical restraints, theft, and other abusive acts. But most of the complaints were not about attendants' violence so much as their neglect of patients and ward conditions. A few years later, a former patient who had also been in the New York State Hospital at Poughkeepsie recalled that the attendants there were more violent toward the patients than those at the South Carolina State Hospital: "I myself was struck at different times at Columbia but [it was] nothing to what I experienced at Poughkeepsie." But, he continued, the New York hospital was much cleaner and more attractive than its South Carolina counterpart. Poughkeepsie was "as neat as a pin." In contrast, the Columbia hospital was a depressing place, "uninviting, dirty . . . the toilet rooms are repugnant."[86] After a visit to the South Carolina State Hospital in 1909, Frederick H. Wines wrote that he was shocked by the attendants' "indolence and indifference" toward the filth and dinginess of the hospital environment.[87]

The investigation of 1909 found the condition of the men's wards, both white and black, to be extremely dirty and unsanitary. Bathrooms were often filthy, toilets overflowing, patients dirty and verminous. One former patient with a bowel disorder stated that the attendants on his ward had left him to lie on the floor in his filth for many hours, and that he had been forced to pay a fellow patient to keep him clean. Attendants in the men's wards sometimes bathed several patients in the same water. Bedbugs and lice were endemic in some wards, partly because attendants often ignored the rule which required new patients to bathe and change their clothing. Tom Doar wrote his sister several months after his admission that he was still wearing the same clothes he was brought to the hospital in: "You see there are so many patients and only a few attendants. . . . [E]very time I want to go to [my] trunk [to get new clothes], they are busy, or doing something." Then he added, "To tell you the truth, you might just as well

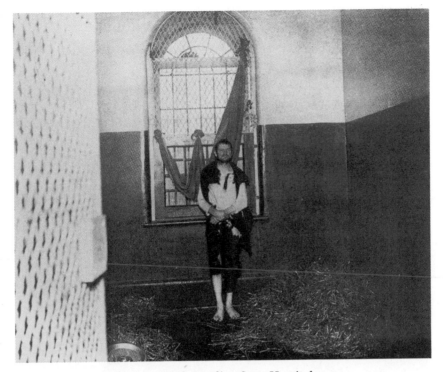

Patient at South Carolina State Hospital, 1909.
(*From* Report of the Legislative Committee on the State Hospital, *1910;*
courtesy South Caroliniana Library, University of South Carolina)

go into a pig pen with your best clothes on as to try to wear them where I
am most of the time."[88]

The 1909 investigation found that the walls had not been whitewashed
for several years and were covered with spit, dirt, and bedbug nests. A
former patient testified that when he complained about the bugs the ward
supervisor, John Mitchell, told him that nothing could be done because
he had no one to do the work. Mitchell later stated that he could have
gotten the bugs out only by neglecting something else. A former attendant
claimed that he had tried to keep his ward as clean as possible, but that
he simply did not have enough help. The physicians agreed. Everyone also
agreed, however, that more attendants alone would not solve problems that
were partly due to the low quality of the personnel. Not surprisingly, the
investigation of 1909 found that conditions in the white women's wards,
which had the most trained nurses, were superior to conditions in the other
wards. Dr. Thompson testified that he could not keep white male nurses
if he forced them to do cleaning. A former white attendant admitted that

he resigned when ordered to whitewash the walls in the white men's wards because he did not think it was his part of his duty.[89]

In 1914, the physician in charge of the black women patients claimed that the problems of his department stemmed largely from the poor quality of the nurses: "If I had the white female [nurses] my results would be better. I have nurses there that cannot read and write their names. . . . [Y]ou know that a negro female is not as intelligent as a white female. . . . I cannot get an intelligent nurse to go there to work."[90] None of the black nurses, of course, had received any formal training at the hospital.

In 1910, the majority report of the legislative committee to investigate the state hospital concluded that the institution had become little more than a custodian for the insane of South Carolina. Since the antebellum period, there had been a marked decline in therapeutic optimism and the employment of moral therapies. Medical therapy became largely a matter of combatting the patients' numerous physical ills. Other state hospitals shared a similar fate. But in many respects, conditions at the South Carolina State Hospital seem to have deteriorated more dramatically than elsewhere.

Evidence concerning occupational and recreational opportunities, use of mechanical restraint, patient-staff ratios, diet, and recovery and mortality rates indicates that the condition of South Carolina's mental patients was among the worst in the nation at the turn of the century. Moreover, conditions for some patients were markedly worse than for others. Black patients were more likely than white patients to be put to work but less likely to be provided recreation. Blacks suffered greater overcrowding, worse sanitary conditions, and higher mortality than whites. In his testimony before the investigation of 1909, Babcock argued that the black patients benefited and white patients suffered from being in the same institution. It is difficult to find any evidence that would substantiate his view.[91]

Discrimination in the care and treatment of patients also extended to whites. Some white patients of a "better class" received preferential treatment in terms of diet, and Babcock unabashedly proclaimed the principle that white women patients were entitled to better care than blacks or white men. For the hospital's more privileged patients, conditions were probably little worse than in many other state mental hospitals. But for the great majority of its patients, the South Carolina State Hospital was unable to fulfill even the minimal expectations of the custodial role. In the words of the majority report of the investigating committee of 1909, "Its custodianship is a menace to the health and life of these afflicted citizens."[92]

Fourteen

THERE IS NOTHING JOYFUL

ABOUT AN ASYLUM

PROGRESSIVISM AND INSANITY

The deteriorating situation at the South Carolina State Hospital attracted little notice until shortly before the First World War. Between 1908 and 1915, however, the institution was the focus of considerable political controversy. By the early years of the new century, the Progressive movement was beginning to make an impact on South Carolina's affairs. The expansion of industry and towns spawned a growing middle class of businessmen and professionals who provided the leadership of the new movement. Legislators influenced by Progressivism battled corruption and pushed for a wide range of political and social reforms, including more humane, efficient, and rational management of state institutions.[1]

One result of these efforts was a damning legislative investigation of the state hospital in 1909. In 1910 Progressive legislators proposed a series of reforms in the care of the insane, including the removal of superintendent Babcock, administrative reorganization, and the establishment of two new mental hospitals — one for each race. A bitter political fight followed in which Babcock's supporters united with anti-Progressive forces to defeat the proposals. In a compromise, the legislature created the State Hospital Commission to buy land and begin developing a second state hospital. Babcock remained as superintendent and was appointed to head the commission. This body purchased a large tract of land at State Park, a few miles from Columbia, but development was slow. The building of a second hospital was hampered by inadequate funding, lack of clear direction, and opposition from Governor Cole Blease and his anti-Progressive supporters. In 1914, conflict between Babcock and Blease led to another legislative investigation at the hospital. Although the inquiry proved an embarrassing defeat for the governor and exonerated Babcock, the superintendent resigned. The Progressives subsequently achieved much of their program for the insane during the governorship of Richard I. Manning III (1915–18). For better or worse, the reforms of the Manning era initiated South Carolina's move back into the American psychiatric mainstream.

Babcock was at the center of the political maelstrom between 1909 and 1914. The degree of his responsibility for the condition of the state hospital was debated vigorously in the press and the legislature. The superintendent was not oblivious to the hospital's deficiencies. More than most of his predecessors he was aware of the manifold needs of mental institutions. His years at McLean had provided him with experience of what was then considered a first-rate mental hospital. He kept informed about the latest ideas about psychiatry through reading, participation in the American Medico-Psychological Association, and occasional visits to other hospitals. He corresponded regularly with other superintendents, especially T. O. Powell of the Georgia State Asylum and P. L. Murphy of the North Carolina State Hospital at Morganton.[2] Babcock's reports frequently drew attention to the need for improvements and suggested various innovations to bring South Carolina up-to-date in the care of the insane. But his criticism of substandard conditions at the hospital, though frequent, was muted and general. Moreover, he seldom went beyond reporting problems. Had he made more of a nuisance of himself in defense of his institution's needs, it might not have deteriorated to the extent that it had by the first decade of the twentieth century. Although he worked extremely hard and seldom took a vacation, his efforts were not always well directed. A fellow psychiatrist who visited the South Carolina State Hospital in 1900 commented that Babcock had failed to make significant progress there because he tended to fritter away time on nonessentials and peripheral interests. "Dr. Babcock's place has disappointed me," he reported. "He has not reached the goal he aimed for when I was there several years ago. . . . [I]f [he] devoted less time to trifles and outside cases his results would be marvelous."[3]

Ironically, Babcock's conscientiousness and sense of duty contributed to his tendency to be diverted by "trifles and outside cases." He found it difficult to say no to those who sought his advice, even when he knew that saying yes was contrary to the interests of the institution and its patients. An example is the issue of outside consultation. Public authorities, physicians, and private individuals often called Babcock out of the state hospital to consult on insanity cases. Eventually, this became a problem, for in 1897 he asked the regents if they approved of his continuing to consult. Although the board gave him permission, two years later Babcock reported that consulting was disrupting his regular work and that the only way to protect the hospital's interests was for the regents to "forbid my seeing patients outside the institution except in consultation with a physician."[4] As we have seen, Babcock's sense of duty also made it extremely difficult for him to refuse admission to any patient and undermined his efforts to relieve overcrowding at the hospital. His determination to extend the service of the hospital to as wide a clientele as possible was laudable in intention but deplorable in effect. Combined with an inadequate physical plant, low state appropriations, and serious administrative and personnel deficiencies, overcrowding contributed to the creation of scandalous conditions by the early years of this century. The critical nature of the situation became apparent to the public in 1909, when the South Carolina General Assembly appointed a committee to investigate allegations of abuses and substandard conditions at the hospital.

The impetus for the 1909 investigation came from a Columbia lawyer, Hunter A. Gibbes. For several months prior to the investigation, Gibbes had been trying to secure the release of certain patients (mainly inebriates and alleged criminals) at the hospital. He saw himself as a champion of patients' rights. Babcock and the regents viewed his actions as mercenary and disruptive. They implied that his main objectives were to extract money from distressed relatives and cause trouble for the physicians. The lawyer's conflicts with the hospital authorities soon broadened to include conditions within the institution.[5] He secured affidavits from several former patients complaining about its facilities and treatment and, armed with this evidence, petitioned the legislature for an investigation. Gibbes's petition accused the hospital's nurses of abusing and neglecting patients and of exploiting patient labor through "practically a system of peonage." He charged that the administration tolerated disgracefully unsanitary and dangerous conditions, that they admitted patients who did not belong in the hospital, and that they refused to discharge a patient who had recovered unless someone agreed in writing to be responsible for the patient's behavior. Gibbes blamed most of the evils he cited on an outmoded system of organization and careless management and argued that a legislative inquiry into conditions at the hospital was needed to provide a salutary corrective.[6] In response to Gibbes's charges, Babcock and the regents also requested an investigation into the hospital's problems.[7]

Following the receipt of the petitions, the legislature passed a resolution establishing a joint committee to investigate the South Carolina State Hospital for the Insane. The committee's deliberations, which lasted for about a month in April and May 1909, were followed with considerable interest by the press. Several members of the committee, including chairman Senator Niels Christensen, were sympathetic to the goals and methods of Progressivism. Shortly before his work on the hospital investigation, Christensen had battled corruption in the state dispensary. Later, he played an important role in the creation of the State Board of Charities and Corrections, the State Training School for the Feeble-Minded, and the State Industrial School for Girls.[8]

Christensen took his charge seriously, and the investigation was typically Progressive in its thoroughness. The committee inspected the state hospital closely, examined its records, and held several days of hearings that produced more than four hundred pages of published testimony. The witnesses included Babcock and the three assistant physicians, several other employees, two former patients, and a former male nurse. Following the hearings, the committee solicited information and advice from many sources. Three outside experts examined the institution and reported on various aspects of its condition: Dr. F. H. Wines, former secretary of the Illinois Board of Public Charities and a recognized authority on issues relating to the care of the insane; Dr. Robert Wilson Jr., chairman of the South Carolina State Board of Health; and Gadsden Shand, a Columbia architect. Members of the committee visited state hospitals in North Carolina, Virginia, Maryland, and New York, as well as the Government Hospital for the Insane in Washington, D.C. The committee also studied reports of many other state hospitals and state boards of charities and information it received from numerous hospital superintendents.[9]

The committee reported in January 1910 that it was unable to agree on a common set of conclusions and recommendations. Four members, including Christensen, issued a majority report; the three other members authored a minority report. Both reports agreed that the hospital was deficient, but they disagreed on the extent, cause, and solution of the deficiencies. The majority sharply condemned conditions and treatment at the hospital. In their view it was a basically custodial institution that made little effort to provide treatment of any kind for the patients. It was run down, severely overcrowded, badly understaffed, and extremely unsanitary, a combination of conditions that produced excessive mortality and below-average recovery rates. The fundamental cause of the hospital's problems, according to the majority, was administrative. The administration was honest but inefficient, economical in intent but wasteful in result. The rules, regulations, and by-laws of the institution were not in line with modern ideas about hospital management and were often ignored. The regents and the superintendent had neglected their duty by failing to inform the legislature of deplorable conditions at the hospital, by neglecting to conduct thorough monthly inspections of the hospital as required by the rules, by not ensuring that repairs they had ordered had been carried out, and by failing to seek adequate appropriations. The majority report conceded that state appropriations had been too low to maintain proper standards of care but blamed the hospital administration for providing inadequate estimates. Since 1900 the general assembly had granted at least the full appropriation for maintenance the hospital had asked for every year but 1905.[10] Responsibility for these administrative failures, the majority concluded, rested largely with the superintendent.[11]

To remedy the most immediate problems at the state hospital, the majority report recommended that the legislature immediately increase the appropriations for maintenance and repairs. As a long-term solution, the majority recommended that the state sell the existing plant in Columbia and erect two new hospitals in the country, one for each race. To accomplish this, the majority urged passage of two bills: one submitting to the voters a bond issue of one million dollars, to be used to purchase land and construct the new plants; and a second directing the governor to appoint a five-man commission to carry out these tasks.[12]

The committee's minority agreed that the hospital was deficient in many respects. But they did not blame the administration for its problems. Babcock and the regents, the minority argued, were hampered by circumstances largely beyond their control, such as poorly designed buildings, inadequate appropriations, and insufficient staff. The elected officials of the state shared responsibility for the hospital's condition, and to criticize the hospital management alone was unfair.[13] The minority also concluded that most of the charges Gibbes had made against the hospital had not been sustained by the investigation. The officers had not generally violated the laws governing the admission and discharge of patients; in the instances in which they did bend the law somewhat, such as in the admission of "idiots, epileptics, inebriates, and dotards," it had been done in "a broad spirit of charity." Some of the charges about unsanitary conditions and the mistreatment, exploitation, and neglect of patients were true. But they were often exaggerated, and insofar as they could be sustained were largely due to lack of money. An example was the low quality of the attendants (or "keepers" as the minority report called them). Given their low pay and the unpleasant nature of their work, they were "as good as could be expected."[14]

The minority conceded that South Carolina lagged behind some other states in providing for the insane, and that efforts should be made to bring the state hospital up to modern humane standards. But paying for the changes would be difficult due to the state's poverty and relatively high taxes. For this reason, they opposed the majority proposal to move the state hospital out of Columbia and create two new hospitals in the country. Instead, the minority urged that the state maintain the existing plant and purchase a farm several miles from the city, where it could place the epileptics, harmless inebriates, and imbeciles or gradually transfer the black insane. The minority argued that their plan was economical and would quickly remedy the two worst problems at the hospital: overcrowding and the lack of means for classifying and separating the patients.[15]

The differences between the minority and majority reports reflected contrasting outlooks on the future social policy of the state. The majority report exuded the Progressives' determination to expose the most embarrassing abuses and a concomitant faith in the possibilities of rational and systematic reform. The minority report was more conservative, cautious, and defensive, less optimistic that systematic changes could produce major improvements. The minority was also concerned about the effect the investigation would have on the state's image: "We are unwilling to publish to the world that South Carolina is negligent in providing for these unfortunate people."[16]

The split within the investigating committee reflected wider political and philosophical divisions among the informed (white) public of South Carolina. The publication of the report set off a heated debate about the seriousness of the situation at the state hospital and the most effective way to deal with it. At the center of the debate stood the enigmatic Babcock. The extent of his responsibility for the hospital's problems became an issue that at times engulfed what the *News and Courier* called "the most essential feature, what should be done to further alleviate conditions [at the state hospital]?" The newspaper urged that the "personal equation . . . be eliminated" and that the legislature act quickly to deal with both existing problems and future needs.[17]

But it was extremely difficult to eliminate the personal equation in a state that put a high premium on matters of personal honor. Babcock viewed the charges the majority report levied against him as an affront to his standing as a physician and a southern gentleman.[18] He had many influential defenders who shared his viewpoint and were determined that he not be made a scapegoat for the state's neglect of the insane. Babcock had some right to feel aggrieved, because he had often pointed out many of the problems cited in the legislative report in his reports. But his critics argued with some justice that he had not done enough to expose the magnitude of the problems or to campaign actively for their amelioration.[19]

A few weeks after the investigating committee issued its report, the judiciary committee of the state senate passed a resolution requesting that Babcock and the regents resign. The resolution quickly aroused sharp rejoinders from Babcock's defenders. The *Columbia Record* claimed that the resolution was part of an unjustified campaign of persecution designed to destroy the superintendent's reputation. Former governor D. C. Heyward protested that Babcock was being unfairly blamed for conditions he had lacked the power to prevent and had labored ceaselessly to alleviate. Paradoxically, Babcock's supporters pictured the superintendent as both indispensable to and overwhelmed by the problems of caring for the state's insane. They praised him as an altruistic gentleman and first-class physician whose undoing was his devotion to his duty and his state. Heyward insisted that Babcock was the only person in the state with the ability to deal with the immensely difficult problems at the state hospital. Yet Heyward also noted that during the early years of his governorship, Babcock was so "physically and mentally worn out by the burdens which rested upon him" that he offered his resignation.[20] Many legislators repeated similar sentiments on the floor of the general assembly.[21] The senate debated the resignation resolution for three stormy days before voting to table it, twenty-seven to nine. The outcome appeared to be a strong vote of confidence in the hospital's officers. But many legislators remained doubtful about the ability of Babcock and the existing regents to deal with the hospital's problems. One senator who supported the majority report remarked that the superintendent and regents "would do themselves a favor not to have charge of any plan we might now institute."[22]

The practical question of what plan to institute was entangled in and complicated by the personal question of Babcock's fate. Both the investigating committee's majority and minority sponsored bills designed to implement their recommendations. The majority brought in two bills. The first appropriated funds to carry out urgently needed improvements at the hospital and to purchase land in the country to which the present institution could ultimately be moved. The second bill proposed to submit a million-dollar bond issue to the voters, to be used for construction of two new rural institutions (one for each race). The bonds were to be paid off by the eventual sale of the existing state hospital. The minority bill proposed to purchase a large tract of land near Columbia to establish a branch of the existing hospital and to increase appropriations to carry out needed improvements at the Columbia plant.[23]

The lengthy debate over the bills and the future of the hospital inevitably centered on its past management. Generally, those who favored the majority's bills wanted to remove Babcock and the regents, whereas supporters of the minority bill defended the beleaguered officers. One advocate of the minority bill protested that he "did not want to see [the hospital's administration] condemned on the testimony of crazy people."[24] Christensen deplored that concern about personalities and reputations tended to obscure the more important issue of the welfare of the state's insane. But the management of the hospital, he insisted, had been inefficient and incompetent, and effective change would require a new administration.[25] Other senators objected to the minority bill on the grounds that it could be viewed as endorsing the present administration of the state hospital. As one put it, "Those who do not come within the personal charm of Dr. Babcock's personality are the ones now to protect the State's interests."[26]

The debate over the bills was also inevitably and inextricably connected with broader political, social, and economic issues. To Christensen and his Progressive colleagues, the state's prestige was at stake. One senator succinctly stated the views of the Progressives: "The name of the people of South Carolina, their reputation for humanity, and correct habits of modern thought . . . is involved in this matter." But the Progressives' plans to modernize and rationalize the care of the insane had to confront a harsh and tenacious aspect of South Carolina life: widespread poverty and an intense opposition to debt and taxes. The *Charleston News and Courier*, although convinced that major improvements were needed at the hospital, dismissed the bond bill as a fantasy that could never secure the approval of two-thirds of the voters.[27] The majority of the general assembly agreed. The house voted down the bond bill by a large majority. Opponents repeatedly stressed their fear that it would increase the state's indebtedness. One legislator declared that a bond issue was not necessary to solve the problems at the hospital. All that the state needed to do was to buy a farm in the country, "separate the races, and build cottages for the negroes out there." With a little money for improvements, the existing hospital would be suitable for the white patients.[28]

Supporters of the Progressives' proposals argued in vain that the present institution was little better than a prison and a deathtrap, and that it would be more humane and cheaper to build new facilities in the country than to remedy the flaws in the existing establishment. Some advocates of the plan to create two new hospitals appealed to racial fears. They pointed out that the minority plan contemplated putting white patients in buildings that had been declared "unfit for negroes," providing "an up-to-date asylum for negroes and a patched-up asylum for the whites."[29]

But none of the arguments of the bond bill's supporters could overcome the fear of debt. Some opponents of the bond issue questioned even the possibility of making significant improvements in the care of the insane, no matter how much the state spent. One representative, who claimed to speak as a "real Farmer," predicted that the million dollars "would be a mere start" and the results would inevitably disappoint: "There is nothing joyful about an Asylum; there never is, but the State cannot help conditions. . . . You cannot make such a place as an Asylum perfect. . . . [T]he State had better go slow and build for the darkies, and the State will have all that is wanted." Like many others, he thought South Carolina was already doing enough for its insane. He recalled that he had gone through the hospital twice and "was much pleased. Every bed had two sheets, everything was clean and the food good." Others in the house agreed; one legislator recalled that a former patient from his district had told him that he lived better at the hospital than at home. The legislator added that "even in a private family things happen that are not pleasant. . . . [H]ow much more liable is this to happen in an asylum?" New buildings would not change anything, predicted another representative, for "it was utterly impossible for [the hospital staff] to keep all the patients in a neat and tidy condition. No one can expect neatness in an asylum."[30]

After the House of Representatives defeated the bond bill, the majority of the investigating committee withdrew their companion bill. The house passed the minority bill without further discussion, but the senate, where Progressive forces were stronger, rejected it. After a few days both houses agreed to a compromise resolution, which established a hospital commission to buy land, draw up plans, and begin the construction of buildings. The commission consisted of the state hospital superintendent, the chairman of the State Board of Health (Dr. Robert Wilson), and three businessmen to be appointed by the governor. The bill empowered them to borrow up to $100,000 to begin the work. The *Charleston News and Courier* praised the compromise as progressive and "not destructive, either of reputations or anything else." The newspaper condemned the state's niggardly treatment of the insane and criticized the hospital's management for not being more aggressive in demanding higher appropriations. But it lauded Babcock as an efficient and conscientious officer and predicted that some-

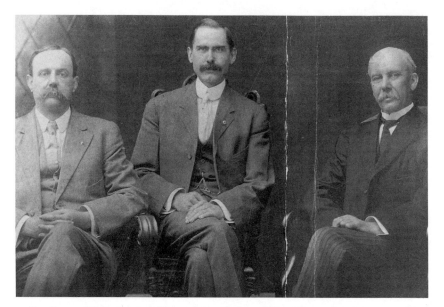

Dr. James W. Babcock (left), with Dr. Robert Wilson Jr. and Col. E. H. Aull,
members of the State Hospital Commission, ca. 1911.
(Courtesy South Caroliniana Library, University of South Carolina)

thing substantial would soon be done to solve the problems at the state hospital.[31]

Events proved the newspaper's prediction unduly optimistic. Despite an increase in state appropriations for maintenance, the condition of the state hospital did not improve significantly during the next few years.[32] In some respects, the situation got worse. Relations among the senior staff became increasingly tense and distant. Babcock was outraged by the attacks on him during the investigation, and he accused some of his subordinates, especially assistant physicians James Thompson and H. H. Griffin, of disloyalty.[33] The superintendent became less involved with the patients than before. As chairman of the new State Hospital Commission, Babcock had to devote much of his time during the next four years to the frustrating task of trying to develop a new hospital at State Park. Hampered by inadequate financial support and a lack of direction, the State Park project made little headway before 1914.[34]

The political climate of the state also inhibited attempts to improve the plight of the insane. Between 1910 and 1914, South Carolina experienced its biggest political upheaval since the Tillman revolution of the 1890s. Once again, the state hospital and its superintendent became the focus of a bitter political conflict. In 1910, Coleman L. Blease, a former Tillman protégé, became governor. Blease's ascent to the governorship alarmed both aristocratic conservatives and middle-class Progressives, for he won overwhelming support from the growing number of textile mill workers and other poor whites. As David Carlton has shown, mill workers voted for Blease not only because he was a racist demagogue but also because he voiced their resentments of the new urban society and its middle-class promoters in business and the professions. The mill workers opposed many of the Progressives' reforms (such as compulsory education and factory regulation) as unjustified government interference in their lives. For several years their support for "Coley" forestalled the Progressives' legislative program. Blease's obstructionism as governor, his coarseness, and his successful appeal to the poor whites frustrated and infuriated the respectable middle class of the towns and most of the state's newspapers, corporations, and traditional political leaders. Between 1910 and 1912, when Blease won reelection, political and class lines hardened and the political temperature rose markedly. Voters went to the polls in unprecedented numbers; in 1912 more than 80 percent of those eligible to vote did so. The ruling Democratic Party, which for years had been marked by shifting coalitions and widespread voter apathy, divided largely along class lines into Bleaseite and anti-Bleaseite factions. By 1912 the anti-Bleaseite camp included Progressives, Bourbon conservatives, and even Blease's former idol Ben Tillman, now a United States senator.[35]

The political warfare of the Blease years had an enormous impact on the state hospital. The governor openly sought state posts for his political supporters and clashed with many state administrators, including Babcock. Blease held a grudge against Babcock for testifying against his friend James Tillman at Tillman's 1903 trial for the murder of N. G. Gonzales, editor of the *State*. Blease later claimed that he intended to remove Babcock for this reason when he became governor but decided not to after hearing Babcock's explanation of his role in the trial. A more likely reason for Blease's forbearance was the superintendent's friendship with Ben Tillman. Blease interfered little in the affairs of the hospital during his first term (1911–12) beyond placing several Bleaseites on its board of regents.[36]

After his reelection in 1912, Blease began interfering more directly in the affairs of the institution. One reason for the change may have been a desire for political revenge. Ben Tillman publicly opposed Blease in 1912, despite an earlier promise of neutrality. Blease was furious at what he saw as Tillman's betrayal, and he decided to seek reprisal by attacking the senator's appointee and friend, Babcock. Following the election, Blease tried to replace Babcock with his family physician, W. G. Houseal, but the senate overwhelmingly refused to confirm Houseal's appointment.[37]

Blease and the Bleaseite regents then began a campaign of harassment designed to force Babcock to resign. They exploited the superintendent's continuing weakness, his relations with his staff. Babcock complained that the regents undermined his authority by encouraging staff complaints and making changes in the senior staff without consulting him.[38] One of the charges the senior staff made against Babcock, and the one that Blease most fully exploited, centered on the second assistant physician, Eleanora B. Saunders. The other assistant physicians complained that Saunders interfered with their departments, was rude, and acted as if she were superintendent; that Babcock favored her over the other assistants; and that he refused to reprimand or control her.

The complaints may have been motivated in part by professional jealousy. Saunders was arguably the most energetic and efficient of the assistant physicians. Her close relationship with Dr. Ernest Cooper, the hospital pathologist, added to the friction. Cooper, who joined the state hospital staff in 1911, had graduated from Johns Hopkins Medical School. There he had learned the techniques of the new scientific medicine, with its emphasis on laboratory analysis. Saunders was eager to apply laboratory methods to psychiatry, and worked closely with Cooper to learn how to perform such things as blood tests and urinalysis. Laboratory medicine was not yet fully accepted by the American medical profession; hostility and skepticism towards its techniques was widespread.

The other assistant physicians at the hospital seem to have shared these views. Perhaps they felt threatened by Cooper's expertise and Saunders's enthusiasm for new ideas. Perhaps they simply resented Saunders's attention to the pathologist. In any event, they charged that the activities of Saunders and Cooper disrupted the harmony of the institution. In response to these complaints, the regents discharged Cooper in July 1913. But he continued to visit the hospital to teach Saunders how to administer the Wassermann test for syphilis. The other physicians complained to the regents that Cooper had no right to come to the institution and insinuated that he and Saunders were involved in a clandestine affair. Cooper's replacement as pathologist, Dr. R. E. Blackburn (who did not know how to perform the Wassermann), accused Saunders of removing materials from the pathology lab without his permission so she could do the tests and charged that Babcock had refused to do anything about it.[39]

Saunders was an unlikely candidate for disciplinary action. The first honor graduate in her class at the Medical College of South Carolina, Saunders had come to the hospital in 1907 to take charge of the white women's wards. Since then, she had worked hard to learn and to implement modern, scientific, and efficient methods in her wards and, when possible, in other wards. Both Babcock and the investigating committee of 1909 praised her energy and devotion to her patients. She was extremely popular with the white women nurses. But her efforts to modernize the hospital did not endear her to her fellow assistant physicians or to the Bleaseite regents. She epitomized in many ways the Progressive outlook Blease's supporters detested. Blease and several of the regents claimed to be scandalized by some of her actions at the hospital, especially her testing of the white women patients for syphilis. The Bleaseite reaction was not unusual. Many people viewed syphilis as a "filthy" disease and a divine punishment for fornication and opposed efforts to prevent or cure it.[40]

Ben Tillman claimed that Blease wanted to oust Saunders and Babcock for political reasons: because they were anti-Blease. There was some truth to the charge. In December 1913, Blease denounced Saunders and Babcock for defying his authority and demanded that the regents get rid of "those people in this institution that are against Blease's administration."[41] The regents first tried to dismiss Saunders in July 1913, at the same time as they fired Cooper. But Babcock appealed to Blease, who recommended that they retain her. Two months later, however, Blease told Babcock that a majority of the regents still wanted to remove her and it would be best if she resigned. Babcock protested that Saunders was the best assistant he had and that he would resign if she was forced out. Blease did not force the issue until November, when he wrote Babcock asking him to "quietly" remove Saunders. The governor explained that he had recently overheard a conversation "engaged in by some ladies" indicating that Saunders had "placed herself in a very unfortunate position" because of her relationship with Cooper.

Babcock replied, correctly, that only the regents could legally dismiss the assistant physicians; he also predicted that Saunders's removal would be followed by "a general exodus of the white women nurses, which will leave unattended nearly six hundred white women patients." Blease ordered Babcock to call a meeting of the board of regents to deal with the matter and retorted that it would be unfortunate if the white women nurses left the hospital, "but if they knew the talk that is going on now, I think the decent women would withdraw, anyhow, if conditions were not changed."[42] Because the regents could have dismissed Saunders themselves, it seems that they were trying to pressure Babcock into removing her, so that they could avoid the appearance of attacking a respectable and popular white woman.

The whole sorry episode exploded at a special meeting of the board of regents held in December 1913. Babcock and Blease were both present as Thompson, Blackburn, H. H. Griffin, and the new assistant physician, W. E. Fulmer, confronted Saunders with charges that she had interfered in their departments. At Babcock's request, Saunders's father, Rep. O. L. Saunders of York, also came to the meeting with his attorney, but the regents barred them from the hearing. Dr. Saunders denied that she had intentionally interfered with anyone else's work, defended her work on syphilis, and claimed that whatever extra work she had done was motivated by a desire to help Dr. Babcock and the patients. She indignantly protested the insinuations of Blease and her accusers that she and Cooper had been sexually involved. At one point, the chairman of the board, Dr. T. R. Carothers, asked Dr. Griffin if Saunders was "a single lady," and Griffin answered, "I suppose she is." Saunders snapped back, "The reference to my being a single woman is an insult. Dr. Griffin knows that I am single." [43]

Blease alternated between appealing for harmony and demanding the resignation of Saunders and other "anti-Bleasites" at the hospital. Babcock stoutly defended Dr. Saunders and asked the board to exonerate her. The regents took no immediate action, but Saunders and Babcock refused to let the matter rest. They claimed that the charges had left a stain on Saunders's reputation. Mr. Saunders demanded that the regents investigate the charges against his daughter so as to clear her "good name." After several weeks, the regents passed several resolutions condemning Dr. Saunders for interfering with her colleagues and suggesting that she resign. The board also reprimanded Babcock for supporting Saunders and denied Mr. Saunders's petition for an investigation on the grounds that no charges had been brought as to her moral character or medical ability. When the regents showed these resolutions to Babcock, he indignantly rejected them and threatened to "refer the matter to another tribunal." [44]

Babcock had already enlisted the support of Tillman, and now asked the senator to push for a legislative investigation of the situation at the hospital. Because the majority of state legislators were anti-Blease, Babcock felt confident a legislative inquiry would exonerate Dr. Saunders. Tillman agreed and told Babcock that if he would "fight with [the] gloves off," he would win. Tillman quickly sent off a letter to a number of state senators accusing Blease and his "underlings and satellites" of trying to remove Babcock so they could manipulate the sale of the State Park property (the land that the hospital commission had bought as the site for a second hospital). Tillman predicted that the "unscrupulous" Bleaseites would try to smear Babcock and Saunders.[45] Whether Tillman intended it or not, one of the recipients of the letter gave a copy to Blease. The governor sent the letter to the general assembly along with a lengthy denial of Tillman's accusations and his own request for an investigation. The revelation and Blease's message created a sensation among the legislators, who quickly appointed an investigating committee. Blease claimed that the furor over his interventions at the state hospital was motivated by political spite, and he was not entirely wrong. The determination of Tillman and other anti-Bleaseites to defend the honor of Babcock and Saunders was quickened by the belief that the investigation provided an opportunity to undermine Blease's political support. The governor's political enemies believed that his attack on Dr. Saunders's character was so unchivalrous that a public disclosure might lead to his impeachment or derail his declared ambition to win a U.S. Senate seat in the 1914 election.[46]

Tillman was so convinced of Blease's vulnerability that he decided to testify on Babcock's behalf. The senator's greatest fear was that the shy Babcock lacked the necessary spirit for what promised to be a nasty encounter. Tillman confided to D. C. Heyward that Babcock was "a man of such refined feeling and so anxious to avoid injuring anything I am afraid he will not fight as he should." The senator continually reminded the superintendent "to fight and strike straight from the shoulder, sparing no one, especially Governor Blease. . . . For God's sake, my friend, stand up and be the man you are, and do not allow these blatherskites and whelps to discredit you, discredit me, and above all, discredit the truth and honorable dealings."[47]

Tillman need not have worried. The investigation was a triumph for the anti-Bleaseites. It opened in the packed chambers of the state supreme court with a much-awaited appearance by Tillman. Then the committee heard from Babcock, Blease, the regents, and the officers who had complained about Saunders. Babcock ably defended Dr. Saunders's honor and medical ability; accused the regents and the governor of trying to force him out and gain control of the hospital; and charged Saunders's accusers of jealousy, incompetence, and disloyalty. He accused Dr. Thompson of scheming for the superintendent's post and suggested that Dr. Griffin had joined the plot to gain revenge for Tillman's dismissal of his father in 1891. Babcock also appealed to his audience's racial prejudices. He insinuated that Griffin was not a gentleman because he had listened to complaints from black attendants about a white woman (Saunders).[48]

Blease's testimony, like the governor himself, was colorful, coarse, and contradictory. He pointed out that the state constitution gave him the power to remove Babcock at any time if he wanted to, and he reminded his audience that Tillman had ousted a political opponent (Peter Griffin) and appointed a political ally and relative (J. W. Bunch) as secretary-treasurer. At the same time, Blease questioned Babcock's fitness for his position and ridiculed his supporters' contention that he was indispensable: "I did not know that he was the only man in the world who could run the Asylum and that when he died all the poor patients would have to be cocained so as to get their treatment in another world." Blease tried to justify the actions against Saunders by suggesting repeatedly that she had compromised herself by her treatment of her colleagues, her relationship with Cooper, and her work on syphilis. On several occasions he (and some of the regents) suggested that working in an insane hospital was something no "decent women" would do: "I am told . . . that women out there . . . handle cases of syphilis and cases of gonorrhea and other diseases which I would not want anybody kin to me that called themselves decent to handle." [49]

Blease's tactic backfired. Saunders successfully portrayed herself as able and dedicated to the welfare of her patients and her accusers as jealous, spiteful, and scurrilous. She immediately became a public heroine and the darling of the anti-Blease press. The investigating committee's report unanimously exonerated Saunders and Babcock, although two of the committee's members were Bleaseites. [50] Based on more than five hundred pages of numbingly repetitive testimony, the report argued that the main cause of the problems and discord at the state hospital was the constitutional proviso that gave the regents rather than the superintendent the power to appoint the hospital's physicians. The result was to prevent the superintendent from exercising effective control and authority over his subordinates. To remedy this source of disharmony, the report recommended that the superintendent be given the power to select and dismiss his staff, subject to the approval of the regents.

The 1914 report, unlike that of 1910, did not include a detailed description of the hospital's conditions, but it was critical of the poor quality of treatment and facilities, particularly for black patients, and the general lack of efficient and modern methods. None of the criticism on this occasion, however, was directed at Babcock. The superintendent, the report claimed, was too overwhelmed by the administrative business of the hospital and the development of State Park to give much attention to matters directly affecting patient care and treatment. The report made a number of recommendations to remedy these deficiencies, which the legislature adopted as concurrent resolutions.[51]

The report was a major political setback for Blease. To his enemies it signified the governor's defeat in what the *Columbia State* dubbed "The War Against the Woman." The newspaper took great delight in noting that Blease had always portrayed himself as the champion of South Carolina womanhood. The negative publicity he received probably contributed to his defeat that summer in his bid to replace Ellison D. "Cotton Ed" Smith in the United States Senate. A few days after the report appeared, the frustrated and embattled governor nearly came to blows in the state house with two of his critics.[52]

Nevertheless, as Blease told the legislature, he was still governor, and the report made him "more determined to exercise" his constitutional powers. He argued that the changes in the hospital's organization contemplated by the concurrent resolutions violated the state constitution and state law and vowed that they would "become a nullity." (A few weeks later, the state attorney general upheld Blease's view.) Blease also made clear that he was determined to get rid of Babcock: "I clearly see from the report that the one thing that it does find is that the institution has not been properly handled. The principal thing I was fighting for . . . was to help the inmates."[53] Although Babcock and Saunders emerged from the investigation in triumph, their position under the Bleaseite board of regents was untenable. Both of them resigned a few weeks later. Babcock opened the state's first private mental hospital (Waverley Sanitarium) near Columbia and became professor of psychiatry at the Medical College of South Carolina. Saunders assisted Babcock at Waverley for a time and later went to the Sheppard and Enoch Pratt Hospital in Maryland.[54]

On the day Babcock resigned, Blease appointed state senator Thomas J. Strait, a former U.S. congressman, as superintendent. Strait was an odd choice in one respect; although he was a Bleaseite, he had been a member of the investigating committee that unanimously exonerated Babcock. Only two weeks before he appointed Strait, the governor had publicly accused him of betrayal. Strait was sixty-eight years old and had no qualifications for the superintendent's job other than being a country physician and sometime political ally of the governor. But Strait's administration lasted only a few months.[55]

The investigation of 1914 and Babcock's departure ended an era in the history of insanity in South Carolina. In the fall of 1914, Richard I. Manning III, a progressive-conservative, was elected governor. Manning's administration represented a watershed in the history of the state. Although many people had voted for him out of disgust with Blease rather than enthusiasm for his program, there was a growing realization among voters that in many respects the state had fallen embarrassingly behind much of the rest of the nation. Manning was able to capitalize on this perception sufficiently to secure the enactment of a number of the Progressives' reforms, including several measures designed to modernize and improve the administration of the state's charitable and penal institutions.

In 1915, the legislature established a central board, the South Carolina State Board of Charities and Corrections, to inspect and recommend changes at such institutions, including the state hospital, the penitentiary, the reformatories, and the almshouses. Most states had long since created a central board or official to supervise such institutions. Soon after it was established, the board began to push for the establishment of a state institution for the feeble-minded. By World War I, the majority of states had already made some institutional provision for the care of idiots and imbeciles. Eugenicists and some mental hygienists were actively publicizing the so-called Menace of the Feeble-Minded and advocating their segregation or sterilization. The idea of segregation won the support of Manning, and in 1918, the legislature established the State Training School for the Feeble-Minded at Clinton.[56]

The Manning administration also implemented major reforms at the state hospital. As soon as he was elected, Manning decided to seek expert advice on dealing with problems at the hospital. He contacted the National Committee on Mental Hygiene (NCMH). The NCMH was a typically progressive organization. Founded in 1909 at the urging of Clifford Beers, a former mental patient, the NCMH was striving to become the national think tank on questions of mental-health policy.[57] On the recommendation of the NCMH, Manning appointed Arthur P. Herring of the Maryland Lunacy Commission to investigate conditions at the hospital and suggest improvements. The governor justified going outside the state for advice on the grounds that he wanted an impartial investigation unclouded by personal and political considerations. The asylum, he told the press, had for too long been a political football. Herring's report, issued in January 1915, repeated most of the criticisms that had been made by the investigations of 1909 and 1914 and made it clear that little had changed during the previous five years. The state hospital, Herring concluded, was deficient in nearly all the essential requirements of an institution for the insane. It was badly overcrowded, severely understaffed, and inefficiently administered.

The buildings were dirty, dilapidated, unsanitary firetraps unfit for human habitation. There was too much use of mechanical restraint and too little effort to engage the patients in occupation and recreation.

To remedy these problems, Herring recommended numerous changes, many of them typical of the progressives' approach to mental-health policy. The facilities at State Park, he argued, should be developed as rapidly as possible, using the black patients' labor. The black patients, along with the idiots, imbeciles, tuberculins, and pellagrins of both races, should be removed to State Park to relieve the overcrowding at Columbia. A psychopathic reception building should be established at the existing hospital, where new patients could be received, thoroughly examined, and if necessary detained for treatment. The Columbia facility should also develop an outpatient department to promote preventive psychiatry. To give the superintendent adequate authority and end the system of divided responsibility, the method of appointing officers should be changed. The superintendent should be appointed by the regents rather than the governor, and the rest of the staff by the superintendent rather than the regents. Herring also recommended additional annual appropriations of $600,000 over five years to pay for more staff, renovations in the buildings at the Columbia plant, and the development of State Park.[58]

Few of Herring's recommendations were new. Most of them had been made by Babcock, the regents, or the previous investigations of the hospital. But the legislature was now ready to make changes it had resisted before and quickly approved Herring's administrative and funding suggestions. Over howls of protest from the Bleaseites, Manning replaced the existing regents and then superintendent Strait. The governor wanted the new superintendent to be a specialist in mental diseases, and he canvassed several national experts for advice. He had chosen Dr. George F. Sargent of the Sheppard and Pratt Hospital in Maryland for the post when a Columbia newspaper pointed out the state constitution required the superintendent to be a citizen of South Carolina. Manning then decided to appoint Dr. C. Frederick Williams, whom he had already chosen as one of the new regents. A Columbia physician in private practice, Williams had formerly served as the state's first health officer. Although not a psychiatrist, he was energetic and a good administrator. He was also sympathetic to progressive currents in the mental-health field and fully in accord with Manning's plans for the state hospital.

One of Williams's first acts as superintendent was to go north and hire experienced psychiatrists as assistant physicians. He then instituted many of the administrative and therapeutic changes Herring's report and earlier investigations had recommended. Mechanical restraint was eliminated by January 1916, hydrotherapy was introduced as a means of calming restless patients, the use of drugs to sedate patients decreased, and the means of occupation and recreation increased. Daily staff meetings were implemented. Methods of examining patients and keeping clinical and other records were modernized. In 1915, most of the black women patients were transferred to the State Park facility, along with about one hundred black men patients. The mortality rate declined from 20.4 percent of the patients under treatment in 1914 to 12.1 in 1916.[59]

Within a few years, the reforms instituted by Manning and carried out by Williams brought practices and conditions at the state hospital into line with those prevailing at other state institutions. In many respects, the state had rejoined the American psychiatric mainstream. Yet the condition of the state's insane remained such as to give little cause for cheer. Although significant improvements were made in the condition of some buildings, the amounts allotted for maintenance increased only slightly.[60] Overcrowding continued to be a serious problem and indeed became critical again in the 1920s.[61]

Moreover, although Manning's reforms affected all the patients, white patients benefited more than black patients. As in other southern states, Progressivism in South Carolina concentrated primarily on improving and uplifting the white population.[62] The State Training School for the Feeble-Minded, for example, restricted its clientele to whites. At the state hospital, accommodations and opportunities for diversion improved more rapidly for whites than blacks. Although mortality rates for patients of both races fell substantially, blacks continued to die at higher rates than whites. In the early 1920s, the death rate for black patients was about twice that of whites. By 1930, the black death rate had fallen to 8.2 percent, but the white rate was 5.0. Williams attributed the difference primarily to the inferior accommodations of the blacks. All of the white patients, he pointed out, had been provided with greatly improved housing. The black patients' quarters had not been improved, making it "impossible under existing conditions to render them the aid they deserve." Inadequate appropriations slowed the development of State Park and the removal of the remainder of the black male patients from the dungeonlike Parker building in Columbia. Williams frequently condemned the buildings allotted to the black patients both in Columbia and at State Park as overcrowded, unsanitary, and poorly ventilated firetraps "hardly fit for human habitation."[63]

Superintendents had been saying much the same for more than sixty years. By the early 1920s, Progressive reforms had eliminated some of the most obvious horrors of the asylum. But much remained to be done to reach the goal of its founders a century earlier: a house of cure for all the insane of South Carolina.

Epilogue

We live in an age that has lost its faith in institutional solutions to the problem of insanity. During the past few decades mental-health policy makers in most Western nations concluded that public mental hospitals were a failure and set in motion the process of deinstitutionalization. But skepticism about institutional solutions is nothing new. In 1831 a South Carolina legislative committee successfully opposed a proposal to establish a state school for the deaf and dumb. The experience of the recently opened lunatic asylum, the committee concluded, showed that "public institutions for the most benevolent purposes do not always succeed."[1]

The bases for these conclusions, however, were markedly different. To late-twentieth-century advocates of deinstitutionalization, mental hospitals had failed largely because they had attracted too many patients of the wrong kind. They had became clogged with the chronically ill, who could derive little benefit from their residence and would be better off in the community. Conversely, the legislative committee of 1831 judged the South Carolina Lunatic Asylum a failure because it had been unable to attract enough patients to justify its existence and pay its way. South Carolina's asylum reformers had predicted that the demand for such an institution would be so great that the fees of wealthy paying patients would subsidize the care of the poor and allow the asylum to support itself without recourse to state aid. To the consternation of legislators already angered by cost overruns in building the asylum, the reformers had overestimated the effective demand for such an institution and had to turn to the state for help.

During the 1840s and 1850s, admissions increased enough to make the asylum largely self-supporting. But for various reasons (mistrust of asylums, cost of care, family pride, advice of physicians, racial exclusion, attitudes of local officials) many potential patients remained in the community, with their families, in poorhouses, or boarded out. Throughout the antebellum period and beyond, asylum advocates deprecated this situation. They were convinced, like asylum reformers elsewhere, that community care was detrimental to the insane, their families, and society. Prompt admission of the insane to an asylum was necessary to maximize their chances of recovery and minimize the dangers their disease posed to themselves and those around them.

Nineteenth-century asylum reformers may have overstated the evils of leaving the insane in the community, as they undoubtedly exaggerated the benefits of institutional care. But, as Andrew Scull argues, late-twentieth-century reformers disillusioned with asylums have promoted highly romanticized notions about the history of noninstitutional care.[2] The evidence concerning the insane outside of asylums in South Carolina defies the sort of easy generalizations that policy makers prefer. The stories of cruel abuse and neglect nineteenth-century reformers marshaled to support asylum care were not merely propaganda; they were real enough. Moreover, the insane who were paupers or slaves and thus under the control of those other than their families must often have fared especially badly. But the evidence is sketchy and decidedly mixed. One can match the horror stories with examples of insane who received kind and sympathetic care in domestic or community settings.

About all one can say with confidence is that from colonial times to the early twentieth century, the insane in the community experienced a wide gamut of care and treatment that was influenced by a complex web of circumstances: class, income, race, status (free or slave), access to medical care, and severity of symptoms all played a part. Physicians and their ideas were important. But so too were the beliefs, attitudes, and resources of families, slave owners, and local officials. Moreover, the insane themselves often helped determine their care and treatment. The exact therapies they received might vary according to how willingly they cooperated with their care givers. The therapies themselves could vary greatly. They might be medical or magical, drastic or moderate, regular or irregular. Many of the insane received no treatment or were dosed with various proprietary medicines, home remedies, or prescriptions from domestic medical manuals. Moreover, medical therapies, both regular and irregular, changed over time. Most drastic in the early nineteenth century, they gradually became more moderate. Yet they tended to retain a certain continuity and consistency based on the idea that mental and other diseases resulted from bodily imbalances that must be combated by regulating the secretions.

The insane who ended up in the South Carolina Lunatic Asylum shared a more uniform experience, although it too varied over time. The aims of those who founded South Carolina's antebellum asylum were paternalistic, in all the ambiguous senses that term conveys. Undoubtedly, the asylum functioned on one level to control the (white) insane and to reeducate them to function in a society in which acceptance of human bondage and male supremacy was a sign of normalcy. But its officers also sought to provide the patients with the most advanced therapeutics and the highest quality care that limited resources and a defective physical plant allowed. The antebellum asylum may never have become the house of cure or happy family that its officers hoped to make it. During the first decade the physicians employed heroic medical therapies and the staff routinely resorted to mechanical restraint, seclusion, and the shower bath to control unruly patients. But the officers implemented a more moderate (although more regimented) regime in the 1840s and 1850s that brought a marked decline in the use of restraint, punishment, and drastic medications. During this period, the South Carolina Lunatic Asylum came closest to fulfilling the ideals of moral treatment, with its emphasis on occupation and amusement in a structured environment. Ironically, one reason for this may have been the relatively low number of admissions during the antebellum period, which kept the patient population small and manageable.

After the Civil War, admissions rose dramatically, and the nature of the asylum and its patient population changed drastically. Its officers did not publicly abandon the asylum's earlier therapeutic and humanitarian goals. Indeed, outwardly, at least, the institution came to resemble a hospital more than ever before. During the 1890s the South Carolina Lunatic Asylum was renamed the South Carolina State Hospital for the Insane. "Attendants" were increasingly referred to as "nurses," and a training school was established to improve their performance. But the inner reality of asylum life was more complex. Like similar institutions elsewhere, the South Carolina State Hospital evolved into a custodial welfare operation with multiple clienteles and functions. It was a poorhouse, nursing home, general hospital, inebriate asylum, and home for the mentally handicapped combined. The complete opening of the institution to blacks and the advent of state maintenance for pauper or beneficiary cases overwhelmed the asylum with a flood of poor patients, many of whom were chronically mentally ill and suffering from various physical disorders. The effect of this influx was exacerbated by the state's economic decline and a series of political revolutions (Reconstruction, Redemption, Tillmanism, Bleaseism) that politicized the asylum. From a largely self-supporting institution, it had become one of the largest single recipients of state aid. As such it was a natural target for patronage-seeking politicians, who were at the same time determined to demonstrate their fiscal conservatism. The chief aim of the superintendents (who changed with every political revolution) became the "study of economy": to care for the patients as cheaply as possible. Despite the superintendents' efforts to limit admissions and return harmless chronic patients to their communities, the patient population grew much faster than the staff and accommodations. Between the 1880s and World War I, per capita expenditures at the South Carolina Lunatic Asylum were at or near the bottom for American state mental institutions. The buildings became increasingly overcrowded, decrepit, and unsanitary. The use of mechanical restraints increased, and efforts to amuse and occupy the patients declined; at the same time the asylum became increasingly dependent economically on patient labor. Mortality grew to scandalous proportions. Except in the white female wards, the training school had little impact on the quality of nursing. That the asylum's black patients fared worst from these conditions is hardly surprising given the simultaneous advent of a white supremacist regime in the state. What is more surprising perhaps is that despite the strong segregationist trend in the state, patients of both races remained in the same institution until after World War I. The horrific conditions in the institution aroused little public concern until they were widely exposed by a Progressive-inspired investigation in 1909. Even then, intense voter opposition to taxes and debt effectively blocked reforms until the administration of Governor Richard I. Manning. Between 1915 and 1918, progressive reformers achieved some improvement in the situation at the state hospital. But it remained a custodial and badly overcrowded institution in which black patients were provided accommodations and care markedly inferior to those of the whites.

In many respects the fate of the insane in South Carolina was not unusual. Slavery before the Civil War and poverty and racialism after it no doubt aggravated the condition of the insane outside of institutions. But by and large, their experience was probably not markedly different from that of the noninstitutionalized insane in other parts of the United States and in Europe. The story of the insane who found their way to the South Carolina Lunatic Asylum between 1828 and the First World War was more complicated. In its aims, methods, organization, and problems, the South Carolina Lunatic Asylum resembled similar institutions in the United States and Europe. Like most of them, it began as a small institution marked by therapeutic optimism and grew into a mammoth custodial warehouse. But the decline in conditions at the South Carolina Lunatic Asylum may have been more extreme than in many other public institutions. The sharp changes in the size, economic status, and racial nature of the patient population between the antebellum and postbellum eras; the state's rapid economic decline; the political bitterness and racial animosities that festered in the wake of defeat, emancipation, and occupation—all combined to produce an environment that was less conducive to public philanthropy than that in places where history moved along in a more benign and less bumpy fashion.

Notes

AR   South Carolina State Hospital, *Annual Report*

CCP   Charleston Commissioners of the Poor, Records, Charleston City Archives

CH   South Carolina State Hospital, Case Histories, South Carolina Department of Archives and History, Columbia

CP   South Carolina State Hospital, Commitment Papers, South Carolina Department of Archives and History, Columbia

DMH   South Carolina Department of Mental Health, Columbia

GAP   Papers of the South Carolina General Assembly, South Carolina Department of Archives and History, Columbia

MBR   South Carolina State Hospital, Minutes of the Board of Regents, South Carolina Department of Archives and History, Columbia

PTR   South Carolina State Hospital, Patients' Treatment Record, South Carolina Department of Archives and History, Columbia

RR   *Reports and Resolutions of the General Assembly of South Carolina*

SCDAH South Carolina Department of Archives and History, Columbia

SCHM *South Carolina Historical Magazine*

SCHS   South Carolina Historical Society, Charleston

SCL   South Caroliniana Library, Columbia

SHC   Southern Historical Collection, University of North Carolina, Chapel Hill

SRR   South Carolina State Hospital, Superintendent's Reports to the Regents, South Carolina Department of Archives and History, Columbia

WHL   Waring Historical Library, Medical University of South Carolina, Charleston

INTRODUCTION

1. C. Vann Woodward, ed., *Mary Chesnut's Civil War* (New Haven, Conn.: Yale University Press, 1981), p. 676.

2. Albert Deutsch, *The Mentally Ill in America: A History of Their Care and Treatment from Colonial Times* (Garden City, N.Y.: Doubleday, Doran, 1937); Gregory Zilboorg, *A History of Medical Psychology* (New York: Norton, 1941); Franz Alexander and Sheldon Selesnick, *The History of Psychiatry* (New York: New American Library, 1966).

3. Erving Goffman, *Asylums* (Garden City, N.Y.: Doubleday, 1961); Thomas Szasz, *Ideology and Insanity* (Garden City, N.Y.: Doubleday, 1970); R. D. Laing, *The Politics of Experience* (New York: Ballantine Books, 1967).

4. On deinstitutionalization, see Andrew Scull, *Decarceration: Community Treatment and the Deviant — a Radical View* (New Brunswick: N.J.: Rutgers University Press, 1984) and *Social Order/Mental Disorder: Anglo-American Psychiatry in Historical Perspective* (London: Routledge, 1989), pp. 300–329; Gerald Grob, *The Mad Among Us: A History of America's Mentally Ill* (New York: Free Press, 1994), pp. 287–309.

5. Michel Foucault, *Madness and Civilization*, trans. Richard Howard (New York: New American Library, 1965).

6. David Rothman, *The Discovery of the Asylum: Social Order and Disorder in the New Republic* (Boston: Little, Brown, 1971) and *Conscience and Convenience: The Asylum and Its Alternatives in Progressive America* (Boston: Little, Brown, 1980); Andrew T. Scull, *Museums of Madness: The Social Organization of Insanity in Nineteenth-Century England* (New York: St. Martin's Press, 1979), *The Most Solitary of Afflictions: Madness and Society in Britain, 1700–1900* (New Haven, Conn.: Yale University Press, 1993) and *Social Order/Mental Disorder*; Richard W. Fox, *So Far Disordered in Mind: Insanity in California, 1870–1930* (Berkeley: University of California Press, 1978).

7. Scull, *Social Order/Mental Disorder*, pp. 31–39.

8. Gerald Grob, *Mental Illness and American Society, 1875–1940* (Princeton, N.J.: Princeton University Press, 1983), pp. 5, ix–xiii, 3–6, and *Mental Institutions in America: Social Policy to 1875* (New York: Free Press, 1973), pp. xi–xiii. See also Gerald Grob, *From Asylum to Community: Mental Health Policy in Modern America* (Princeton, N.J.: Princeton University Press, 1991) and *Mad Among Us*.

9. Nancy Tomes, *A Generous Confidence: Thomas Story Kirkbride and the Art of Asylum Keeping, 1840–1883* (Cambridge: Cambridge University Press, 1984); Ellen Dwyer, *Homes for the Mad: Life Inside Two Nineteenth-Century Asylums* (New Brunswick, N.J.: Rutgers University Press, 1987); Anne Digby, *Madness, Morality, and Medicine: A Study of the York Retreat, 1796–1914* (Cambridge: Cambridge University Press, 1985); S. E. D. Shortt, *Victorian Lunacy: Richard M. Bucke and the Practice of Late Nineteenth-Century Psychiatry* (Cambridge: Cambridge University Press, 1986); Elaine Showalter, *The Female Malady: Women, Madness, and English Culture, 1830–1980* (New York: Pantheon Books, 1985); Roy Porter, *Mind Forg'd Manacles: A History of Madness in England from the Restoration to the Regency* (Cambridge, Mass.: Harvard University Press, 1987); Michael MacDonald,

Mystical Bedlam: Madness, Anxiety, and Healing in Seventeenth-Century England (Cambridge: Cambridge University Press, 1981).

10. Grob, *Mental Institutions in America*, pp. 143, 243–44, and *Mental Illness and American Society*, pp. 22–23, 26, 220–21; Norman Dain, *Concepts of Insanity in the United States, 1789–1865* (New Brunswick, N.J.: Rutgers University Press, 1964), pp. 90–91, 104–8.

11. Grob, *Mental Institutions in America*, pp. 95–96, 190, 195, 342–43, 359–68, and *Mental Illness and American Society*, pp. 25–26, 104, 159–60, 218–20; Dain, *Concepts of Insanity*, pp. 128, 177, 225 n. 2, 242 n. 17.

12. Todd L. Savitt and James Harvey Young, eds., *Disease and Distinctiveness in the American South* (Knoxville: University of Tennessee Press, 1988); Ronald L. Numbers and Todd L. Savitt, eds., *Science and Medicine in the Old South* (Baton Rouge: Louisiana State University Press, 1989); Edward H. Beardsley, *A History of Neglect: Health Care for Blacks and Mill Workers in the Twentieth-Century South* (Knoxville: University of Tennessee Press, 1987). Todd L. Savitt, *Medicine and Slavery: The Diseases and Health Care of Blacks in Antebellum Virginia* (Urbana: University of Illinois Press, 1978); Kenneth F. Kiple and Virginia H. King, *Another Dimension to the Black Diaspora: Diet, Disease, and Racism* (Cambridge: Cambridge University Press, 1981).

13. Works that treat various aspects of insanity in southern history include Samuel B. Thielman, "Southern Madness: The Shape of Mental Health Care in the Old South," in Numbers and Savitt, *Science and Medicine in the Old South*, pp. 256–75; Norman Dain, *Disordered Minds: The First Century of Eastern State Hospital in Williamsburg, Virginia, 1766–1866* (Charlottesville: University Press of Virginia, 1971); Savitt, *Medicine and Slavery*, pp. 248–70; John S. Hughes, "Labeling and Treating Black Mental Illness in America," *Journal of Southern History* 58 (1993): 435–60, and "The Madness of Separate Spheres: Insanity and Masculinity in Victorian Alabama," in *Meanings for Manhood: Constructions of Masculinity in Victorian America*, ed. Mark Carnes and Clyde Griffin (Chicago: University of Chicago Press, 1990); Ronald F. White, "Custodial Care for the Insane at Eastern State Hospital in Lexington, Kentucky, 1824–44," *Filson Club Quarterly* 62 (1988): 303–35, and "A Dialogue on Madness: Eastern State Lunatic Asylum and Mental Health Policies in Kentucky, 1824–1883" (Ph.D. diss., University of Kentucky, 1984).

14. Michael R. Hindus, *Prison and Plantation: Crime, Justice and Authority in Massachusetts and South Carolina, 1767–1878* (Chapel Hill: University of North Carolina Press, 1980); Albert D. Oliphant, *The Evolution of the Penal System in South Carolina from 1866 to 1916* (Columbia, S.C.: The State Co., 1916); David D. Wallace, *The History of South Carolina*, 3 vols. (New York: American Historical Society, 1934), 3:28–37, 423, 444; Robert Mills, *Statistics of South Carolina* (Charleston, 1826), pp. 198–99.

15. This is not to say that control of insane blacks was not an issue, only that the

founders of the South Carolina Lunatic Asylum did not advocate it for that purpose and that it is impossible to argue that it functioned as a method of controlling them in its early decades. Only after the asylum began receiving applications for the admission of blacks from slave owners and free black families did its officers contemplate integrating it, and only after the Civil War did the number of black patients begin to make up a significant proportion of the institution's population.

16. The census of 1840 enumerated 513 lunatics and idiots in South Carolina, of whom about 60 were in the state asylum. In 1850, the census counted 597 insane; the asylum held about 120. J. D. B. De Bow, ed., *Statistical View of the United States, Being a Compendium of the Seventh Census* (Washington, D.C., 1854, reprint, New York: Gordon and Breach Science Publishers, 1970).

17. For examples of historians who have looked extensively at the situation of the insane in the community for one or more of these purposes, see Tomes, *Generous Confidence*; Dwyer, *Homes for the Mad*; Fox, *So Far Disordered in Mind*; John Walton, "Casting Out and Bringing Back in Victorian England: Pauper Lunatics, 1840-1870," in *The Anatomy of Madness*, 3 vols., ed. W. F. Bynum, Roy Porter, and Michael Shepherd (London: Tavistock, 1985), 2:132-46.

18. Works that provide insight into the situation of the insane in community settings include Porter, *Mind Forg'd Manacles*; MacDonald, *Mystical Bedlam*; Samuel B. Thielman, "Community Management of Mental Disorders in Antebellum America," *Journal of the History of Medicine* 44 (1989): 351-74; John S. Hughes, "Commitment Law, Family Stress, and Legal Culture: The Case of Victorian Alabama," in *The Constitution, Law, and American Society: Critical Aspects of the Nineteenth-Century Experience*, ed. Donald Nieman (Athens: University of Georgia Press, 1992); Mary Ann Jimenez, *Changing Faces of Madness: Early American Attitudes and Treatment of the Insane* (Hanover, N.H.: University Press of New England, 1987); Peter Rushton, "Lunatics and Idiots: Mental Disability, the Community and the Poor Law in Northeast England, 1600-1800," *Medical History* 32 (1988): 34-50.

CHAPTER ONE

1. *Journal of the Commons House of Assembly: The Colonial Records of South Carolina*, 13 vols. (Columbia: Historical Commission of South Carolina, 1951-), 6:43-45 (hereafter cited as *Commons Journal*); Thomas Cooper and David J. McCord, eds., *The Statutes at Large of South Carolina*, 10 vols. (Columbia, S.C., 1836-41), 3:647; Leila G. Johnson, "A History of the South Carolina State Hospital" (M.A. thesis, University of Chicago, 1930), pp. 3-4.

2. Peter Wood, *Black Majority: Negroes in Colonial South Carolina* (New York: Norton, 1974), xiii-xiv, xviii, pp. 143, 166, 271-74; John Duncan, "Servitude and Slavery in Colonial South Carolina" (Ph.D. diss., Emory University, 1972), p. 250;

Carl Bridenbaugh, *Myths and Realities: Societies of the Colonial South* (New York: Atheneum, 1965), pp. 62–66.

3. The European and African population of South Carolina was about 6,000 in 1700, 25,000 in 1750, and 150,000 in 1788. Population density was about 9 per square mile on the eve of the Revolution. Robert M. Weir, *Colonial South Carolina* (Millwood, N.J.: KTO Press, 1983), pp. 205–6; Bridenbaugh, *Myths and Realities*, p. 61; Gerald Grob, *Mental Institutions in America: Social Policy to 1875* (New York: Free Press, 1973), p. 4.

4. Albert Deutsch, *The Mentally Ill in America: A History of Their Care and Treatment from Colonial Times* (Garden City, N.Y.: Doubleday, Doran, 1937), p. 39.

5. Roy Porter, *Mind Forg'd Manacles: A History of Madness in England from the Restoration to the Regency* (Cambridge, Mass.: Harvard University Press, 1987), p. 277.

6. James Guignard to Benjamin Rush, May 6, 1810, Manuscript Correspondence of Benjamin Rush, Historical Society of Pennsylvania, vol. 4, p. 97; David D. Wallace, *The History of South Carolina*, 4 vols. (New York: American Historical Society, 1934), 3:49–50. For an example of boarding out from the early nineteenth century, see PTR, 1, Susan Simmons.

7. Robert Pringle to Henry and John Brock, June 28, 1744, in Walter Edgar, ed., *The Letterbook of Robert Pringle* (Columbia: University of South Carolina Press, 1972), p. 714; Anne King Gregorie, ed., *Records of the Court of Chancery of South Carolina, 1671–1779* (Washington, D.C.: American Historical Association, 1950), p. 460.

8. John Belton O'Neall, *Biographical Sketches of the Bench and Bar of South Carolina*, 2 vols. (Charleston, 1859), 2:159–62; See also documents relating to Harriet Bounds, 1830, GAP. Wandering lunatics appear somewhat more frequently in records of other colonies. See Mary Ann Jimenez, *Changing Faces of Madness: Early American Attitudes and Treatment of the Insane* (Hanover, N.H.: University Press of New England, 1987), pp. 40–42; Deutsch, *Mentally Ill in America*, pp. 45–46.

9. The Mason Lee case set an important precedent; afterward, it became extremely difficult to overturn a will on the grounds of mental incompetence. "Heirs at Law of Mason Lee v. Ex. of Mason Lee," Columbia, 1827, in David J. McCord, *Reports of Cases Argued and Determined in the Court of Appeals in South Carolina, 1826–1828* (Columbia, S.C., 1830), pp. 183–97; D. D. McColl, *Sketches of Old Marlboro* (Columbia, S.C.: State, 1916), pp. 5–12.

10. *Charleston Courier*, November 30, 1825.

11. O'Neall, *Biographical Sketches* 2:160–61; Robert Y. Hayne, "Biographical Memoir of David Ramsay," *Analectic Magazine*, September 1815, pp. 223–24; Adam Hodgson, *Remarks During a Journey through North America in the Years 1819, 1820, and 1821* (New York, 1823), p. 131; Walter J. Fraser Jr., *Charleston!*

Charleston!: The History of a Southern City (Columbia: University of South Carolina Press, 1989), pp. 57-58, 77-78, 122-23. For records of early South Carolina Lunatic Asylum patients who had been in jail prior to commitment, see PTR, 1.

12. Cooper and McCord, *Statutes* 3:163-65, 5:570-71.

13. Gregorie, *Records of the Court of Chancery*, pp. 332, 400, 403, 407, 422.

14. H. W. DeSaussure, *Report of Cases Argued and Determined in the Court of Chancery of the State of South Carolina from the Revolution to December 1813, Inclusive* (Columbia, 1817), pp. 116, 136, 144-45; Joseph Manigault to Gabriel Manigault, January 3, 1786, Manigault Family Papers, SCL.

15. Petition de Lunatico, re Catherine Wigfall, April 29, 1806, Court of Chancery and Court of Equity, Petitions and Commissions for Writs to Inquire and Determine Lunacy, Miscellaneous Papers, 1786-1806, SCDAH.

16. St. Philip's Parish, Vestry Minutes, October 9, 1749, SCHS.

17. Gregorie, *Records of the Court of Chancery*, pp. 430, 460; Woodrow W. Harris, " 'Disordered in their Senses': Provisions for Early South Carolina's Mentally Ill," *Psychiatric Forum* 9 (1980): pp. 36-37.

18. Petition of George Gill in behalf of Jacob Castor, 1793, GAP.

19. Grob, *Mental Institutions in America*, pp. 5-10.

20. Barbara Ulmer, "Benevolence in Colonial Charleston," *Proceedings of the South Carolina Historical Association*, 1980, pp. 1-2; Cooper and McCord, *Statutes* 2:116-17, 2:593-98; Michael D. Byrd, "Ye Have the Poor Always with You: Attitudes towards Poor Relief in Colonial Charles Town" (M.A. thesis, University of South Carolina, 1973), pp. 66-72.

21. St. Philip's Parish, Vestry Minutes, April 9, June 11, 1733; St. John's Parish, Berkeley, Vestry Minutes, SCHS, March 17, 1739/40, July 25, 1753; St. John's Parish, Colleton, Vestry Minutes, SCHS, October 8, 1751, March 30, May 20, June 9, 1752; Christ Church Parish, Vestry Minutes, April 15, 1745, May 21, 1746, August 17, 1748, Charleston Library Society; Brent Holcombe, ed., *St. David's Parish, South Carolina, Minutes of the Vestry, 1768-1832* (Easley, S.C.: Southern Historical Press, 1979), April 12, May 3, September 13, 20, 1773; Joseph I. Waring, *A History of Medicine in South Carolina*, 3 vols. (Columbia: South Carolina Medical Association, 1964-71) 1: 48. In 1767, Charleston supported 129 pauper inmates in the workhouse and 67 on outdoor relief. See J. H. Easterby, "Public Poor Relief in Colonial Charleston: A Report to the Commons House of Assembly about the Year 1767," *SCHM* 42 (1941): 83-86.

22. Spartanburg County, Commissioners of the Poor, Minutes, 1796-1827, SCL; *Commons Journal* 14:63; *The Register Book for the Parish Prince Frederick Winyaw* (Baltimore: Williams and Wilkins, 1916), pp. 188-205; Governor's Message no. 1318, 1822, in GAP; Robert Mills, *Statistics of South Carolina* (Charleston, 1826), pp. 348-782.

23. Peter Coclanis, *The Shadow of a Dream: Economic Life and Death in the South Carolina Low Country, 1670-1920* (New York: Oxford University Press, 1989), pp. 49-51; Weir, *Colonial South Carolina*, p. 212; Marion Eugene Sirmans,

Colonial South Carolina: A Political History, 1663–1763 (Chapel Hill: University of North Carolina Press, 1966), p. 226; Charles Woodmason, *The Carolina Backcountry on the Eve of the Revolution; the Journal and Other Writings of Charles Woodmason, Anglican Itinerant*, ed. Richard J. Hooker (Chapel Hill: University of North Carolina Press, 1953), pp. xvi–xvii; Barbara L. Bellows, *Benevolence among Slaveholders: Assisting the Poor in Charleston, 1670–1860* (Baton Rouge: Louisiana State University Press, 1994), chap. 1.

24. St. Philip's Parish, Vestry Minutes, January 6, 1734; Walter J. Fraser Jr., "Controlling the Poor in Colonial Charleston," *Proceedings of the South Carolina Historical Association*, 1980, pp. 13–18; Bellows, *Benevolence among Slaveholders*, chap. 1. The population of Charleston increased from about thirty-five hundred in 1706 to around six thousand by 1740, when it was the fourth largest city in British North America. Fraser, *Charleston!* pp. 26, 55.

25. St. Philip's Parish, Vestry Minutes, November 27, 1738; Ulmer, "Benevolence in Colonial Charleston," p. 3; Byrd, "Ye Have the Poor," pp. 50–58.

26. William Simpson, *The Practical Justice of the Peace and Parish Officer of His Majesty's Province of South Carolina* (Charleston, 1761), p. 263.

27. St. Philip's Parish, Vestry Minutes, August 12, 1754; Harris, "Disordered in Their Senses," p. 39; Waring, *History of Medicine in South Carolina* 1:62; Byrd, "Ye Have the Poor," pp. 71–72.

28. *Commons Journal* 13:74–75, 174, 200, 282; St. Philip's Parish, Vestry Minutes, March 17, 1768.

29. *Rules of the Fellowship Society* (Charleston, 1762), iii–v.

30. Deutsch, *Mentally Ill in America*, pp. 58–61; Nancy Tomes, *A Generous Confidence: Thomas Story Kirkbride and the Art of Asylum Keeping, 1840–1883* (Cambridge: Cambridge University Press, 1984), pp. 22–27; Grob, *Mental Institutions in America*, pp. 16–23. On the development of hospitals in England, see F. F. Cartwright, *A Social History of Medicine* (London: Longman, 1977), pp. 36–39; John Woodward, *To Do the Sick No Harm: A Study of the British Voluntary Hospital System to 1875* (London: Routledge and Kegan Paul, 1974), pp. 1–22.

31. *Rules of the Fellowship Society*, iv–v.

32. David Ramsay, *History of South Carolina*, 2 vols. (Charleston, 1809), 2:363; J. L. E. W. Shecut, *Medical and Philosophical Essays* (Charleston, 1819), p. 28.

33. St. Philip's, Vestry Minutes, December 15, 1766, February 12, March 18, 1750; *South Carolina Gazette*, June 1765; Easterby, "Public Poor Relief," pp. 83–86; Carl Bridenbaugh, *Cities in Revolt: Urban Life in America, 1743–1776* (New York: Knopf, 1955), p. 323.

34. Cooper and McCord, *Statutes* 7:90; *South Carolina Gazette*, April 18, 1768.

35. Robert M. Weir, ed., *The Letters of Freeman: Essays on the Nonimportation Movement in South Carolina* (Columbia: University of South Carolina Press, 1977), pp. 8–9, 34, 114.

36. William Gilmore Simms, "The Morals of Slavery," in *The Proslavery Argument* (Charleston, 1852), p. 255; Bernhard Alexander Uhlendorf, *The Siege of*

Charleston (Ann Arbor: University of Michigan Press, 1938), p. 89; Fraser, *Charleston!* p. 162, pp. 470–71 n. 67.

37. Board of Police Journals, May 18, 24, 1782, SCDAH.

38. G. B. Eckhard, *A Digest of the Ordinances of the City of Charleston, 1783–1844* (Charleston, 1844), p. 203; *South Carolina Gazette and General Advertiser*, May 29, 1784.

39. Eckhard, *Ordinances of the City of Charleston*, p. 204; Minutes, December 29, 1800, September 21, December 14, 1801, CCP; Waring, *History of Medicine in South Carolina* 1:133–34.

40. Most historians of insanity, whether Whig or revisionist, have tended to view the eighteenth century as, in Roy Porter's words, a psychiatric "dark age," marked by brutal and repressive treatment of the insane. Porter argues that treatment of the insane in Georgian England was marked by variety. For views on eighteenth-century care of the insane, see Gregory Zilboorg, *A History of Medical Psychology* (New York: Norton, 1941), pp. 311–18; Franz Alexander and Sheldon Selesnick, *The History of Psychiatry* (New York: New American Library, 1966), pp. 154–56; Deutsch, *Mentally Ill in America*, esp. chaps. 3–4; Foucault, *Madness and Civilization*, trans. Richard Howard (New York: New American Library, 1965), esp. chaps. 2–3; Andrew T. Scull, *Museums of Madness: The Social Organization of Insanity in Nineteenth-Century England* (New York: St. Martin's Press, 1979), esp. pp. 62–65; Michael MacDonald, *Mystical Bedlam: Madness, Anxiety, and Healing in Seventeenth-Century England* (Cambridge: Cambridge University Press, 1981), pp. 11, 230–31; Porter, *Mind Forg'd Manacles*; Dain, "American Psychiatry in the Eighteenth Century," in *American Psychiatry, Past, Present, and Future* (Charlottesville: University Press of Virginia, 1975), pp. 16–17. On the care of the insane in early Massachusetts, see Jimenez, *Changing Faces of Madness*, esp. pp. 49–50.

41. Porter, *Mind Forg'd Manacles*, pp. 19–31, chaps. 2 and 4; Jimenez, *Changing Faces of Madness*, esp. chaps. 1, 3, and 4; Norman Dain, *Concepts of Insanity in the United States, 1789–1865* (New Brunswick, N.J.: Rutgers University Press, 1964), chaps. 1–2. Porter contains the fullest and most balanced discussion of eighteenth-century English perceptions of madness. For the seventeenth-century background, see MacDonald, *Mystical Bedlam*. See Max Byrd, *Visits to Bedlam: Madness and Literature in the Eighteenth Century* (Columbia: University of South Carolina Press, [1974]), and Michael Deporte, *Nightmares and Hobbyhorses: Swift, Sterne and Augustan Ideas of Madness* (San Marino, Calif.: Huntington Library, 1974) for perceptions of madness in Georgian literature. On ancient Greek and medieval views of insanity, see Bennett Simon, *Mind and Madness in Ancient Greece* (Ithaca, N.Y.: Cornell University Press, 1978); Judith S. Neaman, *Suggestion of the Devil* (New York: Anchor Books, 1975); Stanley Jackson, *Melancholia and Depression: From Hippocratic Times to Modern Times* (New Haven, Conn.: Yale University Press, 1986).

42. Eliza Lucas Pinckney to Miss B., 1742, E. Pinckney, ed., *The Letterbook*

of *Eliza Lucas Pinckney* (Chapel Hill: University of North Carolina Press, 1972), p. 46.

43. Joseph Manigault to Gabriel Manigault, January 3, 1786, Manigault Family Papers, SCL; Robert Pringle to Henry and John Brock, June 28, 30, 1744, Edgar, *Letterbook of Robert Pringle*, pp. 714, 722.

44. Robert Pringle to Henry and John Brock, June 28, 30, 1744, Edgar, *Letterbook of Robert Pringle*, pp. 714, 722; Jimenez, *Changing Faces of Madness*, p. 15; Porter, *Mind Forg'd Manacles*, pp. 85–87. On eighteenth-century medical perceptions of melancholia, see Stanley W. Jackson, "Melancholia and Mechanical Explanation in Eighteenth Century Medicine," *Journal of the History of Medicine* 38 (1983): 298–319. On hysteria, see Guenter B. Risse, "Hysteria at the Edinburgh Infirmary," *Medical History* 32 (1988): 1–22.

45. Woodmason, *Carolina Backcountry*, pp. 61–62, and note 51.

46. Porter, *Mind Forg'd Manacles*, pp. 57–58, 66–81; Byrd, *Visits to Bedlam*, pp. 18–19, 46, 68–73; Deporte, *Nightmares and Hobbyhorses*, pp. 38–43.

47. Woodmason, *Carolina Backcountry*, p. 101.

48. Wood, *Black Majority*, pp. 308–26.

49. *South Carolina Gazette*, March 20–27, 1742, January 1–8, 1741.

50. On the Bryan episode, see Edward McCrady, *History of South Carolina under the Royal Government, 1719–1776* (New York: Macmillan, 1899), pp. 238–43; Weir, *Colonial South Carolina*, pp. 186–87; Sirmans, *Colonial South Carolina*, pp. 231–32; David Duncan Wallace, *A Short History of South Carolina* (Chapel Hill: University of North Carolina Press, 1951), p. 184; Fraser, *Charleston!* p. 71.

51. Memorandum, March 11, 1742, Pinckney to Mrs. Cheesman, [March 1742], Pinckney, *Letterbook of Eliza Lucas Pinckney*, pp. 28, 30.

52. *Commons Journal* 3:461–62.

53. Pinckney to Mrs. Cheesman, [March 1742], Pinckney, *Letterbook of Eliza Pinckney*, p. 28.

54. *Commons Journal* 3:461–62; McCrady, *History of South Carolina*, p. 238.

55. John Belton O'Neall, *Annals of Newberry* (Charleston, 1859), pp. 352–53.

56. J. Alexander to Benjamin Rush, July 28, 1810, John Adamson to Benjamin Rush, November 1, 1810, Rush Correspondence, Historical Society of Pennsylvania, Philadelphia (hereafter cited as Rush, Correspondence), 10, 39; Alice D. Izard to Margaret I. Manigault, May 11, June 1, 1815, May 11, 1817, Manigault Family Papers, SCL.

57. South Carolina State Hospital, PTR, 1, Mary Saxon.

58. *Register Book for the Parish Prince Frederick Winyaw*, pp. 188–205; Harris, "Disordered in Their Senses," pp. 37–38.

59. Robert Mills, *Statistics of South Carolina* (Charleston, 1826), pp. 372–73, 528, 547, 626, 348–782; Spartanburg County, Commissioners of the Poor, Minutes, August 5, 1805, August 2, 1819, January 21, 1821, April 8, 1823, SCL; Governor's Message no. 1318, 1822, St. Peter's Parish return. Mills's information concerning the insane and poor was provided by local officials. A few districts provided fairly

specific data about the numbers and care of the poor, the insane, and other dependent groups, but most of the returns were extremely vague, and some districts did not provide any information about the dependent.

60. Weir, *Letters of Freeman*, p. 114.

61. John Hammond Moore, ed., "The Abiel Abbot Journals: A Yankee Preacher in Charleston," *South Carolina Historical Magazine* 68 (1967): 115-17.

62. Cooper and McCord, *Statutes* 3:647; Wood, *Black Majority*, pp. 285-86.

63. St. Philip's Parish, Vestry Minutes, March 17, August 22, 1768; Minutes, 1800-56, CCP.

64. Richard Harrison Shryock, *Medicine and Society in America, 1660-1860* (Ithaca, N.Y.: Cornell University Press, 1975), pp. 12-15; Waring, *History of Medicine in South Carolina* 1:1-5, 16; Hennig Cohen, *The South Carolina Gazette, 1732-1775* (Columbia: University of South Carolina Press, 1953), pp. 40-48.

65. Whitfield J. Bell Jr., "A Portrait of the Colonial Physician," in *Sickness and Health in America*, ed. Judith Walzer Leavitt and Ronald L. Numbers (Madison: University of Wisconsin Press, 1978), pp. 41-47; Paul Starr, *The Social Transformation of American Medicine* (New York: Basic Books, 1982). pp. 37-40; John Duffy, *The Healers: A History of American Medicine* (Urbana: University of Illinois Press, 1979), pp. 26-41; Shryock, *Medicine and Society in America*, pp. 7-8; Waring, *History of Medicine in South Carolina* 1:16; Cohen, *South Carolina Gazette*, pp. 40-42; Suzanne C. Linder, *Medicine in Marlboro County* (Baltimore: Gateway Press, 1980), p. 2.

66. St. Philip's Parish, Vestry Minutes, April 9, 1733, August 8, 1737, May 4, 1741, July 25, 1748, July 17, 1749, May 3, 1750.

67. *South Carolina Gazette*, March 6, 1749; *State Gazette*, August 16, September 21, 1793; Duncan, "Servitude and Slavery," pp. 250-52; Waring, *History of Medicine in South Carolina* 1:57, 78, 113, 140, 143, 152, 154.

68. Alexander Hewett, *An Historical Account of the Rise and Progress of the Colonies of South Carolina and Georgia*, 2 vols. (London, 1779), 2:95, cited in Duncan, "Servitude and Slavery," p. 251.

69. Porter, *Mind Forg'd Manacles*, esp. chap. 4.

70. Deutsch, *Mentally Ill in America*, pp. 59-60, 132-35; Norman Dain, *Disordered Minds: The First Century of Eastern State Hospital in Williamsburg, Virginia, 1766-1866* (Charlottesville: University Press of Virginia, 1971), pp. 28-30, 34; Dain, *Concepts of Insanity*, pp. 4, 9-11; Jimenez, *Changing Faces of Madness*, esp. chap. 4; *Rules of the Fellowship Society*, iii-iv.

71. Jimenez, in *Changing Faces of Madness*, pp. 43-44, argues that Massachusetts settlers seldom employed medical treatment for insanity until the end of the colonial period. She ascribes this to the unsophisticated nature of medical practice in the colonies, yet notes that some members of the colonial medical elite were informed about English remedies for insanity, citing Pennsylvania as an example. South Carolina's medical elite was also well informed about English practice. Reli-

gious differences may have made South Carolinians more receptive than the people of colonial Massachusetts to medical treatments for insanity. The Puritans, who dominated Massachusetts, retained beliefs in possession and exorcism longer than the Anglicans, who dominated South Carolina. See MacDonald, *Mystical Bedlam*, pp. 206–9, for a discussion of the Anglican hierarchy's rejection of supernatural concepts of insanity during the seventeenth century.

72. Pringle to Henry and John Beck, June 28, 1744, Edgar, *Letterbook of Robert Pringle*, p. 714.

73. *Register Book for the Parish of Prince Frederick Winyaw*, July 17, 1766, p. 188.

74. Charles Drayton, Medical Casebook, 1777–1781, Drayton Papers, SCHS.

75. DeSaussure, *Report of Cases Argued*, pp. 394–99; "J. and C. Barlow and S. Pope v. the Committee of Hugh O'Neall, a lunatic," case notes, Thomas Waties Papers, SCL. See also St. Philip's Parish, Vestry Minutes, September 29, 1766.

76. Martin Kaufman, *Homeopathy in America: The Rise and Fall of a Medical Heresy* (Baltimore: Johns Hopkins University Press, 1971), pp. 3–5; Porter, *Mind Forg'd Manacles*, pp. 184–87; Dain, *Disordered Minds*, p. 34; Deutsch, *Mentally Ill in America*, p. 60.

77. Lester S. King, *The Medical World of the Eighteenth Century* (Chicago: University of Chicago Press, 1958), pp. 59–89; Waring, *History of Medicine in South Carolina* 1:4–5; Duffy, *Healers*, pp. 26–28; Dain, *Concepts of Insanity*, p. 10.

78. Waring, *History of Medicine in South Carolina* 1:196; Duffy, *Healers*, pp. 26–28; Charles Rosenberg, "The Therapeutic Revolution," in *The Therapeutic Revolution*, ed. Morris J. Vogel and Charles Rosenberg (Philadelphia: University of Pennsylvania Press, 1979), pp. 6–9.

79. David Ramsay, *A Review of the Improvements, Progress, and State of Medicine in the Eighteenth Century* (Charleston, 1801), pp. 17, 24.

80. Benjamin Rush, *Medical Inquiries and Observations upon the Diseases of the Mind*, 3d ed. (Philadelphia, 1827), pp. 14–25, 183–89; Dain, *Concepts of Insanity*, pp. 15–21.

81. Alice D. Izard to Margaret I. Manigault, January 8, 1809, Manigault Family Papers, SCL; J. Alexander to Benjamin Rush, July 28, 1810, John Adamson to Rush, November 1, 1810, Rush Correspondence, vol. 1, 10, 39.

82. Quoted in Joseph I. Waring, "The Influence of Benjamin Rush on the Practice of Bleeding in South Carolina," *Bulletin of the History of Medicine* 3 (1961): 231, 230–37.

83. Waring, "The Influence of Benjamin Rush," pp. 231–37.

84. On eighteenth-century medical theory and practice regarding insanity, see Porter, *Mind Forg'd Manacles*; Jackson, "Melancholia and Mechanical Explanation," 298–99; Stanley W. Jackson, "Melancholia and the Waning of the Humoral Theory," *Journal of the History of Medicine* 33 (1978): 367–376; Jackson, *Melancholia and Depression*; Eric T. Carlson and Meribeth M. Simpson, "Models of

the Nervous System in Eighteenth-Century Psychiatry," *Bulletin of the History of Medicine* 43 (1969): 101–15; Ida Macalpine and Richard Hunter, *George III and the Mad-Business* (London: Allen Lane, 1969).

85. Woodmason, *Carolina Backcountry*, p. 38; Suzanne C. Linder, *Medicine in Marlboro County* (Baltimore: Gateway Press, 1980), p. 1; Horace F. Rudisill, *Doctors of Darlington County, 1760–1912* (Darlington, S.C.: Darlington County Historical Society, 1962), iii–iv. According to Rudisill, there was only one physician in Darlington as late as 1819.

86. James Guignard to Benjamin Rush, June 21, 1810, Rush Correspondence, vol. 6, 98; Shryock, *Medicine and Society in America*, pp. 4–6; Waring, *History of Medicine in South Carolina* 1:65; Duffy, *Healers*, pp. 52–55.

87. Alice D. Izard to Margaret I. Manigault, May 11, 1815, Manigault Family Papers, SCL; Ramsay, *History of South Carolina* 2:110–11. *South Carolina Gazette*, March 6, 1749, quoted in Duncan, "Servitude and Slavery in Colonial South Carolina," p. 251; Waring, *History of Medicine in South Carolina* 1:49–50; Shryock, *Medicine and Society in America*, pp. 5–6; James Harvey Young, *The Toadstool Millionaires: A Social History of Patent Medicines in America Before Federal Regulation* (Princeton, N.J.: Princeton University Press, 1961), chaps. 1–3.

88. An edition of Buchan was published in Charleston in 1807. Another manual, *The Medical Vade-Mecum*, was published there in 1800. Other early American domestic manuals include Henry Wilkins, *The Family Advisor* (Philadelphia, 1795) and James Ewell, *The Planter's and Mariner's Medical Companion* (Philadelphia, 1807). For discussion of domestic medicine in the eighteenth century, see John B. Blake, "From Buchan to Fishbein: The Literature of Domestic Medicine," in *Medicine Without Doctors: Home Health Care in American History*, ed. Guenter B. Risse, Ronald L. Numbers, and Judith Walzer Leavitt (New York: Science History Publications, 1977), pp. 11–15, 18–19; Ginnie Smith, "Prescribing the Rules of Health: Self-Help and Advice in the Late Eighteenth Century," in *Patients and Practitioners: Lay Perceptions of Medicine in Pre-industrial Society*, ed. Roy Porter (London: Cambridge University Press, 1985), pp. 249–82; King, *Medical World of the Eighteenth Century*, pp. 34–38; Starr, *Social Transformation of American Medicine*, pp. 32–37.

89. John Wesley, *Primitive Physick*, 24th ed. (Philadelphia, 1795), pp. 44, 56, 60–61.

90. William Buchan, *Domestic Medicine* (Charleston, 1807), pp. 274–93; Dain, *Concepts of Insanity*, pp. 38–40; Porter, *Mind Forg'd Manacles*, pp. 169–71.

91. St. Philip's Parish, Vestry Minutes, September 2, 1751.

92. Joshua Gordon, Witchcraft Book, 1784, SCL; *South Carolina Gazette*, March 12, 1754; *Commons Journal* 13:74; E. Don Herd Jr., *The South Carolina Upcountry, 1540–1980* (Greenwood, S.C.: Attic Press, 1980), pp. 133–51; John Hawkins, "Magical Medical Practise in South Carolina," *Popular Science Monthly*, 1907, pp. 165–74; Herbert M. Morais, *The History of the Negro in Medicine* (New York: Publishers Co., 1967), pp. 11, 12–16; Starr, *Social Transformation of Ameri-*

can Medicine, pp. 30-33, 47-49; Porter, *Mind Forg'd Manacles*, pp. 173-74; MacDonald, *Mystical Bedlam*; Wood, *Black Majority*, pp. 116-17, 120; Margaret Washington Creel, *"A Peculiar People": Slave Religion and Community Culture Among the Gullahs* (New York: New York University Press, 1988), pp. 56-58; Young, *Toadstool Millionaires*, p. 18. For a discussion of slave conjuring and healing on South Carolina low-country plantations in the nineteenth century, see Charles Joyner, *Down By the Riverside: A South Carolina Slave Community* (Chicago: University of Illinois Press, 1984), pp. 145-53. See also Julia F. Morton, *Folk Remedies of the Low Country* (Miami: E. A. Seaman Publishing, 1974), pp. 14-16. On the religio-magical tradition, see Keith Thomas, *Religion and the Decline of Magic* (New York: Schocken Books, 1971).

93. The literature on moral treatment is vast. For varying interpretations of its early history, see Porter, *Mind Forg'd Manacles*, pp. 187-228; Andrew Scull, "Moral Treatment Reconsidered: Some Sociological Comments on an Episode in British Psychiatry," in *Madhouses, Mad-Doctors, and Madmen: The Social History of Psychiatry in the Victorian Era*, ed. Andrew Scull (Philadelphia: University of Pennsylvania Press, 1981), pp. 105-20; William F. Bynum, "Rationales for Therapy in British Psychiatry," in Scull, *Madhouses*, pp. 35-57.

94. Philippe Pinel, *A Treatise on Insanity*, trans. D. D. Davis (Sheffield, 1806); Samuel Tuke, *Description of the Retreat, an Institution near York for Insane Persons of the Society of Friends* (York, 1813). On the York retreat, see Digby, *Madness, Morality, and Medicine: A Study of the York Retreat, 1796-1914* (Cambridge: Cambridge University Press, 1985).

95. Thomas G. Morton, *History of the Pennsylvania Hospital* (Philadelphia, 1895), pp. 148-50; L. H. Butterfield, *Letters of Benjamin Rush*, 2 vols. (Princeton, N.J.: Princeton University Press, 1951), 1:528, 2:799; Rush, *Medical Inquiries and Observations*, pp. 173-79, 202-41.

96. Deutsch, *Mentally Ill in America*, pp. 95-106; Dain, "American Psychiatry," pp. 24-25; Grob, *Mental Institutions in America*, pp. 47-48; Norman Dain and Eric T. Carlson, "Milieu Therapy in the Nineteenth Century: Patient Care at the Friends' Asylum, Frankford, Pennsylvania, 1817-1861," *Journal of Nervous and Mental Diseases* 131 (1960): 277-78.

97. David Ramsay, *An Eulogium upon Benjamin Rush, M.D.* (Philadelphia, 1813), p. 41.

98. Alice D. Izard to Margaret I. Manigault, June 1, 1815, Manigault Family Papers, SCL; Pennsylvania Hospital, Insane Patients at 8th Street Hospital, 1790-1841, Pennsylvania Hospital Archives; Grob, *Mental Institutions in America*, pp. 16-21; Deutsch, *Mentally Ill in America*, pp. 58-61; Morton, *History of the Pennsylvania Hospital*.

CHAPTER TWO

1. Daniel Trezevant, *Letters to His Excellency Governor Manning on the Lunatic Asylum* (Columbia, S.C., 1854; reprint, New York: Arno Press, 1973), p. 4; William Crafts, *A Selection in Prose and Poetry from the Miscellaneous Writings of the Late William Crafts, to Which Is Prefixed, A Memoir of His Life* (Charleston, 1828), xxvi; *Charleston Courier*, August 3, 1822; John Belton O'Neall, *Biographical Sketches of the Bench and Bar of South Carolina*, 2 vols. (Charleston, 1859), 2:160-61; James Woods Babcock, "Public Charity in South Carolina," *Handbook of South Carolina: Resources, Institutions, and Industries of the State* (Columbia, S.C., State, 1907), pp. 45-46; P. B. Waters, *A Genealogical History of the Waters and Kindred Families* (Atlanta: Foote and Davis, 1902), p. 118; Leila G. Johnson, "A History of the South Carolina State Hospital" (Master's thesis, University of Chicago, 1930), pp. 20-26; Barbara Bellows, " 'Insanity is the Disease of Civilization': The Founding of the South Carolina Lunatic Asylum," *SCHM* 82 (1981): 263-72.

2. Michael Hindus, *Prison and Plantation: Crime, Justice and Authority in Massachusetts and South Carolina, 1767-1878* (Chapel Hill: University of North Carolina Press, 1980), pp. 210-13, 216; Gerald Grob, *Mental Institutions in America: Social Policy to 1875* (New York: Free Press, 1973), pp. 36, 48-50, 85, 108-9, 174-76.

3. Trezevant, *Letters to His Excellency*, p. 4.

4. O'Neall, *Biographical Sketches* 2:159-62.

5. Trezevant, *Letters to His Excellency*, pp. 3-4; Crafts, *Selection from the Miscellaneous Writings*, xxvi; Waters, *Genealogical History*, p. 118.

6. William Freehling, *Prelude to Civil War: The Nullification Controversy in South Carolina, 1816-1836* (New York: Harper and Row, 1966), p. 13.

7. Crafts, *Selection from the Miscellaneous Writings*, introduction; O'Neall, *Biographical Sketches* 2:160-61; *South Carolina Gazette*, May 7, 1828; *Dictionary of American Biography*, s.v. "Crafts, William Jr." (New York: Scribner's, 1946-58); file on William Crafts, SCL; Charles Fraser, *Reminiscences of Charleston* (Charleston, 1854), pp. 82-85; Hugh S. Legare, "The Fugitive Writings of William Crafts," *Southern Review* 1 (1828): 503-29; Michael O'Brien, *A Character of Hugh Legare* (Knoxville: University of Tennessee Press, 1985), pp. 134-35; *Biographical Directory of the South Carolina House of Representatives*, ed. Walter B. Edgar, 4 vols. (Columbia: University of South Carolina Press, 1974-84), 4:131-33.

8. Lacy K. Ford Jr., *The Origins of Southern Radicalism: The South Carolina Upcountry, 1800-1860* (New York: Oxford University Press, 1988), p. 19; Rachel N. Klein, *Unification of a Slave State: The Rise of a Planter Class in the South Carolina Back Country, 1760-1808* (Chapel Hill: University of North Carolina Press, 1990); David Duncan Wallace, *The History of South Carolina*, 4 vols. (New York: American Historical Society, 1934) 2:360-74; Yates Snowden, *The History of South Carolina*, 5 vols. (New York: Lewis Publishing, 1920), 1:511-17.

9. Crafts, *Selection from the Miscellaneous Writings*, xxvi–xxvii; Charles Wiltse, *The New Nation, 1800–1845* (New York: Hill and Wang, 1961), chap. 2.

10. *Southern Patriot*, November 25, 1818; *Charleston Courier*, August 3, 1822; A. G. Smith, *Economic Readjustment of an Old Cotton State, South Carolina, 1820–1860* (Columbia: University of South Carolina Press, 1958), pp. 4–6; Ford, *Origins of Southern Radicalism*, p. 16; Gene Waddell and Rhodi W. Liscombe, *Robert Mills' Courthouses and Jails* (Easley, S.C.: Southern Historical Press, 1981), pp. 1–2; David Kohn, ed., *Internal Improvements in South Carolina, 1817–1828* (Washington, D.C.: privately printed, 1938); Freehling, *Prelude to Civil War*, p. 26, chap. 4.

11. Special Committee Report on the Resolutions Relative to Lunatics, [1818], GAP; *RR*, 1818, p. 80; *Charleston City Gazette*, Dec. 14, 1818.

12. Kohn, *Internal Improvements*, report no. 1, 1819; Ford, *Origins of Southern Radicalism*, pp. 14–15; Freehling, *Prelude to Civil War*, pp. 25–48; Smith, *Economic Readjustment*, pp. 6–18.

13. Journal of the South Carolina House of Representatives (hereafter cited as House Journal), 1819, pp. 46, 90, 116–17, SCDAH; Medical Society of South Carolina, Minutes, November 16, 1820, WHL. The vote on the asylum bill of 1819 was sixty-two to thirty-six.

14. Smith, *Economic Readjustment*, p. 7; Freehling, *Prelude to Civil War*, pp. 26–27, 36, 45; *Charleston City Gazette*, Dec. 14, 1818; House Journal, 1818, pp. 116–17; *Charleston Courier*, December 8, 1819, December 15, 1820; *Biographical Directory of the House of Representatives of South Carolina* 1:304–5; Medical Society of South Carolina, Minutes, November 16, 1820, typescript, WHL.

15. Trezevant, *Letters to His Excellency*, p. 4; Crafts, *Selection from the Miscellaneous Writings*, 1828, xxvii; O'Neall, *Biographical Sketches* 2:160–61; Journal of the Senate of South Carolina (hereafter cited as Senate Journal), 1821, pp. 3, 15, 196, 214, 248, SCDAH; House Journal, 1821, pp. 106, 175, 212; *Charleston City Gazette*, December 11, 1821.

16. Smith, *Economic Readjustment*, pp. 7–13; Freehling, *Prelude to Civil War*, pp. 26–27; *Charleston Courier*, December 15, 1820.

17. *Southern Times and State Gazette*, August 17, 1838; Trezevant, *Letters to His Excellency*, p. 4; *Union Daily Times*, October 16, 1969, clipping in WHL file on James Davis; *Cyclopedia of Eminent Men of the Carolinas*, s.v. "James Davis" (Madison, Wis., 2 vols., 1892), 1:355.

18. Anne Royall, *Mrs. Royall's Southern Tour* (Washington, D.C., 1831), p. 63; Thomas Cooper, *Tracts on Medical Jurisprudence* (Philadelphia, 1819), pp. 355–56; James Moultrie, *Memorial on the State of Medical Education in South Carolina* (Charleston, 1836), p. 4; Dumas Malone, *The Public Life of Thomas Cooper* (New Haven, Conn.: Yale University Press, 1926), pp. 233, 279–81; Daniel Hollis, *The University of South Carolina*, vol. 1, *South Carolina College* (Columbia: University of South Carolina Press, 1951–56).

19. The physicians included Edward Fisher, Daniel Trezevant, and Samuel

Percival; the lawyers, William F. Desaussure and John J. Chappell; and planters John and Thomas Taylor Jr. All served on one or more of the commissions and boards which oversaw the building of the asylum, brought it into operation, and governed it during its first years. Wallace, *History of South Carolina* 2:400, 404, 3:55; Thomas Cooper and David J. McCord, *The Statutes-at-Large of South Carolina*, 10 vols. (Columbia, S.C., 1836–41), 6:168; House Journal, 1822, p. 177, 1823, p. 197; Babcock, "Public Charity in South Carolina," p. 50.

20. White's involvement in the asylum movement may have been related to an event which shocked all of Charleston: the murder in 1815 of David Ramsay by an alleged lunatic. White arrived at the scene just after Ramsay had been shot, and later recorded the event in his journal. See *National Cyclopedia of American Biography*, s.v. "John Blake White," (J. R. White, n.p., 1893; reprint, Ann Arbor, Mich.: University Microfilms, 1967), 3:21–22; Special Committee on Lunatics, [1818]; William Gilmore Simms, ed., *The Charleston Book* (Charleston, 1845), pp. 131–32; Paul R. Weidner, ed., "The Journal of John Blake White," *SCHM* 43 (1942): 162; Robert Y. Hayne, "Biographical Memoir of David Ramsay," *Analectic Magazine*, 1815, pp. 223–24; *Charleston Courier*, May 9, 1815; *Southern Patriot*, May 6, 9, 10, 15, 1815.

21. *Biographical Directory of the Senate of South Carolina, 1776–1985*, ed. N. Louise Bailey, Mary L. Morgan, Carolyn R. Taylor, 3 vols. (Columbia: University of South Carolina Press, 1974); *RR*, 1818, p. 80; Cooper and McCord, *Statutes* 6:168; Senate Journal, 1826, pp. 9, 17, 137; Report of Special Committee Relative to the Lunatic Asylum, 1826, GAP; *National Cyclopedia of American Biography*, s.v. "John Lyde Wilson," 12:164–65; *Pendleton Messenger*, December 13, 1826; *Charleston Courier*, December 2, 1825; Report of the Commissioners appointed to superintend the work done on the Lunatic Asylum, [1826], GAP.

22. William Crafts, *Oration on the Occasion of Laying the Corner Stone of the Lunatic Asylum at Columbia, July, 1822* (Charleston, 1822), pp. 12–13.

23. Special Committee on Lunatics, [1818]. Currie used the term "labouring poor" instead of "man." Roy Porter, *English Society in the Eighteenth Century* (Harmondsworth, England: Penguin Books, 1990).

24. Crafts, *Oration*, pp. 15–21.

25. Ibid., pp. 6–14, 21–22; Special Committee on Lunatics, [1818]. On antebellum reform, see Ronald Walters, *American Reformers, 1815–1860* (New York: Hill and Wang, 1978); Alice F. Tyler, *Freedom's Ferment: Phases of American Social History to 1860* (Minneapolis: University of Minnesota Press, 1944); David Brion Davis, ed., *Ante-Bellum Reform* (New York: Harper and Row, 1967); Constance McGovern, *Masters of Madness: Social Origins of the American Psychiatric Profession* (Hanover, N.H.: University Press of New England, 1985), pp. 33–34, 42–43.

26. *AR*, 1842, p. 18.

27. The original members of the asylum commission were John L. Wilson, James Davis, Dr. Edward Fisher, and Thomas Taylor Jr. The governor, Thomas

Bennett, and the intendant of Charleston, Elias Horry, were also named as ex-officio members. When Wilson became governor in 1822, he took Bennett's place on the commission, and William Crafts was appointed to fill Wilson's seat. At the same time, a seventh commissioner, James Gregg, was added to the board. These men apparently served until the asylum was finished, with the exception of Wilson, who was replaced by Governor Richard I. Manning in 1824, and Crafts, who died in 1826. See Cooper and McCord, *Statutes*, 6:168; *RR*, 1822, pp. 101, 103-4.

28. The school for the deaf and dumb was not established until 1848. The *Charleston Courier* predicted in December 1821 that the projected school might fail because of "the alledged [sic] difficulty of procuring adequate teachers." *Charleston Courier*, December 12, 1821.

29. Joint Committee of the Senate, Report on the Lunatic Asylum and the School for the Deaf and Dumb, and Abstract of Proceedings of the Board of Commissioners for Building a Lunatic Asylum and a School for the Deaf and Dumb, 1822, GAP; *RR*, 1822, pp. 103-4; Cooper and McCord, *Statutes* 6:168; Petition of Benjamin Williams to the State of South Carolina, 1822, GAP.

30. Senate Committee Report on the Lunatic Asylum, 1822, GAP.

31. Mills had spent a good deal of time in Philadelphia, and was familiar with the Friends' Retreat at Frankford, opened in 1817 and modeled on the York Retreat. Indeed, he drew the plans for the central heating system at the Frankford Retreat. The South Carolina Lunatic Asylum Commission purchased a book on English hospitals for Mills which was probably Samuel Tuke's *Practical Hints on the Construction and Economy of Pauper Lunatic Asylums*, published in 1815. Another possibility is a book that in some respects influenced Tuke: William Stark's *Remarks on the Construction of Public Hospitals for the Cure of Mental Derangement* (Glasgow, 1810). On Mills's design and the influences on it, see John M. Bryan and Julie M. Johnson, "Robert Mills' Sources for the South Carolina Lunatic Asylum, 1822," *Journal of the South Carolina Medical Association* 75 (1979): 264-68; John Bryan, ed., *Robert Mills, Architect* (Washington, D.C.: American Institute of Architects Press, 1989), pp. 85-88. Mills briefly described the asylum in *Statistics of South Carolina* (Charleston, 1826), pp. 213, 704-5. The *Charleston Courier*, February 19, 21, 1824, contains a detailed description of the asylum, probably written by Mills.

32. *RR*, 1822, p. 103; House Journal, 1823, p. 187; Report of the Commissioners of the Lunatic Asylum, 1823, GAP; Report of the Special (House) Committee on the Lunatic Asylum, 1824, GAP; *Charleston Courier*, August 3, 1822, February 19, 1824.

33. Reports of the Commissioners of the Lunatic Asylum, 1823, 1824, GAP; Report of the Committee on the Lunatic Asylum, [1823?], GAP; Governor's Message no. 1381, Richard I. Manning, 1825, GAP. The total cost of the asylum's construction is unclear. Various contemporary estimates put it at between $80,000 and $100,000. Special appropriations for the asylum between 1821 and 1827 totaled

almost $77,000, but other funds from the general appropriation for public buildings appear to have been used as well. Robert Mills, the architect of the asylum, wrote in 1826 that it had cost $91,000 to that point. See Reports of the Comptroller-General, in *RR*, 1822–1827; Robert Mills, *Statistics of South Carolina* (Charleston, 1826) p. 85.

34. House Journal, 1827, pp. 194–95.

35. Report of the Commissioners of the Lunatic Asylum, 1824, GAP.

36. Report of the Commissioners of the Lunatic Asylum, 1823, 1824, GAP; Report of the Committee on the Lunatic Asylum on the Report of the Commissioners for Building the Same, [1823?], GAP; Report of the Special (House) Committee on the Lunatic Asylum, 1824, GAP; Waddell and Lipscombe, *Robert Mills' Courthouses and Jails* pp. 1–6.

37. Report of the Special (House) Committee on the Lunatic Asylum, 1824, GAP; Report of the Commissioners of the Lunatic Asylum, 1824, GAP.

38. *Charleston Courier*, November 27, 1824; Laura A. White, *Robert Barnwell Rhett* (New York: Century, 1931), p. 7 n. 15; *National Cyclopedia of American Biography*, s.v. "John Lyde Wilson," 12:164–65; David Duncan Wallace, *South Carolina: A Short History* (Chapel Hill: University of North Carolina Press, 1951), p. 411.

39. *Charleston Southern Patriot*, December 9, 1825; Freehling, *Prelude to Civil War*; White, *Robert Barnwell Rhett*, pp. 11–12.

40. *Pendleton Messenger*, December 13, 1826; *Charleston Mercury*, December 4, 1826; *Charleston Southern Patriot*, December 4, 18, 1826; *Charleston Courier*, December 18, 1824, December 24, 1825; Freehling, *Prelude to Civil War*, chaps. 2, 4; Ford, *Origins of Southern Radicalism*, pp. 117–18; Smith, *Economic Readjustment*, chap. 1.

41. *Charleston Courier*, April 5, 1826, December 17, 1827; Special (House) Committee on the Lunatic Asylum, 1824, GAP; John H. Moore, ed., "Jared Sparks visits South Carolina," *SCHM* 71 (1971): 150–60; House Journal, 1825, pp. 36–37.

42. House Journal, 1826, pp. 75, 240–41; Senate Journal, 1826, pp. 9, 17, 137; Report of the Commissioners of the Lunatic Asylum, [1826], GAP; *Pendleton Messenger*, December 13, 1826; *Charleston Courier*, December 15, 1826.

43. Wilson to John Belton O'Neall, December 3, 1824, cover letter filed with Report of the Commissioners of the Lunatic Asylum, 1824, GAP.

44. Wilson to John Belton O'Neall, December 3, 1824, cover letter filed with Report of the Commissioners of the Lunatic Asylum, 1824, GAP; Thomas D. Clark, ed., *South Carolina: The Grand Tour* (Columbia: University of South Carolina Press, 1973), pp. 97–98, 120; Royall, *Mrs. Royall's Southern Tour*, p. 62; Herbert B. Adams, *The Life and Writings of Jared Sparks*, 2 vols. (Boston, 1893), 1:441–42; Report of the Commissioners of the Lunatic Asylum, [1826], GAP; *Charleston Courier*, February 19, 1824, April 5, 1826, December 17, 1827; *Pendleton Messenger*, December 13, 1826; Senate Journal, 1826, p. 137; Governor's Message no. 1381, Richard I. Manning, 1825, GAP; Woodrow W. Harris, "Footprints at

the Asylum: Nineteenth Century Visitors at the South Carolina Lunatic Asylum," *Psychiatric Forum* 13 (1984-85): 7-21.

45. House Journal, 1827, p. 196.

46. Apparently the other districts did not reply, or the results were unsatisfactory, for in 1824 the legislature again asked the commissioners of the poor to report their idiots and lunatics. The returns of this survey do not seem to have survived. Robert Mills tried to include the numbers of insane, idiotic, blind, and deaf and dumb in the state his *Statistics of South Carolina* (1826), but only a few local authorities provided him with specific numbers. *RR*, 1818, p. 80, 1824, p. 121; House Journal, 1827, pp. 194-97; Joint Committee of the Senate on the Lunatic Asylum, 1822, GAP; Governor's Message no. 1318, Thomas Bennett, 1822; Reports from Commissioners of the Poor in Obedience to the Act of 1821, GAP; Mills, *Statistics of South Carolina*, pp. 348-782.

47. Special Committee on Lunatics, 1818, GAP; *Charleston Courier*, February 21, 1824.

48. Crafts, *Oration*, pp. 15-16.

49. Special Committee on Lunatics, [1818], GAP; Crafts, *Oration*, pp. 12-16; *Pendleton Messenger*, May 20, 1829, Feb. 11, 1829.

50. Governor's Message no. 1318, Thomas Bennett, 1822; Charles Rosenberg, *The Care of Strangers: The Rise of America's Hospital System* (New York: Basic Books, 1987), pp. 18-22; John Woodward, *To Do the Sick No Harm: A Study of the British Voluntary Hospital System to 1875* (London: Routledge and Kegan Paul, 1974), chap. 4.

51. Special Committee on Lunatics, [1818], GAP; *Columbia Telescope*, January 30, 1829; see also Thomas W. Moore, "On Mania" (Medical thesis, Medical College of South Carolina, 1829), pp. 16-17, WHL. *Pendleton Messenger*, February 6, 1828.

52. House Journal, 1826, pp. 240-41, 1827, pp. 195-96.

53. *Columbia Telescope*, January 30, 1829.

54. Report of the Trustees to Effect the Operation of the Lunatick Asylum, c. 1827, GAP; *Pendleton Messenger*, February 6, 1828.

55. *Charleston Courier*, December 17, 1827.

56. House Journal, 1827, pp. 195-96; see also House Journal, 1825, pp. 36-37.

57. House Journal, 1827, pp. 196-97; Cooper and McCord, *Statutes* (1827) 6:322-24.

CHAPTER THREE

1. William Gilmore Simms, "The Morals of Slavery," in *The Proslavery Argument* (Charleston, 1852), pp. 226-27. Patient statistics come from SCSH, Admission Book, 1828-1874, and *AR*, 1829-1850. The totals derived from these for particular years do not always agree, but do not vary significantly.

2. PTR, 1, Andrew Stephenson.

3. Thomas Cooper and David J. McCord, *The Statutes-at-Large of South Carolina*, 10 vols. (Columbia, S.C., 1836-41), 6:322-24; Senate Journal, 1827, pp. 267-68; MBR, February 2, 1828; *AR*, 1829.

4. MBR, January 29, 1829. The original regents were B. F. Taylor, W. F. DeSaussure, William C. Preston, Abram Blanding, Dr. Daniel H. Trezevant, D. J. McCord, E. W. Johnstone, Dr. Edward Fisher, and Prof. Robert Henry. Taylor and Fisher resigned at the first meeting and Thomas Cooper and Dr. Samuel Cooper replaced them. Other prominent Columbians who served as regents of the antebellum asylum included the physician and scientist Robert Wilson Gibbes, Rev. Peter Shand, Andrew Wallace, and several professors from South Carolina College, including Maximilian Laborde, Francis Lieber, and William H. Ellett.

5. The acting physicians during Davis's illnesses were Daniel Trezevant, Samuel Percival, and M. H. DeLeon. See DMH, SCSH, list of regents and physicians at end of vol. 1 of Orders for Commitment, Detention and Discharge, 1828-1877, SCDAH.

6. *Columbia South Carolinian*, March 18, 1873, obituary of Daniel H. Trezevant; Robert M. Myers, *The Children of Pride: A True Story of Georgia and the Civil War* (New Haven, Conn.: Yale University Press, 1972), p. 1704; file on Daniel H. Trezevant, WHL.

7. *AR*, 1829; MBR, March 17, 1828, April 3, June 5, July 2, 1830, February 5, November 5, 29, 1831; PTR, 1, George Duff, John McConnell, John Carlisle, William Ross, Albert Gallatin.

8. MBR, December 1836; William S. Hall, "John Waring Parker, M.D., First Medical Superintendent—South Carolina State Hospital," *Journal of the South Carolina Medical Association* 69 (1973): 381-89.

9. MBR, 1828-1836; *AR*, 1829; *Columbia Telescope*, January 30, 1829; House Journal, 1826, p. 241; Hall, "John Waring Parker"; Nancy Tomes, *A Generous Confidence: Thomas Story Kirkbride and the Art of Asylum Keeping, 1840-1883* (Cambridge: Cambridge University Press, 1984), pp. 84-85; Gerald Grob, *Mental Institutions in America: Social Policy to 1875* (New York: Free Press, 1973), pp. 133-34; Andrew T. Scull, *Museums of Madness: The Social Organization of Insanity in Nineteenth-Century England* (New York: St. Martin's Press, 1979), pp. 154-58.

10. MBR, 1828-1836.

11. *AR*, 1829; MBR, November 29, 1831, March 17, 1828-April 4, 1840; House Journal, 1830, pp. 114, 125; SRR, January 14, 1837.

12. Cooper and McCord, *Statutes* 6:382-83.

13. *South Carolina State Gazette*, March-June 1828; *Charleston Mercury*, March-June 1828; *Columbia Telescope*, January 9, 30, 1829.

14. *Camden Journal*, April 19, 1828.

15. SCSH, Admission Book, 1828-1874, DMH, SCDAH, p. 1; PTR, 1; *Charleston Mercury*, November 28, 1828; *Pendleton Messenger*, December 10, 1828; MBR, July 5, December 12, 1828; *AR*, 1831. The number of admissions during this period

was somewhat larger than the admission book reveals, because a few patients for whom case records exist do not appear in the admission book.

16. Cooper and McCord, *Statutes* 6:322–24, 6:383.

17. *Pendleton Messenger*, May 20, 1829, reprinted from *Charleston Mercury*.

18. *Columbia Telescope*, January 30, 1829; see also *Pendleton Messenger*, February 11, 1829. See also William Gilmore Simms, "Lunatic Asylum," *Magnolia; or Southern Apalachian* 1, n.s. (1842): 394.

19. *Pendleton Messenger*, May 20, 1829, reprinted from *Charleston Mercury*; *Biographical Directory of the South Carolina House of Representatives* (Columbia: University of South Carolina Press, 1974–84), 4:154–56; John Belton O'Neall, *Biographical Sketches of the Bench and Bar of South Carolina*, 2 vols. (Charleston, 1859), 1:243–52. Desaussure was a Trustee of the College of Charleston, the Charleston Orphan House, and the Columbia Academy, as well as one of the founders of the South Carolina College.

20. John Belton O'Neall, *Annals of Newberry* (Charleston, 1859), pp. 252–53; O'Neall, *Biographical Sketches* 2:159–62; PTR, 1, Rebecca O'Neall.

21. Thomas Y. Simons, *Observations on Mental Alienation and Medical Jurisprudence* (Charleston, 1828), p. 7.

22. MBR, May 1, 1847.

23. Thomas W. Moore, "On Mania" (Medical thesis, Medical College of South Carolina, 1829), pp. 16–17, WHL.

24. Samuel Henry Dickson, *Essays on Pathology and Therapeutics*, 2 vols. (New York, 1845), 2:380.

25. Simms, "Lunatic Asylum," p. 394; *AR*, 1842, pp. 20–22.

26. Arthur Lynah, "Dissertation on Insanity" (Medical thesis, Medical College of South Carolina, 1847); Camden M. Boykin, "Mania" (Medical thesis, Medical College of South Carolina, 1841), pp. 9–10. See also William C. Miller, "Remarks on Insanity" (Medical thesis, Medical College of South Carolina, 1845).

27. MBR, May 7, 1842; *AR*, 1842; Reports of the Committee on the Lunatic Asylum, 1859c, 1859, GAP. See also the *Charleston Courier*, December 5, 1840; Simms, "Lunatic Asylum," pp. 394–95; *Charleston Medical Journal* 7 (1852): 693–94; House Journal, 1833, pp. 134–37; Reports of the Legislative Committees on the Lunatic Asylum, *RR*, 1835–1848.

28. Henry H. Townes to Rachel Townes, May 6, May 18, 1835, Henry Townes to George F. Townes, May 11, July 18, 1835, Henry H. Townes to John Townes, August 29, 1835, Townes Family Papers, SCL.

29. Henry H. Townes to Rachel Townes, July 20, 1835, Townes Family Papers, SCL.

30. John C. Calhoun to Armistead Burt, May 18, 1838, John C. Calhoun Papers, Manuscript Department, Perkins Library, Duke University.

31. John C. Calhoun to Armistead Burt, May 27, 1838, Manuscript Department, Perkins Library, Duke University. The published papers of John C. Calhoun contain several letters relating to the illness of Patrick Calhoun, including some from

members of the Townes family. See Clyde N. Wilson, ed., *The Papers of John C. Calhoun* (Columbia: University of South Carolina Press, 1981), 14:292–93, 305, 311–12, 354, 499, 593.

32. PTR, 2, Patrick Calhoun; John C. Calhoun to Mrs. Anna Maria Calhoun Clemson, March 18, 1839, in Wilson, *Papers of John C. Calhoun*, 14:593. See also Charles M. Wiltse, *John C. Calhoun, Nullifier, 1829–1839* (New York: Bobbs-Merrill, 1949), pp. 312–13. Wiltse states mistakenly that Patrick recovered without being sent to the asylum.

33. Theodore S. Gourdin to R. F. W. Allston, February 7, 1848, Theodore S. Gourdin Papers, SCHS.

34. R. F. W. Allston to Theodore S. Gourdin, Feb. 21, 1848, Theodore S. Gourdin Papers, SCHS.

35. MBR, March 7, May 2, 1829, April 3, 1830; SCSH, Admission Book, 1828–1874; James Woods Babcock, "The State Hospital for the Insane, Columbia, South Carolina," in *The Institutional Care of the Insane in the United States and Canada*, ed. Henry M. Hurd, 4 vols. (Baltimore: Johns Hopkins Press, 1916–17), 3:593.

36. SCSH, Admission Book, 1828–1874; PTR, 1. It is impossible to be precise about the number of pauper patients admitted during the first year. Some patients were not designated paying or pauper in the admission book, although Davis often mentioned the patient's status in his case record. To confuse things more, some of the patients in the physicians' case records are not listed in the admission book.

37. AR, 1828; MBR, November 29, December 22, 1828, February 4, 1832; Report of the Trustees of the Lunatic Asylum, 1827, GAP.

38. *Charleston Mercury*, November 27, 1829; *Pendleton Messenger*, December 9, 1829; Report of the Trustees of the Lunatic Asylum, 1827. Cooper and McCord, *Statutes* (1829) 6:382–83; *AR*, 1830, GAP.

39. Cooper and McCord, *Statutes* (1831) 6:437.

40. *AR*, 1847, pp. 8–9, 1842, p. 23.

41. CCP, Minutes, November 16, 1824, May 8, 1828, July 16, 1829; Robert Mills, *Statistics of South Carolina*, pp. 431–32.

42. CCP, Minutes, 1828–34, list inside front cover of state grants to the city for transient paupers, 1784–1828; CCP, Minutes, February 28, April 10, 24, May 8, 1828. The amount of the state grant to Charleston for transient paupers dropped from twelve thousand dollars in 1825 to four thousand dollars in 1828.

43. Quoted in *Pendleton Messenger*, June 23, 1830.

44. MBR, May 19, 1832.

45. CCP, Minutes, January 26, 1832.

46. Ibid., June 24, 28, November 30, 1832, February 7, 21, 1833; MBR, November 3, 1832.

47. Harriet Martineau, *Retrospect of Western Travel*, 2 vols. (London, 1838), 1:293–94; CCP, Minutes, May 4, 1836, January 8, 1840, August 31, 1842, January 3, 1844; CCP, Letter Book, August 1835, April 26, 1836, June 20, 1837, January 8, 1838.

48. *AR*, 1829; MBR, June 7, 1828, April 4, June 6, 1829.

49. *AR*, 1832, in GAP; *AR*, 1829; MBR, November 29, 1828.

50. Harriet Martineau, *Society in America*, 2 vols. (New York, 1837), 2:291–92; MBR, January 5, February 2, March 2, 1839, November 2, 1844; SRR, February 2, 1839; *AR*, 1844, p. 4.

51. PTR, 1, Jefferson; MBR, June 27, November 28, 1828, April 4, June 6, October 3, 1829; *AR*, 1829; Babcock, "State Hospital," pp. 602–3.

52. PTR, 2, David I. Duncan. Duncan was readmitted in 1850. See Admission Book, 1828–1874.

53. Simms, "Lunatic Asylum," p. 395.

54. *RR*, 1848, p. 77; Report of the House Committee on the Lunatic Asylum, December 16, 1847, GAP.

55. Parker reported the number of black admissions since 1848 as thirty in *AR*, 1858, pp. 12–13; SCSH, Admission Book, 1828–1874, shows only twenty-six black (slave or colored) admissions between 1848 and 1860, but a few may not be listed as black.

56. SCSH, Admission Book, 1828–1874; *AR*, 1858, pp. 12–13.

57. *AR*, 1860, p. 13.

58. *AR*, 1849, pp. 3, 5, 1850, p. 12, 1851, p. 8, 1853, p. 24, 1858, pp. 12–13; 1860, p. 13; *RR*, 1849, p. 236; MBR, December 23, 1848, November 6, 1858, November 5, 1859, August 4, September 17, 1860. During the Civil War, the regents decided not to admit any blacks. In 1863, Parker apologized to the board for receiving a slave woman. MBR, September 5, 1863. On the connections between the economic, political, and racial situation in antebellum South Carolina and the state's policies toward blacks, see William Freehling, *Prelude to Civil War: The Nullification Controversy in South Carolina, 1816–1836* (New York: Harper and Row, 1966), chap. 2; George C. Rogers Jr. *Charleston in the Age of the Pinckneys* (Norman: University of Oklahoma Press, 1969), pp. 141–49; Marina Wikramanyake, *A World in Shadow: The Free Black in Antebellum South Carolina* (Columbia: University of South Carolina Press, 1973); John Barnwell, *Love of Order: South Carolina's First Secession Crisis* (Chapel Hill: University of North Carolina Press, 1982), pp. 32–33.

59. "Proceedings of the Association," *American Journal of Insanity* 12 (1855): 43.

60. Grob, *Mental Institutions in America*, pp. 243–55; Todd L. Savitt, *Medicine and Slavery: The Diseases and Health Care of Blacks in Antebellum Virginia* (Urbana: University of Illinois Press, 1978), pp. 258–79; Norman Dain, *Disordered Minds: The First Century of Eastern State Hospital in Williamsburg, Virginia, 1766–1866* (Charlottesville: University Press of Virginia, 1971), p. 19, and *Concepts of Insanity in the United States, 1789–1865* (New Brunswick, N.J.: Rutgers University Press, 1964), pp. 107–8.

61. *AR*, 1829–1860. See the following chapter for a fuller discussion of the nature of the antebellum patient population.

62. Freehling, *Prelude to Civil War*, p. 121; Lacy K. Ford, *The Origins of South-*

ern Radicalism: The South Carolina Upcountry, 1800–1860 (New York: Oxford University Press, 1988), pp. 18–20.

63. Senate Journal, 1831, pp. 65–66, 1830, pp. 117, 125, 127; House Journal, 1830, pp. 102, 114, 125, 161, 209.

64. *AR*, 1832.

65. *AR*, 1829; MBR, April 3, 1830, February 4, 1832.

66. *AR*, 1830.

67. MBR, January 1, 1831.

68. MBR, November 29, 1831.

69. *RR*, 1832, p. 11; Cooper and McCord, *Statutes* 6:437.

70. PTR, 1, Daniel McHenry.

71. Mortality statistics were irregularly reported until the later 1840s and are not available for every year. *AR*, 1842, p. 24; SRR, September 1, October 13, 27, November 3, 10, 1832, October 1833; MBR, January 7, 1832; House Journal, 1833, p. 135; SCSH, Admission Book, 1828–1874.

72. House Journal, 1833, pp. 134–37; Senate Journal 1835, p. 121; *RR*, 1834, p. 4, 1835, p. 32.

73. See *RR*, Reports of the House and Senate Committees on the Lunatic Asylum and Comptroller General's Reports, 1835–1856; Leila G. Johnson, "A History of the South Carolina State Hospital" (M.A. thesis, University of Chicago, 1930). p. 43, table 3.

CHAPTER FOUR

1. Albert Deutsch, *The Mentally Ill in America: A History of Their Care and Treatment from Colonial Times* (Garden City, N.Y.: Doubleday, Doran, 1937), p. 106; Norman Dain, *Concepts of Insanity in the United States, 1789–1865* (New Brunswick, N.J.: Rutgers University Press, 1964), p. 128; Gerald Grob, *Mental Institutions in America: Social Policy to 1875* (New York: Free Press, 1973), pp. 96, 344.

2. The Kentucky Asylum was a custodial institution in its early years, according to Ronald F. White, "Custodial Care for the Insane at Eastern State Hospital in Lexington, Kentucky, 1824–44," *Filson Club Quarterly* 62 (1988): 303–35. See also his dissertation, "A Dialogue on Madness: Eastern State Lunatic Asylum and Mental Health Policies in Kentucky, 1824–1883" (Ph.D. diss., University of Kentucky, 1984).

3. On the influence of the corporate asylums on the founders of the state asylums, see Andrew Scull, "The Discovery of the Asylum Revisited," in *Madhouses, Mad-Doctors, and Madmen*, ed. Andrew Scull (Philadelphia: University of Pennsylvania Press, 1981), chap. 6; Grob, *Mental Institutions in America*, chaps. 2, 3.

4. Statistics of paying and pauper admissions were not always included in the annual reports, nor is patient status always recorded in the asylum's admission book.

5. Petition of Citizens of Anderson District praying that John King, a Lunatic, may be Supported at the Expence of the District, 1831, GAP; Report of the Pendleton Delegation on the Memorial of Sundry Citizens of that District respecting John King a Lunatic, 1831, GAP; *RR*, 1831, p. 60.

6. SRR, November 7, 9, 1833, January 20, 1834, March 5, June 4, 1836, June 6, 1838, February 9, 1839, May 25, 1844, May 20, 1848, December 11, 1852; MBR, June 6, 1829, February 6, 1830, May 1, 1830; John C. Calhoun to Armistead Burt, July 2, 1838, John C. Calhoun Papers, Manuscript Department, Perkins Library, Duke University.

7. *AR*, 1842, pp. 16-17.

8. Crafts, *Oration*, pp. 12-16; Special Committee on Lunatics, [1818], GAP; Deutsch, *Mentally Ill in America*, chap. 8.

9. *Pendleton Messenger*, May 20, 1829; see also ibid., February 11, 1829; *AR*, 1829.

10. *AR*, 1829.

11. *AR*, 1842, p. 24.

12. According to a letter in the *Pendleton Messenger*, Davis visited most of the asylums as far north as New York. The institutions were not named, but they probably included the Friends Retreat at Frankford, Pennsylvania, perhaps the lunatic department of the Pennsylvania Hospital in Philadelphia, the Bloomingdale Asylum in New York, and perhaps the Hartford Retreat in Connecticut. Because the asylums Davis visited were described as "Northern," he probably did not visit any of the existing southern asylums such as the Eastern Virginia Asylum at Williamsburg, the Western Virginia Asylum at Staunton, and the Kentucky and Maryland asylums. MBR, March 17, November 29, 1828; *Pendleton Messenger*, May 20, 1829.

13. *Pendleton Messenger*, May 20, 1829, reprinted from *Charleston Mercury*. See also *South Carolina State Gazette*, March 22, 1828.

14. Samuel Tuke, *Description of the Retreat* (York, 1813).

15. *AR*, 1829.

16. *AR*, 1829, 1830; *Pendleton Messenger*, May 20, 1829.

17. SRR, July 14, 1832; see also SRR, September 1, 1832, July 19, 1834, August 17, 1834.

18. *AR*, 1830, pp. 1-2.

19. MBR, November 29, 1828, May 1, 1830, April 2, 1831; House Journal, 1833, p. 136.

20. Robert Gardiner Hill, *Total Abolition of Personal Restraint in the Treatment of the Insane* (London [1839]), p. 21; see also Hill's *Lunacy: Its Past and Present* (London, 1870), esp. pp. 33-38; John Conolly, *The Treatment of the Insane Without Mechanical Restraint* (London, 1856), pp. 178-79. For a detailed account of Hill's work, see Justin A. Frank, "Non-Restraint and Robert Gardiner Hill," *Bulletin of the History of Medicine* 41 (1967): 140-60.

21. Grob, *Mental Institutions in America*, pp. 206-11; Nancy Tomes, "The Great Restraint Controversy: A Comparative Perspective on Anglo-American Psy-

chiatry in the Nineteenth Century," in *The Anatomy of Madness*, ed. W. F. Bynum, Roy Porter, and Michael Shepherd (London: Tavistock, 1985), 3:190-225.

22. The medical officers of the South Carolina Lunatic Asylum did not participate regularly in the meetings of Association of Medical Superintendents of American Institutions for the Insane (AMSAII). But Parker attended the meetings in 1846 and 1851. MBR, April 4, 1846, April 23, 1851; John Curwen, *History of the Association of Medical Superintendents of American Institutions for the Insane* (n.p., 1875), pp. 10-11, 22-26. On the superintendents' debate over nonrestraint, see Grob, *Mental Institutions in America*, pp. 206-10.

23. *AR*, 1844, 1.

24. *AR*, 1847, in *RR*, p. 112.

25. Ibid.; *AR* 1850, in *RR*, p. 54; *AR* 1853, pp. 18-19, 25; *AR* 1857, p. 7; *AR*, 1858, in *RR*, p. 232; SRR, June 17, 1854.

26. William Bynum, "Rationales for Therapy in British Psychiatry, 1780-1835," in Scull, *Madhouses*, pp. 41-44.

27. *AR*, 1829; On American physicians' attempts to reconcile medical and moral approaches, see Dain, *Concepts of Insanity*, pp. 13-14.

28. *AR*, 1829-1831; MBR, 1828-1836. For a discussion of Davis's therapeutics in the wider context of antebellum asylum medicine, see Samuel Thielman, "Madness and Medicine: Trends in American Medical Therapeutics for Insanity, 1820-1860," *Bulletin of the History of Medicine* (1987) 61:35-37, and "Madness and Medicine: The Medical Approach to Madness in Antebellum America, with Particular Reference to the Eastern Lunatic Asylum of Virginia and the South Carolina Lunatic Asylum" (Ph.D. diss., Duke University, 1986).

29. PTR, 1, Warren Williams.

30. One of Davis's pupils, Josiah C. Nott, was for a time enthusiastic about some aspects of Broussais's system; indeed, it was Nott who performed the postmortem referred to in the text. Nott was especially attracted by the fact that Broussais emphasized moderate, topical bleeding with leeches or cups rather than general bleeding. The problem in making any such connections, as John Harley Warner notes, was that there were often substantial gaps between the therapeutic theories individual physicians held and their therapeutic principles and practices. Moreover, Broussais's influence concerning bleeding in insanity was ambivalent. He criticized the kind of drastic bleeding Rush recommended but also blasted Pinel for deemphasizing bloodletting for insanity too much. John Harley Warner, *The Therapeutic Perspective: Medical Practice, Knowledge, and Identity in America, 1820-1885* (Cambridge, Mass.: Harvard University Press, 1986), esp. pp. 2-6, 37-57; F. J. V. Broussais, *On Irritation and Insanity*, trans. Thomas Cooper (Columbia, S.C., 1831), pp. 268-73; Hardy Wickwar and Charles S. Bryan, "Broussais in Columbia, South Carolina—1831," *Journal of the South Carolina Medical Association* 77 (1981): 615-22; Thielman, "Madness and Medicine: The Medical Approach," pp. 107-8. On Nott, see Reginald Horsman, *Josiah Nott of*

Mobile: Southerner, Physician, and Racial Theorist (Baton Rouge: Louisiana State University Press, 1987).

31. PTR, 1, Eliza Fanning, Peter Savanna, Rachel Ward, James Flournoy, Edward Clanahan, Nathaniel Snow, Edward Rains, Joseph Bowie, Samuel Irwin. For a discussion of the use of bleeding by antebellum asylum physicians, see Thielman, "Madness and Medicine: Trends," pp. 35–37, and "Madness and Medicine: The Medical Approach," pp. 108-16. The gradual decline of bleeding in American medicine is chronicled in Leon S. (Charles) Bryan Jr., "Bloodletting in American Medicine, 1830-1892," *Bulletin of the History of Medicine* 38 (1964): 516–29.

32. PTR, 1, David McMillan, William Ross, John Pearson, Eliza Fanning, Spencer Mann, Elizabeth Caldwell, John Adams. The changing medical therapeutics of antebellum alienists is discussed in Thielman, "Madness and Medicine: Trends," pp. 25–46. For general discussions of heroic medicine in the antebellum era, see William G. Rothstein, *American Physicians in the Nineteenth Century: From Sects to Science* (Baltimore: Johns Hopkins University Press, 1972); John S. Haller Jr., *American Medicine in Transition, 1840–1910* (Urbana: University of Illinois Press, 1981); Warner, *Therapeutic Perspective*, esp. chap. 2; Charles Rosenberg, "The Therapeutic Revolution," in *the Therapeutic Revolution*, ed. Morris J. Vogel and Charles Rosenberg (Philadelphia: University of Pennsylvania Press, 1979).

33. PTR, 1, Rachel Hair, Rebecca O'Neall, James McMillan, Edmund Caldwell, Samuel Irwin; Haller, *American Medicine in Transition*, pp. 68–90.

34. PTR, 1, James Flournoy; see also ibid., Edward Rains, John Stokes, Ann Thompson.

35. PTR, 1, James Craig, Rachel Hair, Alexander Howell.

36. Warner, *Therapeutic Perspective*, chap. 3. See also John Harley Warner "The Idea of Southern Medical Distinctiveness: Medical Knowledge and Practice in the Old South," in *Science and Medicine in the Old South*, ed. Ronald L. Numbers and Todd L. Savitt (Baton Rouge: Louisiana State University Press, 1989), pp. 179-206. For a general discussion of medical treatment of insanity in the antebellum south, see Samuel B. Thielman, "Southern Madness: The Shape of Mental Health Care in the Old South," in Numbers and Savitt, *Science and Medicine in the Old South*, pp. 256-75.

37. PTR, 1, John Stokes. See also PTR, 1, Morris Fitzgerald, Elizabeth Allen.

38. PTR, 1, Elizabeth Caldwell; see also PTR 1, S. J. Mann, Alfred Frisbee, Samuel McCants.

39. PTR, 1, Stephen Parkman.

40. PTR, 1, Archibald Baynard; see also PTR, 1, John Carlisle, Mary Keadle, Cynthia Peach, Alexander Horn.

41. PTR, 1, Mary (Polly) Saxon.

42. PTR, 1, Nathaniel Snow; see also PTR, 1, Mary Donn.

43. PTR, 1, Allen Griffin.

44. PTR, 1, Polly Saxon.

45. PTR, 1, James McMillan, Allen Griffin; see also PTR, 1, Joseph Bowie; Haller, *American Medicine in Transition*, pp. 92–93.

46. PTR, 1, Polly Saxon.

47. PTR, 1, James Craig, Joseph Bowie.

48. Rothstein, *American Physicians*, pp. 50–52; Warner, *Therapeutic Perspective*, pp. 116–25. PTR, 1, Samuel Irwin, John Truitt, Elizabeth Marshall.

49. *AR*, 1850, pp. 9–11, 1859, pp. 12–13. Parker occasionally referred in his case book to an "Old Record" and to a "receipt book" that contained greater details about some patients' treatment. But these apparently have not survived.

50. PTR, 2, Robert Mayrant, Densby Dorn, Walter McLintock, Stephen Monk, Peter McMakin, A. S. Queen, Daniel Fisher.

51. PTR, 1, John Townes; for similar examples, see PTR, 1, Susan Kennedy, Benjamin Jenkins; PTR, 2, Josephine Catonet, Samuel Thomas, Rachel Hair, E. N. McFaddin, Mary Wiss.

52. PTR, 2, Francis Adams.

53. PTR, 1, James Nauher.

54. PTR, 2, James Nauher, M. I. Inhan; see also PTR, 2, Sarah Simmons, Catherine White, John Hurst, Ausibel Morgan, Mary Highland, Mary Wilcox, Sarah Boone, Georgia Robert, Mary Burger.

55. *AR*, 1842, pp. 19–20.

56. *AR*, 1847, pp. 5–6; Thielman, "Madness and Medicine: Trends," and "Madness and Medicine: The Medical Approach."

57. PTR, 1, Sally Owens.

58. PTR, 2, Mary Couterier.

59. PTR, 2, Densby Dorn, A. C. Shesgreen, Moses Hollis, Alexander Branyan, Sarah Cornelius; see also PTR, 2, Margaret Means, Georgia Robert, Susan Wray, Elizabeth Horsley, Elizabeth Douglas.

60. *AR*, 1847, p. 10.

61. *AR*, 1857, p. 7.

62. *AR*, 1859, p. 11.

63. PTR, 2, John Cline.

64. PTR, 3, John Smith. See also Thomas Faysoux, Martin Cox.

65. PTR, 3, Robison Marsh, John Mayo; see also PTR, 3, Betsy Sears, V. R. Gary, Jane Hadden, Caroline Barnett.

66. Thielman, "Madness and Medicine: Trends," pp. 33–46; Warner, *Therapeutic Perspective*, chap. 4.

67. This figure is based on the annual reports for 1829, 1830, 1832, and 1833. Those for 1831 and 1834 did not mention the number of cures.

68. *AR*, 1855, in *RR*, pp. 155–58, 1852, pp. 12–16.

69. On recovery rates and the problems of assessing them, see William Lloyd Parry-Jones, *The Trade in Lunacy: A Study of Private Madhouses in England in the Eighteenth and Nineteenth Centuries* (London: Routledge and Kegan Paul,

1972), pp. 198–206; Anne Digby, *Madness, Morality, and Medicine: A Study of the York Retreat, 1796–1914* (Cambridge: Cambridge University Press), 1985, pp. 121–24; Ellen Dwyer, *Homes for the Mad: Life Inside Two Nineteenth-Century Asylums* (New Brunswick, N.J.: Rutgers University Press, 1987), pp. 149–56; Grob, *Mental Institutions in America*, pp. 68–69, 182–185.

70. Christopher C. G. Memminger, quoted in Anne Scott, *The Southern Lady: From Pedestal to Politics, 1830–1930* (Chicago: University of Chicago Press, 1970), pp. 16–17. For an overview of the position of women in the antebellum South, see Scott, pp. 3–45; Catherine Clinton, *The Plantation Mistress: Woman's World in the Old South* (New York: Pantheon Books, 1982).

71. Elaine Showalter, *The Female Malady: Women, Madness, and English Culture, 1830–1980* (New York: Pantheon Books, 1985), pp. 28, 48–50, 74–83; Andrew T. Scull, *Museums of Madness: The Social Organization of Insanity in Nineteenth-Century England* (New York: St. Martin's Press, 1979), chap. 4. Showalter's view that nineteenth-century asylums were particularly repressive toward women is questioned by Nancy Tomes, "Historical Perspectives on Women and Mental Illness," in *Women, Health and Medicine in America*, ed. Rima D. Apple (New Brunswick, N.J.: Rutgers University Press, 1990), pp. 143–71.

72. PTR, 2, Martha Smith; PTR, 1, Josephine Catonet.

73. PTR, 1, Rachel Seybert.

74. PTR, 1, Josephine Catonet.

75. PTR, 2, M. I. Inhan.

76. PTR, 1, Patrick Flanagan, Thomas Martin.

77. PTR, 1, G. F. Williams.

78. See, for example, PTR, 1, 2, Matthew Talbot. During the 1850s, Parker obliquely accused Trezevant of discharging as cured patients who were still insane and dangerous. But at the time the two were in conflict over their respective spheres of authority. See SRR, August 11, September 4, 1855, August 23, November 1, 1856, February 14, 1857.

79. *AR*, 1857, p. 6, 1829, 1842, pp. 11–13, 20, 1847, in *RR*, p. 104.

80. Report of the Committee on the Lunatic Asylum, c. 1859, GAP.

81. *AR*, 1842, p. 23; *AR*, 1830; Cooper and McCord, *Statutes* 6:437.

82. *AR*, 1842, p. 23, 1847, in *RR*, 104, 1848, p. 8.

83. PTR, 1, Eliza Fanning.

84. PTR, 1, 1828–37, Elizabeth Marshall, William Ross. See also PTR, 1, Ezekiel Harris, Elizabeth Caldwell, William Gee, Shelton Lofton.

85. *AR*, 1844, p. 11; PTR, 1, Mrs. Nancy Hair; PTR, 2, A. N. Knight, Martha Smith; PTR, 3, Ann Lanagan; SRR, October 23, 1847, May 30, August 1, 1857.

86. PTR, 1, John Parr, Stephen P. Monk; MBR, June 2, July 1, 1837, May 6, 1843, October 18, 1851; SRR, March 20, 1849, January 20, 1855.

CHAPTER FIVE

1. *AR*, 1829, 1830; *Pendleton Messenger*, May 20, 1829, reprinted from *Charleston Mercury*.

2. *AR*, 1844, p. 1.

3. "Pet" to her Sister, November 1854, Porcher-Gregg Family Papers, SCL.

4. Andrew C. Moore to his Mother, February 24, 1855, John Thomas Moore Papers, SCL.

5. MBR, May 12, 1853.

6. PTR, 2, Georgia W. Robert.

7. H. H. Townes to Rachel Townes, May 6, May 18, July 20, 1835, H. H. Townes to George F. Townes, May 11, 1835, September 8, 1836, H. H. Townes to John Townes, August 29, 1835, Townes Family Papers, SCL.

8. Mary P. Allston to Theodore S., William, and Samuel Gourdin, June 24, [July?] 10, December 23, 1848, J. W. Parker to Theodore S. Gourdin, January 7, 1849, July 3, 1850, R. F. W. Allston to Theodore S. Gourdin, December 12, 1850, Theodore S. Gourdin Papers, SCHS; PTR, 2, Mary P. Allston.

9. PTR, 1, John Hollingsworth.

10. SRR, May 27, 1837, July 11, 1839.

11. SRR, September 1, Oct. 13, 27, November 3, 10, 1832; MBR, January 7, 1832; House Journal, 1833, p. 135.

12. PTR, 1, Patrick Hayes; SRR, August 25, September 1, 1832, April 7, October 19, November 9, 1833; *AR*, 1829.

13. SRR, June 23, August 25, 1832; PTR, 1, Maria Schmidt, Christian Rumph; PTR, 2, Zachariah Goodson.

14. PTR, 1, John Stokes.

15. SRR, June 30, July 7, 21, August 25, 1832.

16. PTR, 1, Rachel Seybert.

17. PTR, 1, Maria Schmidt.

18. SRR, August 17, 1833; PTR, 1, Stephen P. Monk.

19. SRR, June 23, July 7, 21, September 1, 8, 1832, February 23, March 2, 30, 1833; PTR, 1, Harriet J. Gray, Christian Rumph, Rachel Seybert, Edward Clanahan, Polly Griffin, Rachel Hair, Micajah Ford.

20. *AR*, 1851, pp. 8–9.

21. SRR, July 6, 1851; *AR*, 1851, pp. 8–9.

22. SRR, June 25, 1836.

23. SRR, March 22, 1834.

24. SRR, May 18, 1833, March 22, 1834.

25. PTR, 1, John Hollingsworth. See also PTR, 1, Edward Clanahan.

26. SRR, July 9, 1836; PTR, 1, Christian Rumph.

27. *AR*, 1842, p. 19; *AR*, 1844, p. 1.

28. SRR, April 30, 1837, June 2, 1838, May 19, 1849. See also SRR, December 19, 1836, January 26, 1850.

29. *AR*, 1859, p. 12.

30. Gerald Grob, *Mental Institutions in America: Social Policy to 1875* (New York: Free Press, 1973), pp. 176-78; Andrew T. Scull, *Museums of Madness: The Social Organization of Insanity in Nineteenth-Century England* (New York: St. Martin's Press, 1979), pp. 198-203; Charles Rosenberg, *The Care of Strangers: The Rise of America's Hospital System to 1875* (New York: Basic Books 1987), pp. 34-38.

31. MBR, January 5, March 17, 1828, February 5, April 2, August 6, 1831.

32. *AR*, 1847, in *RR*, pp. 108, 112-13, 1850, in *RR*, p. 54, 1852, p. 13.

33. MBR, November 2, 1850.

34. *AR*, 1844, pp. 11-13, 1849, in *RR*, p. 230, 1851, p. 12. In the 1870s, one of the regents complained that locals often came to the asylum to take flowers from the garden and greenhouse. MBR, July 13, 1876.

35. *AR*, 1849, in *RR*, p. 227.

36. SRR, May 26, 1855; *AR*, 1852, pp. 12, 18; Trezevant, *Letters to His Excellency*, pp. 45-46.

37. MBR, April 3, 1841, January 5, 1850; *Acts Concerning the Lunatic Asylum of South Carolina; and By-Laws for Its Government* (Columbia, 1850), p. 16.

38. *AR*, 1844, pp. 10-11, 1852, p. 18.

39. *AR*, 1851, p. 12, 1852, p. 18. The case history of Robison Marsh illustrates some of the problems visits by relatives might create. After a visit from his father, Marsh became highly excited for several days, destroyed his furniture and dishes, and continually denounced his father. PTR, 3, Robison P. Marsh.

40. *AR*, 1842, pp. 3-11, 16, 22-23.

41. Samuel Tuke, *Description of the Retreat* (York, 1813), pp. 160-61; George Man Burrows, *An Inquiry into Certain Errors Relative to Insanity* (London, 1820), pp. 223, 230; Grob, *Mental Institutions in America*, p. 180; Norman Dain, *Concepts of Insanity in the United States, 1789-1865* (New Brunswick, N.J.: Rutgers University Press, 1964), p. 184; Nancy Tomes, *A Generous Confidence: Thomas Story Kirkbride and the Art of Asylum Keeping, 1840-1883* (Cambridge: Cambridge University Press, 1984), p. 48.

42. MBR, May 2, August 1, September 6, 1829, August 4, 1838, May 14, 1842, November 10, 1844; *AR*, 1842, pp. 8-9, 23, 1844, pp. 1-2, 6-7.

43. Helen Kohn Hennig, *Columbia: 1786-1936* (Columbia, S.C.: R. L. Bryan, 1936), p. 150; E. B. Hort to Thomas Kirkbride, April 29, 1850, Kirkbride Correspondence, General, Pennsylvania Hospital Library, Philadelphia (hereafter cited as Kirkbride Correspondence). Hort had made Kirkbride's acquaintance during a visit to the Pennsylvania Hospital in 1848. See John W. Parker to Kirkbride, July 8, 1848, in same correspondence.

44. *AR*, 1847, in *RR*, pp. 110, 1848, p. 10, 1850, p. 55, 1856, p. 11, 1857, p. 7.

45. *AR*, 1852, p. 4.

46. *AR*, 1842, pp. 7, 16, 22, 1844, pp. 1-2; MBR, January 4, 1830, June 3, 1832, February 7, 1846.

47. In 1853, 12.5 percent of the patients were foreign born; in 1859, the percent-

age was 14.9. As in the North, most immigrant patients were Irish. *AR*, 1853, pp. 27-31, 1859, pp. 16-21, 23; U.S. Bureau of the Census, *A Century of Population Growth* (Baltimore: Genealogical Publishing, 1967), p. 128. U.S. Bureau of the Census, *Statistics of the United States in 1860* (New York: Arno Press, 1976), xx. For discussion of immigrant patients in nineteenth-century American asylums, see Grob, *Mental Institutions in America*, pp. 230-36; Dain, *Concepts of Insanity*, pp. 99-104; David Rothman, *The Discovery of the Asylum: Social Order and Disorder in the New Republic* (Boston: Little, Brown, 1971), pp. 283-87.

48. *AR*, 1842, pp. 15-17, 1848, pp. 2, 4-9, 1851, pp. 3-4, 1852, pp. 4, 8-9, 1853, p. 5; *House Journal*, 1842, p. 17; *RR*, 1842, p. 99, 1848, p. 77; MBR, October 7, 1848.

49. *AR*, 1829; MBR, January 4, 1830, February 4, 1832.

50. *AR*, 1844, pp. 3-5; 1842, pp. 9-10.

51. House Journal, 1833, p. 135, 1834, pp. 164-65; MBR, March 7, May 2, 1829, January 4, 1830, February 4, 1832; *AR*, 1832.

52. In 1842, the regents stated that the asylum owned "60 to 70 acres," but in 1853, Trezevant reported the acreage as 55. House Journal, 1833, p. 135; John M. Galt, *The Treatment of Insanity* (New York, 1846), pp. 557-58; *AR*, 1842, p. 10 note, 1853, p. 9.

53. *AR*, 1844, p. 2; MBR, February 4, 1843, March 1, 1845, January 5, 1850, February 3, 1855, June 7, July 5, 1856; *AR*, 1857, p. 6; Report of the Committee on the Lunatic Asylum, c. 1859, GAP.

54. SRR, January 27, 1838; *AR*, 1857, p. 6.

55. PTR, 1, Peter Nightime, Jacob Paul.

56. *AR*, 1842, p. 26.

57. *AR*, 1844, pp. 7-8; PTR, 1, Peter Nightime.

58. *AR*, 1844, pp. 7-8; *AR*, 1847, pp. 97-101. On Lieber, see Frank Freidel, *Francis Lieber, Nineteenth Century Liberal* (Baton Rouge: Louisiana State University Press, 1947).

59. *AR*, 1844, p. 2, 1855, p. 21, 1857, p. 6; MBR, February 3, 1855, June 7, July 5, 1856; Report of the Committee on the Lunatic Asylum, c. 1859.

60. *AR*, 1847, in *RR*, pp. 97-101; SRR, September 30, 1837; PTR, 1, Maria Schmidt; *AR*, 1855, in *RR*, p. 159.

61. *AR*, 1847, in *RR*, pp. 105-6, 1842, pp. 22-23.

62. John W. Parker to R. F. W. Allston, April 16, 1860, R. F. W. Allston Papers, SCHS; Report of the Committee on the Lunatic Asylum, 1859, GAP; *AR*, 1850, pp. 18-19, 1853, pp. 25-26, 1855, in *RR*, pp. 159-60, 1857, pp. 4, 6, 1859, pp. 12-13, 1860, in *RR*, p. 263; MBR, April 1, 1854; SRR, May 6, 1854; John W. Parker to R. D. Bacot, September 9, 1861, Bacot Family Papers, SCL.

63. *AR*, 1855, in *RR*, p. 159.

64. *AR*, 1847, in *RR*, p. 109.

65. SRR, July 14, 1832, February 16, May 25, 1833, July 19, August 9, September 27, 1834, May 23, 1835.

66. *AR*, 1844, pp. 2–3.

67. *AR*, 1847, in *RR*, pp. 109–10, 1849, in *RR*, pp. 233, 1850, in *RR*, p. 55.

68. *AR*, 1857, p. 6.

69. *AR*, 1847, in *RR*, pp. 105–6.

70. *AR*, 1852, p. 12.

71. *AR*, 1855, pp. 19–20; 1857, pp. 6–7, 1859, p. 12.

72. *AR*, 1831, 1842, p. 7, note; 1847, in *RR*, p. 108, 1848, p. 7, 1849, in *RR*, p. 232, 1852, p. 7, 1860, in *RR*, p. 268; *Acts Concerning the Lunatic Asylum*, p. 14.

73. *AR*, 1842, pp. 6–7, 1844, pp. 5–6, 1847, in *RR*, p. 108, 1848, p. 7, 1850, in *RR*, p. 55.

74. *AR*, 1847, in *RR*, p. 108, 1848, p. 7.

75. PTR, 1, Jonas Robertson, PTR, 2, Susan Walsh.

76. *AR*, 1844, pp. 5–6.

77. John W. Parker to Thomas S. Kirkbride, August 7, 1858, July 19, 1859, Kirkbride Correspondence. On the problems northern institutions had in obtaining and retaining competent attendants, see Grob, *Mental Institutions in America*, pp. 211–19; Tomes, *Generous Confidence*, pp. 181–85; Ellen Dwyer, *Homes for the Mad: Life Inside Two Nineteenth-Century Asylums* (New Brunswick, N.J.: Rutgers University Press, 1987), pp. 163–85.

78. MBR, August 1, September 21, 1829, April 1, 1854, October 4, 1856; SRR, October 25, 1837, August 17, 1838, April 4, 1840, May 1, 1852, April 22, 1854, August 11, 1855; *AR*, 1852, pp. 11–12.

79. SRR, May 1, 1852, August 11, 1855, April 26, 1834, January 14, November 4, 1837, August 1, 1840, December 31, 1842, November 4, 1847, April 22, 1854; *AR*, 1848, p. 7; MBR, April 4, December 5, 1829, July 2, August 7, 1830, January 1, 1831.

80. MBR, November 4, 1847.

81. *AR*, 1856, p. 11; MBR, May 1, 1858; SRR, September 6, 1856.

82. SRR, April 27, 1844, June 10, August 5, 1848.

83. *AR*, 1842, p. 7.

84. Out of thirteen attendants listed in the 1850 census, ten were natives of Ireland. In the 1860 census, eighteen of twenty-four attendants were from Ireland. Only two of the attendants listed in the 1850 census were still working at the asylum in 1860. United States, 7th Census, 1850, 8th Census, 1860, Population Schedules for Richland Co.; J. F. Williams, *Old and New Columbia* (Columbia, S.C.: Epworth Orphanage Press, 1929), pp. 91–92.

85. *AR*, 1848, p. 7, 1860, in *RR*, p. 268; MBR, March 4, 1854, October 4, December 6, 1856, January 10, 1857, November 6, 1858, March 5, 1859.

86. John W. Parker to Thomas Kirkbride, August 7, 1858, Kirkbride Correspondence — General; MBR, March 17, 1828. In 1860 the South Carolina Lunatic Asylum employed twenty-three attendants at $200, and two others, probably part time, received $120 and $108, respectively. Two were paid $400 and one, the chief attendant, $700. *AR*, 1860, in *RR*, p. 268.

87. *AR*, 1847, in *RR*, p. 108, 1849, in *RR*, p. 232, 1851, p. 9, 1852, pp. 13, 19, 1853, p. 26, 1854, in *RR*, p. 124, 1857, p. 8, 1858, in *RR*, p. 235.

88. *AR*, 1853, p. 20, 1848, p. 7, 1849, in *RR*, p. 232, 1850, in *RR*, p. 55, 1851, p. 9, 1852, pp. 12-13, 1854, in *RR*, p. 121, 1855, in *RR*, pp. 154, 161, 1856, p. 11, 1857, p. 8, 1859, p. 13, 1860, in *RR*, p. 262.

CHAPTER SIX

1. *AR*, 1853, p. 11.

2. *AR*, 1853, p. 16; Daniel Trezevant, *Letters to His Excellency Governor Manning on the Lunatic Asylum* (Columbia, S.C., 1854; reprint, New York: Arno Press, 1973), p. 3.

3. *AR*, 1852, p. 8, 1851, pp. 6-7, pp. 11, 16-17; MBR, May 22, 1850; Trezevant, *Letters to His Excellency*, pp. 10-24.

4. *AR*, 1848, pp. 3-4, 1849, in *RR*, 1849, pp. 229-30, 1850, in *RR*, pp. 50-51, 1851, p. 6. MBR, June 7, 1856, May 2, 1857.

5. Trezevant, *Letters to His Excellency*, p. 40.

6. Ibid., pp. 40-42.

7. *AR*, 1849, in *RR*, pp. 230-31, 1851, pp. 6-7, 1852, p. 9; Trezevant, *Letters to His Excellency*, pp. 8-9, 18-19, 25, 40-42.

8. *AR*, 1853, p. 16.

9. *AR*, 1853, pp. 11, 15-16. Trezevant, *Letters to His Excellency*, p. 35; *AR*, 1849, in *RR*, p. 230, 1851, p. 6.

10. Frank Freidel, *Francis Lieber, Nineteenth Century Liberal* (Baton Rouge: Louisiana State University Press, 1947), pp. 259-61; SRR, April 14, 1846; Francis Lieber to Dorothea Dix, November 5, 1846, April 18, 1851, Dix Papers, Houghton Library, Harvard University; Lieber to G. S. Hilliard, May 1851, in T. S. Perry, ed., *The Life and Letters of Francis Lieber* (Boston, 1882), pp. 253-54.

11. Francis Lieber to Dorothea Dix, November 12, 1851, quoted in Freidel, *Francis Lieber*, p. 259; Lieber to G. S. Hilliard, May 1851, in Perry, *Life and Letters of Francis Lieber*, pp. 253-54; Lieber to Hilliard, August 11, 1850, Dix to Lieber, June 23, 1850, Francis Lieber Papers, SCL; John Barnwell, *Love of Order: South Carolina's First Secession Crisis* (Chapel Hill: University of North Carolina Press, 1982), pp. 11-13, 22-23, 26-27.

12. Thomas Kirkbride, *On the Construction, Organization, and General Arrangements of Hospitals for the Insane* (Philadelphia, 1854); Nancy Tomes, *A Generous Confidence: Thomas Story Kirkbride and the Art of Asylum Keeping, 1840-1883* (Cambridge: Cambridge University Press, 1984), pp. 6, 141-47, 265-66; Harold Coolidge, "The Kirkbride Plan: Architecture for a Treatment System that Changed," *Hospital and Community Psychiatry* 27 (1976): 473-74.

13. Wade Hampton Jr. to Thomas Kirkbride, August 22, 1853, John W. Parker to Thomas Kirkbride, July 12, 1854, Kirkbride Correspondence—General; Report

of the Committee on the Lunatic Asylum, 1853, GAP; Report of the Committee on the Lunatic Asylum and Medical Accounts, 1853, GAP.

14. Harold Coolidge, "The Kirkbride Plan: Architecture for a Treatment System that Changed," *Hospital and Community Psychiatry* 27 (1976): 473-77; Tomes, *Generous Confidence*, pp. 141-46.

15. *AR*, 1853, p. 12.

16. *AR*, 1853, pp. 12-13, 1855, pp. 8-9; MBR, January 8, February 19, April 3, November 17, 1853, February 4, 1854; John W. Parker to Thomas Kirkbride, July 12, 1854, Kirkbride Correspondence—General. The original asylum building designed by Mills had used the single range. The wings added later used the double range.

17. John W. Parker to Thomas Kirkbride, July 12, 1854, Kirkbride Correspondence—General; *AR*, 1855, p. 22.

18. Thomas S. Kirkbride, *Letter to the Regents of the South Carolina Hospital for the Insane* (n.p., 1854).

19. Francis Lieber to Dorothea Dix, February 2, 1854, Dix Papers, Houghton Library, Harvard University.

20. MBR, February 4, 1854.

21. MBR, November 20, 1852, January 28, 1854; *AR*, 1852, pp. 4-5, 10-11, 1853, pp. 3-8; Report of the Committee on the Lunatic Asylum, 1852, GAP.

22. *AR*, 1854, in *RR*, p. 119.

23. *AR*, 1854, in *RR*, pp. 118-19; MBR, January 28, November 11, 1854.

24. *AR*, 1853, pp. 14-15, 1855, p. 7; *Daily South Carolinian*, August 12, 21, 25, September 8, 13, 16, 1854; Trezevant, *Letters to His Excellency*.

25. *House Journal*, 1853, pp. 25-27, 1854, p. 24; MBR, April 13, May 10, 1853.

26. James M. Gaston, *An Essay on the Action and Reaction of the Mind and Body as Affecting Insanity* (Columbia, 1853), pp. 25-26.

27. Report of the Committee on the Lunatic Asylum, [1854], GAP. (incorrectly dated as 1853 in SCDAH index). Report of the Committee on the Lunatic Asylum and Medical Accounts, [1854], GAP (dated as c. 1852 in SCDAH index); *Report of the Committee on the Lunatic Asylum* (Columbia, 1855), pp. 3-4; *RR*, 1854, pp. 270-71. In the summer of 1853 the chairman of the House Committee on the Asylum, Wade Hampton Jr., wrote to Kirkbride to solicit his opinions concerning the design and location of a new building for the South Carolina Lunatic Asylum. Kirkbride made suggestions and sent some books on the construction of asylums. During the session of 1853, legislators frequently referred to Kirkbride's expertise. Wade Hampton Jr. to Kirkbride, August 22, 1853, Kirkbride Correspondence—General.

28. *RR*, 1854, pp. 270-71; MBR, September 27, October 6, November 17, 1855, June 7, July 5, 1856; *AR*, 1855, pp. 4, 7-16; Report of the Special Joint Committee on the Lunatic Asylum, [1855], GAP; Report of the Committee on the Lunatic Asylum and Medical Accounts, 1855, GAP.

29. *RR*, 1856, pp. 342-43; MBR, January 10, February 7, March 7, 1857; Parker to Thomas Kirkbride, April 26, 1857, Kirkbride Correspondence—General.

30. Francis Lieber to Dorothea Dix, February 2, 1854, Dix Papers, Houghton Library, Harvard University.

31. *AR*, 1853, p. 14; MBR, February 4, 1854. In 1855 the regents asked Trezevant to alter his annual report in a part relating to their position on removal. MBR, November 3, 1855.

32. *AR*, 1853, p. 19.

33. *AR*, 1853, p. 14.

34. Trezevant, *Letters to His Excellency*, p. 56.

35. *AR*, 1855, in *RR*, pp. 152-154. On Worcester and Massachusetts' policies toward its insane during this period, see Gerald Grob, *The State and the Mentally Ill: A History of Worcester State Hospital in Massachusetts* (Chapel Hill: University of North Carolina Press, 1966), pp. 145-60, and *Mental Institutions in America: Social Policy to 1875* (New York: Free Press, 1973), pp. 259-60.

36. Julian A. Selby, *Memorabilia and Anecdotal Reminiscences of Columbia, South Carolina* (Columbia, 1905), pp. 20-21.

37. *AR*, 1856, pp. 7-8; Selby, *Memorabilia*, 20-21.

38. *AR*, 1844, pp. 8-9; "Lunatic Asylums in the United States," *American Journal of Insanity* 2 (1845): 145-75, esp. p. 160; "American Insane Hospital Reports," *American Journal of the Medical Sciences* 28, n.s. (1854): 488.

39. *AR*, 1850, in *RR*, pp. 52-53, 1852, p. 17.

40. MBR, April 4, 1846, April 23, 1851. On the early history of AMSAII, now the American Psychiatric Association, see John Curwen, *History of the Association of Medical Superintendents of American Institutions for the Insane* (n.p., 1875), esp. pp. 10-11, 22-26; Grob, *Mental Institutions in America*, esp. pp. 132-39; Constance M. McGovern, *Masters of Madness: Social Origins of the American Psychiatric Profession* (Hanover, N.H.: University Press of New England, 1985).

41. *AR*, 1850, in *RR*, p. 53; 1852, p. 17, 1854, in *RR*, p. 124, 1855, p. 22; 1871, pp. 24-25.

42. MBR, August 5, 1854; SRR, August 11, September 4, 1855, August 23, November 1, 1856, February 14, 1857.

43. MBR, June 2, 1855; *AR*, 1855, pp. 5-6.

44. Trezevant's 1856 report was not printed with the asylum's annual report for that year, but it was included in the *Reports and Resolutions of the General Assembly*. *AR*, 1856, in *RR*, pp. 137-59; MBR, February 4, November 18, December 2, 23, 1854, January 6, 10, 1855, June 7, 1856.

45. *AR*, 1856, p. 5; MBR, May 5, June 2, November 17, 1855, November 19, December 8, 1856, January 10, February 7, 1857; SRR, February 14, 1857.

46. *AR*, 1856, in *RR*, pp. 158-59. Trezevant continued to be a leading figure of the Columbia medical establishment. In the 1860s he served as president of the Columbia Medical Society, and after the Civil War he authored a pamphlet that ac-

cused Sherman of ordering the burning of the city. Controversy continued to dog him. In October 1865 he took out an advertisement to contradict stories that he had refused to attend blacks. *Columbia Daily Phoenix*, May 23, October 1, 1865.

47. *AR*, 1858, in *RR*, p. 33.

48. *AR*, 1860, in *RR*, pp. 261–62.

49. John W. Parker to Dorothea Dix, March 15 [1859], December 28, 1859, April 9, 1860, Dix Papers, Houghton Library, Harvard University.

50. Helen Marshall, *Dorothea Dix, Forgotten Samaritan* (New York: Russell and Russell, 1937), p. 195; Freidel, *Francis Lieber*, p. 261; Grob, *Mental Institutions in America*, p. 108.

51. Freidel, *Francis Lieber*, p. 261; SRR, April 14, 1846. On Dix, see Marshall, *Dorothea Dix*; Dorothy C. Wilson, *Stranger and Traveler: The Story of Dorothea Dix, American Reformer* (Boston: Little, Brown, 1975).

52. Francis Lieber to G. S. Hilliard, May 1851, in Perry, *Life and Letters of Francis Lieber*, pp. 253–54.

53. A. R. Young to Rev. and Mrs. Cornish, February 5, 1859, John Hamilton Cornish Papers, SCL.

54. Report of the Committee on the Lunatic Asylum, 1859, GAP; Benjamin F. Perry to Elizabeth F. Perry, December 8, 1859, Benjamin F. Perry Papers, SCL. Marshall, *Dorothea Dix*, p. 195; MBR, December 3, 1859.

55. *AR*, 1858, in *RR*, pp. 228, 234, 1859, pp. 10–11, 1860, in *RR*, p. 260; Report of the Committee on the Lunatic Asylum, 1859, GAP. Report of the Committee on the Lunatic Asylum and Medical Accounts, 1859, GAP.

56. Report of the Committee on the Lunatic Asylum and Medical Accounts, *RR*, 1858, pp. 307–8; MBR, November 5, 1859, January 21, 1860; *AR*, 1859, pp. 10–11, 1860, in *RR*, pp. 262–263; John W. Parker to Dorothea Dix, March 15 [1859], November 12, 1859, Dix Papers, Houghton Library, Harvard University; Report of the Committee on the Lunatic Asylum, 1859, GAP; Report of the Committee on the Lunatic Asylum and Medical Accounts, 1859, GAP.

57. MBR, April 7, 10, November 3, 1860; *AR*, 1860, in *RR*, pp. 256, 260.

58. Wilson, *Stranger and Traveler*, pp. 259–260; Marshall, *Dorothea Dix*, p. 196. Both biographers imply incorrectly that the asylum received $155,000.

59. John W. Parker to Dorothea Dix, January 31, 1861, Dix Papers, Houghton Library, Harvard University; MBR, October 26, 1861.

CHAPTER SEVEN

1. Dorothea Dix, *On Behalf of the Insane Poor* (New York: Arno Press, 1971), p. 22.

2. *AR*, 1842, pp. 11–13.

3. *AR*, 1847, pp. 7–9, 1842, p. 29, pp. 12–13, 20–21.

4. See Andrew T. Scull, *Museums of Madness: The Social Organization of Insanity in Nineteenth-Century England* (New York: St. Martin's Press, 1979), p. 262, for a reminder about the dangers of romanticizing community care in the past.

5. J. D. B. De Bow, *Statistical View of the United States, Being a Compendium of the Seventh Census* (Washington, D.C., 1854; reprint, New York: Gordon and Breach Science Publishers, 1970), pp. 60, 76-77, 93-94, 112-13; Report of House Committee on the Lunatic Asylum, *RR*, 1840; *AR*, 1842, p. 16, 1850, p. 9.

6. Pennsylvania Hospital, Insane Patients at the 8th Street Hospital, 1790-1841; Institute of Pennsylvania Hospital, Medical Registers, 1:1841-50, 2:1851-65, 3:1866-83; Pennsylvania Hospital, Admissions to Hospital for the Insane, 1841-1860, item no. 183; Pennsylvania Hospital, Medical Register, Male Department, 1:1859-1874, Pennsylvania Hospital Archives, Philadelphia; *Charleston Courier*, December 12, 1821, letter re Bloomingdale Asylum in New York.

7. Mitchell King Diary, March 17, 1855, King Papers, SHC; A. W. Higgins, "Diseases of the Mind" (Medical thesis, Medical College of South Carolina, 1854).

8. David Rothman, *The Discovery of the Asylum: Social Order and Disorder in the New Republic* (Boston: Little, Brown, 1971), pp. 137-38; Barbara G. Rosenkrantz and Maris A. Vinovskis, "Caring for the Insane in Ante-Bellum Massachusetts: Family, Community, and State Participation," in *Kin and Communities: Families in America*, ed. Allan J. Lichtman and Joan R. Challinor (Washington, D.C.: Smithsonian Institution Press, 1979), pp. 191-93; Nancy Tomes, *A Generous Confidence: Thomas Story Kirkbride and the Art of Asylum Keeping, 1840-1883* (Cambridge: Cambridge University Press, 1984), pp. 90-91.

9. *AR*, 1847, pp. 7-9; 1842, pp. 15, 19-21.

10. Simon Abbott, *The Southern Botany Physician* (Charleston, 1844), pp. 281-82; J. Hume Simons, *The Planter's Guide and Family Book of Medicine* (Charleston, 1848), p. 101; Scull, *Museums of Madness*, p. 64; Roy Porter, *Mind Forg'd Manacles: A History of Madness in England from the Restoration to the Regency* (Cambridge, Mass.: Harvard University Press, 1987), esp. chaps. 1, 2; Norman Dain, *Concepts of Insanity in the United States, 1789-1865* (New Brunswick, N.J.: Rutgers University Press, 1964), pp. 37-41.

11. PTR, 1, Andrew Stephenson, David McMillan, Edmund Caldwell, Cynthia Peach, Edward Clanahan, Allen Griffin, John King, James Flournoy.

12. SRR, August 1, 1857; PTR, 3, John Wells, J. N. Mayo.

13. CH, 15, nos. 7444, 7673, 13, no. 6426; CP, no. 11332. The case histories and commitment papers of the late nineteenth and early twentieth centuries contain numerous similar examples.

14. Platts v. Kinard and others, Barnwell Equity Court, Reports and Minutes, February 1835, SCL.

15. York County, Sessions Journal, 1840-1860, November 12, 1846, April 7, 1852, SCL. York County, Court of Equity Reports, 1840-1851, July 4, 1846, SCL; York County, Court of Equity Minutes, 1848-1859, June 25-26, 1852, SCL.

16. PTR, 1, Agnes Allen. See also PTR, 1, Betsy Cockrel, Matthew Talbot,

James Cloud, William McCaw; PTR, 2, A. J. Brevard, Mary Couterier; PTR, 3, Nancy Hocott.

17. PTR, 2, Mary P. Allston; Letters re Mary P. Allston, 1848–1850, Theodore S. Gourdin Papers, SCHS.

18. *AR*, 1842, pp. 20–21.

19. John C. Calhoun to Armistead Burt, May 18, 27, 1838, John C. Calhoun Papers, Manuscript Department, Perkins Library, Duke University (hereafter cited as John C. Calhoun Papers).

20. Undated letter from Mr. Robert at the end of PTR, 3. See also PTR, 2, Georgia W. Robert.

21. PTR, 1, Susan R. Simmons.

22. John Andrew Rice, *I Came Out of the Eighteenth Century* (New York: Harper and Brothers, 1942), pp. 117–21. I would like to thank Tom Johnson of the South Caroliniana Library for bringing my attention to this source.

23. PTR, 1, Susan R. Simmons, Andrew Stephenson, PTR 2, Harriet Broughton.

24. CCP, Minutes, June 22, July 20, Aug. 31, 1842.

25. PTR, 2, Harriet Broughton.

26. In 1864, the committee of Jane C. Miller, a lunatic under the supervision of the equity court, paid Levi Stone of Spartanburg sixty-five dollars to board Miller and her child for the year. Care in the asylum as a private patient would have cost several times that amount. Spartanburg Court of Equity, Minutes, 1860–72, August 9, 11, 1866, SCL.

27. Spartanburg County, Court of Equity Decrees, 1841–69, June 8, 1846, pp. 29–30, June 1853, p. 108, SCL.

28. Union County, Court of Equity Minutes, 1842–52, August 29, 1843, January 3, 1844, pp. 42–45, SCL.

29. On the issue of insanity among slaves see Todd L. Savitt, *Medicine and Slavery*, pp. 248–52; William Postell, *The Health of Slaves on Southern Plantations* (Gloucester, Mass: Peter Smith, 1971), pp. 86–87; Wood, *Black Majority*, pp. 285–86. On the controversy over medical treatment of slaves in general, see these works as well as Robert W. Fogel and Stanley L. Engermann, *Time on the Cross* (Boston: Little, Brown, 1974), pp. 117–21; Richard Sutch, "The Care and Feeding of Slaves," in *Reckoning with Slavery*, ed. Paul A. David, Herbert Gutman, Richard Sutch, Peter Termin and Gavin Wright (New York: Oxford University Press, 1976), pp. 233, 282–84.

30. William Gilmore Simms, "The Morals of Slavery," in *The Proslavery Argument* (Charleston, 1852), pp. 226–28; Review of Samuel Cartwright, "Diseases and Peculiarities of the Negro Race," *Charleston Medical Journal and Review* 6 (1851): 643–52; "Negro-Mania," *Southern Quarterly Review* 5 (1852): 165; Solon Robinson, "Negro Slavery at the South," *De Bow's Review* 7 (1844): 206–25; John S. Haller, "The Negro and the Southern Physician," *Medical History* 16 (1972): 238–53; Savitt, *Medicine and Slavery*, pp. 248–49; Dain, *Concepts of Insanity*, pp. 104–

8. The argument that blacks were less susceptible to mental disorders than whites predated its use in proslavery argument. See David Ramsay, *History of South Carolina*, 2 vols. (Charleston, 1809), 2:92–93. Although Ramsay was no apologist for slavery, Simms appears to have copied his arguments almost word for word.

31. John C. Calhoun, *Works*, 6 vols., ed. Richard K. Cralle (New York, 1856), 5:337–39; Edward Jarvis, "Insanity among the Colored Population of the Free States," *American Journal of the Medical Sciences* 7 (1844): 71–83, and "Insanity among the Colored Population of the Free States," *American Journal of Insanity* 8 (1852): 268–82.

32. "Reflections on the Census of 1840," *Southern Literary Messenger* 9 (1843): 34–49; "Vital Statistics of Negroes in the U.S.," *De Bow's Review* 21 (1856): 408–10; Albert Deutsch, "The First U.S. Census of the Insane and Its Use as Pro-Slavery Propaganda," *Bulletin of the History of Medicine* 15 (1945): 469–82; Dain, *Concepts of Insanity*, pp. 104–8; William S. Jenkins, *Pro-Slavery Thought in the Old South* (Chapel Hill: University of North Carolina Press, 1935), pp. 246–47; George Frederickson, *The Black Image in the White Mind* (New York: Harper and Row, 1971), pp. 50–51. The census of 1850 revealed an even lower incidence of insanity among blacks in South Carolina. The number of insane and idiotic blacks enumerated in 1850 was 124, or 1 to 3,177 of the population. De Bow *Statistical View of the United States*, p. 94.

33. Harriet Martineau, *Society in America*, 2 vols. (New York, 1837), 2: 291–92. On the contemporary concern over the condition of the insane in England, see Peter McCandless, "Insanity and Society: A Study of the English Lunacy Reform Movement, 1815–1870" (Ph.D. diss, University of Wisconsin, 1974); Scull, *Museums of Madness*.

34. Martineau, *Society in America* 2:291–92.

35. Simms, "Morals of Slavery," pp. 225–28.

36. James H. Easterby, ed., "Charles Cotesworth Pinckney's Plantation Diary, April 6–December 15, 1818," *SCHM* 41 (1940): 139; M. D. McCleod, "Hints on the Treatment of Negroes" (Medical thesis, Medical College of South Carolina, 1850), pp. 2–3, 10–13, WHL; James O. Breeden, ed., *Advice Among Masters* (Westport, Conn.: Greenwood Press, 1980), pp. 191–92; Kenneth F. Kiple and Virginia H. King, *Another Dimension to the Black Diaspora: Diet, Disease, and Racism* (London: Cambridge University Press, 1981), pp. 168–69.

37. Frances Anne Kemble, *Journal of a Residence on a Georgia Plantation in 1838–1839* (New York: Alfred A. Knopf, 1964; reprint, Athens: University of Georgia Press, 1984), p. 149.

38. John H. Tucker to R. F. W. Allston, January 27, 1818, R. F. W. Allston Papers, SCHS; Savitt, *Medicine and Slavery*, p. 252; Postell, *Health of Slaves*, pp. 86–87; James M. Clifton, ed., *Life and Labor on Argyle Island: Letters and Documents of a Savannah River Rice Plantation, 1833–1867* (Savannah, Ga.: Beehive Press, 1978), pp. xxxiv–xxxv.

39. Kemble, *Journal*, p. 230.

40. A. P. Merrill, "An Essay on Some of the Distinctive Peculiarities of the Negro Race," *Memphis Medical Recorder* 4 (1855): 4, cited in Haller, "Negro and the Southern Physician," p. 251.

41. Kiple and King, *Another Dimension*, pp. 131, 173.

42. Daniel Drake, "Diseases of the Negro Population," *Southern Medical and Surgical Journal* 2, n.s. (1845): 341–43.

43. Samuel Cartwright, "Diseases and Peculiarities of the Negro Race," *De Bow's Review* 11 (1851): 331–36; Cartwright, "Diseases and Peculiarities," 643–52.

44. James T. Smith, "Review of Dr. Cartwright's Report on the Diseases and Physical Peculiarities of the Negro Race," *New Orleans Medical and Surgical Journal* 7 (1851–52): 233, 229–37; Review of "Samuel A. Cartwright, 'Diseases and Physical Peculiarities of the Negro Race,'" *Charleston Medical Journal and Review* 6 (1851): 829–43; "Cartwright on the Diseases and Peculiarities of the Negro Race," *Charleston Medical Journal and Review* 7 (1852): 89–98; "Dr. Cartwright and Ourselves," *Charleston Medical Journal and Review* 7 (1852): 719–20; Warner, "Southern Medical Reform," p. 223, and "Southern Medical Distinctiveness," pp. 199–203; Kiple and King, *Another Dimension*, pp. 179–83; Haller, "Negro and the Southern Physician," pp. 247–253.

45. Thomas Ssasz, in "The Sane Slave," *American Journal of Psychotherapy* 25 (171): 228–39, argues that Cartwright's work was part of an attempt to medicalize slave unhappiness and rebelliousness as symptoms of mental disorder.

46. Thomas B. Chaplin, Plantation Journal, December 12, 28, 1848, January 17, 19, 20, 27, March 16, 1849, SCHS. Chaplin's journal has been published, along with an excellent biography, in Theodore Rosengarten, *Tombee: Portrait of a Cotton Planter* (New York: McGraw-Hill, 1987). See pp. 448, 450–53, and 461 for Peter's case.

47. Medical Account Books of Drs. Andrew Hasell (1830–56) and E. B. and A. B. Flagg (1847–53, 1850–54), SCHS; Medical Account Book of Dr. I. L. Lee, (1860–61), WHL; Day Book of Dr. William L. Jenkins, (1840–52), WHL; George P. Rawick, ed., *The American Slave: A Composite Autobiography*, 19 vols. (Westport, Conn.: Greenwood Publishing, 1972), vols. 2 and 3, *South Carolina Narratives*, vol. 2, pt. 1, pp. 27, 63, 105, 125, 150, 167, 305, pt. 2, pp. 31, 38, 210, vol. 3, pt. 3, pp. 81, 87, pt. 4, pp. 46–47, 73, 103, 156; *South Carolina State Gazette*, June 28, 1828, advertisement for "Hospital for Negroes"; *Charleston Medical Journal and Review* 7 (1852): 94, 724, ibid. 12 (1857): 134, ibid. 15 (1860): 850–51; H. W. Moore, "A Thesis on Plantation Hygiene" (Medical thesis, Medical College of South Carolina, 1856), pp. 5, 24–25; Thomas Affleck, "On the Hygiene of Cotton Plantations and the Management of Negro Slaves," *Southern Medical Reports* 2 (1850): 429–36; Clifton, *Life and Labor*, xxxiii–xxxiv; Drew Gilpin Faust, *James Henry Hammond and the Old South: A Design for Mastery* (Baton Rouge: Louisiana State University Press, 1982), pp. 77–78; Kiple and King, *Another Dimension*, pp. 166–68; Savitt, *Medicine and Slavery*, pp. 248–54; Postell, *Health of Slaves*, pp. 87, 129–38; Martha C. Mitchell, "Health and the Medical Profession in the

Lower South, 1845-1860," *Journal of Southern History* 10 (1944): 435-36; Fogel and Engermann, *Time on the Cross*, pp. 117-121; J. H. Easterby, ed., *The South Carolina Rice Plantation as Revealed in the Papers of R. W. F. Allston* (Chicago: University of Chicago Press, 1945), pp. 30, 157-58, 254, 348.

48. W. T. Wragg, "Remarkable Case of Mental Alienation," *American Journal of Insanity* 3 (1846): 67-72.

49. The care of insane slaves and free blacks in Charleston's poorhouse and public hospital is discussed in chapter 8.

50. Clifton, *Life and Labor*, p. 98; Kiple and King, *Another Dimension*, pp. 163-65.

51. Faust, *James Henry Hammond*, pp. 77-79, 81.

52. Kemble, *Journal*, pp. 255-57, 74-77, 363-64.

53. Pierce Mason Butler, MS, c. 1845, list of slaves with character assessment, SCL.

54. S. A. Townes to George Townes, April 24, 1835, Townes Family Papers, SCL.

55. William Gilmore Simms, "Lunatic Asylum," *Magnolia, or Southern Apalachian* (December 1842): p. 395; John H. Tucker to R. F. W. Allston, January 27, 1818, R. F. W. Allston Papers, SCHS.

56. Report on the Colored Insane, 1847, p. 3, GAP.

57. Easterby, *South Carolina Rice Plantation*, p. 137.

58. Thomas B. Chaplin, Plantation Journal, March 16, 1849, SCHS.

59. For the history of free blacks in antebellum South Carolina, see Marina Wikramanayake, *A World in Shadow: The Free Black in Antebellum South Carolina* (Columbia: University of South Carolina Press, 1973); Michael P. Johnson and James L. Roark, *Black Masters: A Free Family of Color in the Old South* (New York: Norton, 1984), and *No Chariot Let Down: Charleston's Free People of Color on the Eve of the Civil War* (New York: Norton, 1984). See Ira Berlin, *Slaves Without Masters: The Free Negro in the Antebellum South* (New York: Oxford University Press, 1974) for a history of free blacks in the Old South. According to Berlin, South Carolina had one of the "mildest free Negro codes" (p. 195). See also Robert S. Starobin, ed., *Denmark Vesey: The Slave Conspiracy of 1822* (Englewood Cliffs, N.J.: Prentice-Hall, 1970), esp. pp. 135-37; R. Y. Hayne, *Report of the Proceedings of the City Authorities of Charleston* (Charleston 1837), pp. 11-12; John Lofton, *Insurrection in South Carolina: The Turbulent World of Denmark Vesey* (Yellow Springs, Ohio: Antioch Press, 1964), pp. 196-97.

60. It is not possible to determine the exact number of free blacks admitted to the South Carolina Lunatic Asylum between 1850 and 1865, because the admission book does not list any of the blacks as free, only as slave or colored. If we assume that those listed with a surname were free, the number was six. SCSH, Admission Book, 1828-1874.

61. Roper Hospital, Case Book No. 2, microfilm, WHL; See Savitt, *Medicine*

and Slavery, pp. 252–79, for the situation of insane free blacks in antebellum Virginia.

62. "Proceedings of the Association," *American Journal of Insanity* 12 (1855): 43; Dain, *Concepts of Insanity*, pp. 107–8, and *Disordered Minds: The First Century of Eastern State Hospital in Williamsburg, Virginia, 1766–1866* (Charlottesville: University Press of Virginia, 1971), p. 19; Savitt, *Medicine and Slavery*, p. 277; Gerald Grob, *Mental Institutions in America: Social Policy to 1875* (New York: Free Press, 1973), pp. 250–55. John Galt, the superintendent of the Eastern Virginia Lunatic Asylum, was the most outspoken advocate of admitting blacks to existing asylums. See John M. Galt, "Asylums for Colored Persons," *Psychological Journal* 1 (1853): 78–88. Most public institutions in antebellum America refused to accept blacks. See Frederickson, *Black Image*, pp. 17–22.

63. Johnson and Roark, *Black Masters*, pp. 212–22.

64. Report on Colored Insane, 1847, p. 3, GAP.

65. York County, Sessions Journal, 1840–1860, April 7, 1852, SCL; York County, Court of Equity Minutes, 1848–1859, June 25–26, 1852, SCL.

66. Union County, Session Journal, 1853–1870, Spring Term, 1856, p. 63, SCL.

67. CP, no. 2979; CH, 3, no. 2745; J. Scott, *Random Recollections of a Long Life* (Columbia, 1884), p. 59.

68. CP, no. 3284.

69. Documents relating to Harriet Bounds, 1830, GAP; *RR*, 1830, p. 55; *AR*, 1830, pp. 5–6.

CHAPTER EIGHT

1. *Pendleton Messenger*, May 20, 1829, reprinted from *Charleston Mercury*.

2. *AR*, 1842, p. 23, 1847, pp. 8–9.

3. *AR*, 1842, pp. 23, 1847, pp. 8–9; SRR, March 20, 1849.

4. CP, no. 3204; CCP, Minutes, February 21, 1833, Letter Book, August 1835, February 1840, March 5, 1853; Williamsburg County, Board of Commissioners, Minutes, January 1874, February 1874, December 1874, February 1875, March 1875, SCL; Newberry County, Board of Commissioners, Minutes, 1868–1875, SCL; Spartanburg County, Board of Commissioners, Minutes, October 22, 1881, January 3, November 14, 1882, SCDAH; York County, Board of County Commissioners, Minutes, February 10, March 31, 1871, SCL; Greenville County, Board of County Commissioners, Minutes, April 1875–Oct. 1879, SCDAH.

5. CCP, Minutes, February 1853.

6. York County, Board of Commissioners, Minutes, November 4, 1869, SCDAH; CP, nos. 3204, 3257, 3475, 3274.

7. CCP, Minutes, August 17, 1842, October 17, 1849, February 1853.

8. CP, no. 3720. See also nos. 3291, 3349, 3466, 3599, 11890; Union County, Sessions Journal, Grand Jury Presentments, October 1879, SCL.

9. CCP, Minutes, January 3, 17, 1844, Letter Book, January 12, 1844.

10. CCP, Letter Book, November 18, 25, 26, 1850, May 10, 1853.

11. CCP, Minutes, August 17, 1842.

12. CCP, Letter Book, January 28, February 13, 28, April 21, 1846.

13. York County, Session Journal, Spring Term, 1859, pp. 298, 301-3, SCL. For other examples, see Union County, Session Journals, March Term, 1841, February 1877, March, October 1879, March 1895, SCL; Kershaw County, Session Journal, Spring Term, 1842, p. 23, SCL.

14. CCP, Minutes, May 2, 1833, May 18, June 1, 1836, May 31, June 14, November 15, 1837; Charleston City Council, Proceedings, June 27, November 6, 1837, Special Collections, Small Library, College of Charleston.

15. CP, nos. 3257, 3894, 2898, 2902, 3068.

16. Casey was sent to the asylum two years later. CCP, Minutes, January 20, 1840, July 7, 1841, June 22, July 20, 1842, Letter Book, January 20, 1840, April 14, 1842.

17. CCP, Minutes, August 17, 1842.

18. CCP, Minutes, February 7, 1833.

19. Papers relating to Harriet Bounds, 1830, pp. 44-45, GAP.

20. Georgetown County, Journal of Probate Judge, May 3, 1881, February 11, 1885, SCL; CP, nos. 3504, 4436; see also CP, no. 5365.

21. PTR, 2, Thomas Hartwell.

22. MBR, August 1, 1885; CH, 3, no. 2654, 4, nos. 2988, 2953.

23. Robert Mills, *Statistics of South Carolina* (Charleston, 1826), pp. 362, 431-32, 453, 528, 679. *RR*, 1878, pp. 392-93; CP, no. 3475; *Camden Journal*, March 17, May 12, August 30, 1828. The counties' changing poor relief methods can be followed by perusing the Grand Jury Presentments of the County Sessions Courts. Many of these records are available at SCL and SCDAH.

24. Spartanburg County, Commissioners of the Poor, Minutes, 1796-1824, SCL; Spartanburg County, Board of Commissioners, Minutes, January 7, 1879, SCDAH; Lancaster County, Commissioners of the Poor, Minutes, January 17, August 1, 1853, January 7, 1861, March 6, 1868, SCDAH.

25. Anderson County, Board of Commissioners, Minutes, July 3, 1890, SCDAH; York County, Board of Commissioners, Minutes, August 6, November 4, 1869, October 12, 1871, SCL; Union County, Sessions Journal, February 1877, October 1879, March 1879, March 1895, SCL; CH, 15, no. 7587.

26. Greenville County, Sessions Journal, Grand Jury Presentment, Fall Term 1854, Fall Term 1841.

27. Barnwell County, Sessions Journal, Grand Jury Presentments, October 27, 1847, March 29, 1848, October 27, 1851, October 28, 1853, October 21, 1858, October 20, 1866, March 20, 1867, SCDAH; Barnwell County, Sessions Journal, Grand Jury Presentments, May Term 1874, January Term 1875, May Term 1875, May Term 1876, SCL. See also Edgefield County, Sessions Journal, Grand Jury Presentments, February Term 1869, July Term 1870, SCL; Newberry County, Ses-

sions Journal, Grand Jury Presentments, September 1870, February 1878, June 1882, SCL.

28. Newberry County, Board of Commissioners, Minutes, March 8, 1870, SCL; Barnwell County, Sessions Journal, Minutes, Grand Jury Presentments, May Term 1876; Edgefield County, Sessions Journal, Grand Jury Presentments, June 1877, SCL; CP, nos. 4272, 4366.

29. *AR*, 1847, in *RR*, pp. 102, 105; CP, nos. 8902, 9123.

30. PTR, 1, Cynthia Peach; CP, no. 4210, 5882, 7102, 14215, 15225, 15812; CH, 14, no. 6730 and 15, no. 7590.

31. CP, no. 3349. See also no. 3291. There are many similar examples in the case histories and commitment papers.

32. Georgetown County, Journal of Probate Judge, February 11, 1885, SCL.

33. CH, 17, no. 8428; see also Chester County, Court of General Sessions, Minutes, 1854–1859, Fall Term 1857, SCL.

34. The minutes of the Charleston Commissioners of the Poor report the number of insane confined in the lunatic wards in most but not all of the years from 1800 to 1856. Between 1809 and 1821, the number was usually between ten and twenty. Between 1828 and 1847, it was usually between twenty and thirty. Between 1848 and 1855 (the last year the insane were under the care of the commissioners), the number ranged between thirty and forty-eight. CCP, Minutes, 1800–1856, May 14, 1810, April 2, 1821, February 21, 1822; G. B. Eckhard, *Digest of the Ordinances of the City of Charleston 1783–1844*, pp. 82, 149, 204–6; *A Collection of the Ordinances of the City Council of Charleston from 1818 to 1823* (Charleston, 1823), p. 23; Mills, *Statistics of South Carolina*, pp. 431–32.

35. CCP, Minutes, 1800–1856.

36. Eckhard, *Ordinances of the City of Charleston*, pp. 203–06; CCP, Minutes, July 10, 1815, November 28, 1822.

37. CCP, Minutes, Rules and Regulations of the Medical Department of the Poor House, April 1821; CCP, Minutes, April 25, May 31, 1832. The Charleston poorhouse was an object of considerable civic pride, and many of the city's leading citizens served as its commissioners. Several visitors left descriptions of the institution. Rev. Abiel Abbott of Massachusetts and gadabout Mrs. Anne Royall commended its facilities and the treatment of its inmates. English writer Harriet Martineau was less impressed. See Moore, "Abiel Abbot Journals," pp. 115–17; Anne Royall, *Mrs. Royall's Southern Tour* (Washington, D.C., 1831), p. 25; Harriet Martineau, *Retrospect of Western Travel* 2 vols. (London, 1838), 1:293–94; For the history of the antebellum Charleston poorhouse, see Barbara L. Bellows, *Benevolence among Slaveholders: Assisting the Poor in Charleston, 1670–1860* (Baton Rouge: Louisiana State University Press, 1993).

38. CCP, Minutes, May 21, 1829, February 28, 1828, October 15, 1851, October 27, 1852

39. CCP, Hospital Register, 1841–1856.

40. CCP, Minutes, 1800–1856, esp. March 24, 1842, April 14, 1850, February

1853; *RR*, 1822, exhibit 16; Benjamin J. Klebaner, "Public Poor Relief in Charleston, 1800–1860," *SCHM* 55 (1954): 210–15.

41. Moore, "Abiel Abbot Journals," p. 115; CCP, Minutes, February 1853.

42. CCP, Minutes, February 21, 1822, August 20, 1828, January 15, July 16, September 24, 1829, February 4, August 5, 1840, February 5, 1841, February 26, 1846; CCP, Letter Book, letter to Hon. Henry L. Pinckney, mayor, July 28, 1838; Charleston City Council, Proceedings, January 7, 1839, typescript of reports from Charleston City Council, Small Library, College of Charleston, Special Collections.

43. CCP, Minutes, August 5, 12, 1840.

44. CCP, Minutes, February 28, April 10, 24, May 8, 1828, August 12, 1840, 1834–40, front page, 1847–52, back page.

45. CCP, Minutes, August 17, 1842, January 22, February 20, 1840, April 6, 1848, January 23, April 3, 6, 17, 1850. CCP, Letter Book, October 23, 30, November 3, 21, 1832, February 6, March 24, 1835.

46. CCP, Minutes, January 26, 1832.

47. CCP, Letter Book, December 17, 1852.

48. CCP, January 9, March 16, September 28, October 12, 15, 1853; SRR, February 25, 1854.

49. CCP, Minutes, November 21, 1821, August 12, 1840; CCP, Letter Book, May 5, 1839.

50. CCP, Minutes, November 12, 1853; see also ibid., September 9. 1857.

51. CCP, Hospital Register, 1841–1856. Before 1841 it is not possible to break down admissions to or residents of the lunatic wards by race. But the records confirm the presence of black patients throughout the period 1800–1856. At least forty-one more admissions to the lunatic wards between 1841 and 1856 are listed as foreign born, twenty-three of them Irish. Thus, about 75 percent of the admissions to the poorhouse lunatic wards betweeen 1841 and 1856 were blacks or immigrants. But the commissioners did not show the same concern about the immigrant as about the black insane in their institution.

52. CCP, Minutes, March 6, 1820, letter from City Council.

53. CCP, Minutes, September 28, 1802, May 12, 1805, July 18, 1808, July 19, September 7, 1812, April 19, May 24, June 28, August 9, 1813, January 24, 1814, January 14, September 16, 1816, January 20, 1817, March 6, December 4, 1820, February 28, May 8, June 19, 1828, April 24, 1844, September 18, 1850; Walter J. Fraser Jr., *Charleston!: The History of a Southern City* (Columbia: University of South Carolina Press, 1989), p. 201; Michael P. Johnson and James L. Roark, *Black Masters: A Free Family of Color in the Old South* (New York: Norton, 1984), pp. 40, 108; Abiel Abbot described Aaron Thompson when he visited the poorhouse in 1819. See Moore, "Abiel Abbot Journals," p. 116.

54. CCP, January 4, 1816.

55. CCP, Minutes, March 6, May 21, 1820, January 1, 1816, January 24, 1814.

56. CCP, Minutes, February 19, March 5, 1821, July 16, 1829, August 17, 1842;

see also March 6, 1820; Johnson and Roark, *Black Masters*, pp. 40, 108, 110–11, 145; Fraser, *Charleston!* p. 201. John Lofton, *Insurrection in South Carolina: The Turbulent World of Denmark Vesey* (Yellow Springs, Ohio: Antioch Press, 1964), pp. 147, 181.

57. CCP, Minutes, September 9, June 2, 16, 1847. See also May 31, July 5, 1822, September 18, 1823, May 19, 1831, November 8, 1843, April 24, 1844, September 6, 20, 1848.

58. CCP, Letter Book, September 23, 1823; CCP, Minutes, January 4, 1816, March 6, December 4, 1820, May 31, July 5, September 18, 1822, September 18, 1823, May 19, 1831, September 9, 1846, September 6, 20, 1848.

59. CCP, Minutes, December 4, 1820, April 2, 1821, May 21, 1821.

60. CCP, Minutes, April 24, 1844, April 29, 1824, January 15, 1829, May 19, 1831, March 29, 1836, June 23, 1841. For the general policies of the city toward relief of blacks in the nineteenth century, see Benjamin J. Klebaner, "Public Poor Relief in Charleston, 1800–1860," *SCHM* 55 (1954): 215–16; Carol Haber and Brian Gratton, "Old Age, Public Welfare, and Race: The Case of Charleston, South Carolina, 1800–1949," *Journal of Social History* (Winter 1987): 265–66.

61. CCP, Minutes, November 8, 1843.

62. CCP, Minutes, September 18, 1823, May 8, June 19, 1828, January 15, June 14, 18, 1829, September 20, 1837, June 23, 1841, February 26, October 7, 1846, Letter Book, September 23, 1823; Henry L. Pinckney, *Report: Containing a Review of the Proceedings of the City Authorities* (Charleston, 1838), pp. 39–41; Charleston City Council, Proceedings, September 29, November 29, 1837; *Charleston Courier*, September 20, 1839, Mayor's Report; R. Y. Hayne, *Report; Containing a Review of the Proceedings of the City Authorities* (Charleston, 1837), pp. 32–33.

63. CCP, Minutes, December 10, 1842; Michael P. Johnson and James L. Roark, *No Chariot Let Down: Charleston's Free People of Color on the Eve of the Civil War* (New York: Oxford University Press, 1984), pp. 10–12. On South Carolina's increasing concern with the defense of slavery, see William Freehling, *Prelude to Civil War: The Nullification Controversy in South Carolina, 1816–1836* (New York: Harper and Row, 1966); John Barnwell, *Love of Order: South Carolina's First Secession Crisis* (Chapel Hill: University of North Carolina Press, 1982), pp. 32–33.

64. Freehling, *Prelude to Civil War*, pp. 49–65, 113; Lofton, *Insurrection*, pp. 182, 196–97; Starobin, *Denmark Vesey*, pp. 135–37; Stephen A. Channing, *Crisis of Fear* (New York: Norton, 1974), pp. 26–27, 38–39, 64–66.

65. Pinckney, *Report*, pp. 39–40; Eckhard, *A Digest of the Ordinances of the City of Charleston*, pp. 205–6.

66. CCP, Minutes, September 18, 1850; see also March 6, 1820. Two years later, Agnes was admitted to the state asylum. See SCSH, Admission Book, 1828–1874.

67. *Ordinances of the City of Charleston from 1854 to 1859* (Charleston, 1859), pp. 28, 33–34; *Charleston Yearbook*, 1880, pp. 50–57, 1886, pp. 88–90; CCP, November 5, 1855, January 2, 1856; Roper Hospital, Case Book No. 2, 1859–

62, WHL; *Annual Report of the City Registrar, 1876* (Charleston, 1877), p. 17; Joseph I. Waring, *Roper Hospital: A Brief History* (Charleston: Board of Commissioners of Roper Hospital, 1964), n.p.; Kenneth Severens, *Charleston Antebellum Architecture and Civic Destiny* (Knoxville: University of Tennessee Press, 1988), pp. 160–66.

68. U.S., 8th Census, 1860, 9th Census, 1870, Population Schedules for City of Charleston, SCDAH; U.S., 10th Census, 1880, Social Statistics, Schedules for Charleston County, SCDAH; for the years 1899 to 1905, the *Charleston Yearbook* provides psychiatric admissions and discharges at the City Hospital for each year. Not enough records survive to provide annual statistics on patient movements.

69. Report of the Committee on the Lunatic Asylum, c. 1857, GAP.

70. *Charleston Yearbook*, 1883, p. 115.

71. *Annual Report of the City Registrar, 1867* (Charleston, 1868), p. 90; *Annual Report of the Officers of the City Government, 1870* (Charleston, 1871), p. 20; *Charleston Yearbook*, 1883, 1899–1905; CH, 6–31. Insufficient records survive to provide more than occasional statistics of patient outcomes.

72. CH, 16, no. 8425; see also CH, 6, no. 3550; *Charleston Yearbook*, 1890, p. 88.

73. *Annual Report of the City Registrar for 1866*, p. 46; *Annual Report of the City Registrar, 1867*, p. 90.

74. Commissioners of the City Hospital, Minute Book, April 14, May 4, May 19, June 29, December 7, 1880, Charleston City Archives; *Charleston Yearbook*, 1883, p. 112.

75. CP, no. 5425; CH, 10, no. 4807; *Charleston Yearbook*, 1880, p. 88. See CH, 6–31. According to the federal census of 1880 two of the thirty-seven insane patients in the City Hospital required mechanical restraint in the form of straitjackets; four others were kept in solitary confinement. U.S., 10th Census, 1880, Social Statistics, Schedules for Charleston County. As late as 1901, the rules and regulations of the City Hospital referred to the rooms for the insane patients as "cells." Charleston City Hospital, *Rules and Regulations, Adopted August 6, 1901* (Charleston, 1901), p. 19.

76. *Charleston Yearbook*, 1902, p. 210; *Annual Report of the Department of Health, 1905* (Charleston, 1906), p. 20.

77. Olin B. Chamberlain, "Analysis of the Psychiatric Cases in Roper Hospital in 1921 and 1922," manuscript, WHL, pp. 1–2, 6; Waring, *Roper Hospital.*

78. Olin B. Chamberlain, "Adequate Facilities for Psychiatric Cases in a General Hospital," manuscript, p. 4, WHL.

79. *Charleston News and Courier*, November 24, 1985, pp. 3E, 12E.

80. PTR, 1, James Adams, Allen Griffin, Patrick Hayes; Ann King Gregorie, *A History of Sumter County* (Sumter: Library Board of Sumter County, 1954), p. 182; SRR, April 17, 1847. See also PTR, 1, Edward Rains, Andrew Venable; CP,

nos. 3122, 3599. The opening of the state penitentiary after the Civil War brought increased numbers of criminal lunatics to the state asylum.

81. CP, no. 2749. The legal papers charging him with lunacy are attached to the commitment papers.

82. PTR, 1, Alexander Horn, Andrew Venable, Edward Rains, John Carlisle. The other four seem to have been in jail only briefly before their commitment.

83. PTR, 1, Patrick Hayes, Anne McCord, A. Wilcox, John Hollingsworth; PTR, 2, George Shephard, Thomas Cartwright; PTR, 3, James Miller, David Simpson, Bennet Wallace, Peter Murphy; CP, nos. 2694, 2914, 3530, 3538, 3350, 3830; Gregorie, *History of Sumter County*, p. 182; SRR, April 17, 1847.

84. *AR*, 1873-74, p. 41.

85. CH, vols. 15-17, 19-27, 29-31. The number of patients who came to the asylum via jails is likely to have been higher than these numbers indicate. The case histories used were erratically kept and some contain little or no information about the patients' situation previous to commitment.

86. CH, vols. 15-17, 19-27, 29-31. An examination of commitment papers for one year, 1896, revealed similar racial and gender percentages among those admitted from jail. But it also indicated that the number of admissions via jail was higher than what the case records reveal. CP, 1896, nos. 7573-7916.

87. Affidavit of B. W. Anderson in CP, no. 10901. See also CP, nos. 3599, 4941, 8463, 8568, 9982, 10007, 12972, 13328, 13372, 13573, 14056, 14606, 15576, 15676, 15688, 15762, 16281.

88. F. H. Creech to J. W. Babcock, December 30, 1903, in CP, no. 11506.

89. George S. McCravy to J. W. Babcock, June 2, 1893, in CP, no. 6750.

90. CP, no. 3183. see also CP, nos. 4141, 4205, 5193, 5194. There are many similar examples in the commitment papers and case histories.

91. Newberry County, Board of Commissioners, Minutes, June 11, 1872, SCL; Spartanburg County, Board of Commissioners, Minutes, September 5, 1877, SCL.

92. CH, 14, no. 6750.

93. Williamsburg County, Board of Commissioners, Minutes, September 15, October 6, November 30, December 18-29, 1874, SCL.

94. CH, 8, no. 4165, 16, no. 7476; CP, nos. 3122, 6750.

95. Edgefield County, Session Journal, Fall Term 1824, Spring Term 1825, Spring Term 1845, June Term 1869, Fall Term 1869, June Term 1877, SCL.

96. Barnwell County, Session Journal, April 4, 1842, SCDAH; Greenville County, Sessions Journal, October Term. 1837, SCDAH; Kershaw County, Sessions Journal, Spring Term 1842, SCDAH.

97. Barnwell County, Sessions Journal, November 4, 1839, April 4, 1842, October 30, 1844, October 21, 1857, August 12, 1870, SCDAH. See also Marlboro County Sessions and Common Pleas Court, Minutes, Fall Term 1838, SCL; Edgefield County, Sessions Journal, Fall Term 1824, June Term 1869, SCL.

98. CP, no. 7604; CH, 9, no. 4533; CH, 17, nos. 8623, 8627.

99. *Report, Legislative Committee to Investigate the State Hospital for the Insane* (Columbia, S.C.: Gonzales and Bryan, 1910), p. 21.

CHAPTER NINE

1. *AR*, 1842, pp. 19–21.

2. CP, no. 5593.

3. CP, 1884, nos. 4138–4423, 1889, nos. 5344–5656, 1894, nos. 6922–7247. Some of the commitment papers were missing for each year. The question about medical treatment was dropped when the form was revised in 1894.

4. Mr. A. Coward to Mrs. C. H. Jenkins, March 19, 1897, Micah Jenkins Papers, SCL.

5. CP, no. 4443; CH, 29, no. 14370.

6. Moore, "On Mania," p. 13.

7. CCP, April 14, 1850.

8. CP, nos. 4487, 4265, 4307, 4358, 4369, 4479, 4561, 4962, 5107, 6966, 7010, 7036, 7156, 3029.

9. CH, 15, no. 7706.

10. Letter from Mr. Robert re Mrs. Georgia Robert, at end of PTR, 3.

11. *AR*, 1842, pp. 19–20; *Charleston Courier*, January 6, 1838, January 16, 1841; *Charleston Mercury*, June 4, 1839; William C. Miller, "Remarks on Insanity" (Medical thesis, Medical College of South Carolina, 1845), WHL; Norman Dain, *Concepts of Insanity in the United States, 1789–1965* (New Brunswick, N.J.: Rutgers University Press, 1964), chap. 6.

12. Eli Geddings, *Valedictory Address to the Graduating Class of the Medical College of the State of South Carolina* (Charleston, 1852), p. 20; Evelyn A. Woods and Eric T. Carlson, "The Psychiatry of Philippe Pinel," *Bulletin of the History of Medicine* 35 (1961): 14–25; Thomas W. Moore, "On Mania" (Medical thesis, Medical College of South Carolina, 1829), pp. 14–16; N. W. Herring, "Delerium Tremens" (Medical thesis, Medical College of South Carolina, 1841), pp. 18–19, both WHL.

13. David Ramsay, *History of South Carolina*, 2:116–20; David Ramsay, *An Eulogium upon Benjamin Rush* (Philadelphia, 1813), pp. vi–vii, 41–46; Brunhouse, *David Ramsay*, pp. 13, 144–45, 151, 162; Waring, "Influence of Benjamin Rush in South Carolina," pp. 230–37; Medical Society of South Carolina, Minutes, June 1, 1805, WHL; Rush, *Diseases of the Mind*, pp. 14–25, 183–89.

14. Thomas Y. Simons, *Observations on Mental Alienation* (Charleston, 1828), pp. 22–25. On Simons, see Joseph I. Waring, *A History of Medicine in South Carolina*, 3 vols. (Columbia: South Carolina Medical Association, 1964–71), 2:295.

15. Moore, "On Mania," pp. 11–13; see also J. Rice Roger, "Dissertation on Insanity" (Medical thesis, Medical College of South Carolina, 1846); W. Agnew, "An Inaugural Dissertation on Insanity" (Medical thesis, Medical College of South Carolina, 1846).

16. Moore, "On Mania," pp. 10–12; see also A. W. Higgins, "Diseases of the Mind" (Medical thesis, Medical College of South Carolina, 1854).

17. Henry D. Holland, "An Inaugural Dissertation on Melancholia and Hypochondriasis" (Medical thesis, Medical College of South Carolina, 1829).

18. J. L. E. W. Shecut, *Medical and Philosophical Essays* (Charleston, 1819), pp. 128, 237–38, 257.

19. Suzanne C. Linder, *Medicine in Marlboro County* (Baltimore: Gateway Press, 1980), p. 8.

20. John Harley Warner, *The Therapeutic Perspective: Medical Practice, Knowledge, and Identity in America, 1820–1885* (Cambridge, Mass.: Harvard University Press, 1986), pp. 40–50.

21. F. J. V. Broussais, *On Irritation and Insanity*, trans. Thomas Cooper (Columbia, 1831), pp. vi, 268–73; Hardy Wickwar and Charles S. Bryan, "Broussais in Columbia, South Carolina—1831," *Journal of the South Carolina Medical Association* 77 (1981): 615–22.

22. Warner, *Therapeutic Perspective*, pp. 2–3, 37–57; Rosenberg, "Therapeutic Revolution," pp. 5–14.

23. Rosenberg, "Therapeutic Revolution," pp. 5–20; Warner, *Therapeutic Perspective*, pp. 17–36; Martin Kaufman, *Homeopathy in America: The Rise and Fall of a Medical Heresy* (Baltimore: Johns Hopkins University Press, 1971), pp. 5–14, 62.

24. Earle's main conclusions were reprinted in the *Southern Medical and Surgical Journal* 10 (1854): 499–501.

25. Samuel Henry Dickson, *Pathology and Therapeutics* (New York, 1845), pp. 381–82, and *Elements of Medicine* (Philadelphia, 1855), p. 652. On Dickson, see Waring, *History of Medicine in South Carolina* 2:222–26. Students at the Medical College of South Carolina reflected Dickson's ambivalence about therapeutics for mental disorders. See Higgins, "Diseases of the Mind," pp. 30–31. See also William Veitch, "Remarks On Insanity" (Medical thesis, Medical College of South Carolina, 1857), pp. 19–20, 27.

26. PTR, 1, Allen Griffin, Stephen Monk; PTR, 2, Densby Dorn. See also PTR, 1, Andrew Stephenson, Rebecca O'Neall, John King; PTR, 2, Susan Dawson, T. H. George, Mary Couterier.

27. PTR, 2, Walter McKlintock; CCP, Minutes, May 21, 1829, January 3, 1844, November 23, 1846, April 14, 1850, December 17, 1852, February 2, 1853; SRR, February 25, 1854.

28. W. T. Wragg, "Remarkable Case of Mental Alienation," *Am. J. Ins.* 3 (1846): 67–72.

29. Kenneth F. Kiple and Virginia H. King, *Another Dimension to the Black Diaspora: Diet, Disease, and Racism* (Cambridge: Cambridge University Press, 1981), pp. 178–79; John S. Haller Jr., "The Negro and the Southern Physician: A Study of Medical and Racial Attitudes," *Medical History* 16 (1972): 243–48.

30. CCP, February 1853.

31. Roper Hospital, Case Book No. 2, 1859–62, microfilm, WHL.

32. CP, no. 4221. On the decline of bleeding for insanity during the antebellum period, see Thielman, "Madness and Medicine: Trends" for the decline of bleeding in American medicine generally, see Leon S. (Charles) Bryan Jr., "Bloodletting in American Medicine, 1830–1892," *Bulletin of the History of Medicine* 38 (1964): 516–29.

33. CP, no. 3294.

34. CP, no. 6148.

35. CP, no. 3029.

36. CP, nos. 3108, 2806, 3516, 4271, 4450, 4692. See Dain, *Concepts of Insanity*, chap. 6, for discussion of how general practitioners' treatment of insanity changed during the later nineteenth century.

37. Elizabeth B. Keeney, "Unless Powerful Sick: Domestic Medicine in the Old South," in *Science and Medicine in the Old South*, ed. Ronald L. Numbers and Todd L. Savitt (Baton Rouge: Louisiana State University Press, 1989), pp. 276, 281–82; Kaufman, *Homeopathy in America*, pp. 15–16; James Cassedy, "Why Self Help? Americans Alone with their Diseases, 1800–1850," in *Medicine Without Doctors: Home Health Care in American History*, ed. Guenter B. Risse, Ronald L. Numbers, and Judith Walzer Leavitt (New York: Science History Publications, 1977), pp. 31–39.

38. *Charleston Courier*, April 5, 1843.

39. Carol Bleser, *The Hammonds of Redcliffe* (New York: Oxford University Press, 1981), p. 101; Drew Gilpin Faust, *James Henry Hammond and the Old South: A Design for Mastery* (Baton Rouge: Louisiana State University Press, 1982), pp. 78–81.

40. On the various challenges to regular medicine in nineteenth-century America, see Norman Gevitz, ed., *Other Healers: Unorthodox Medicine in America* (Baltimore: John Hopkins University Press, 1988); Risse et al., *Medicine Without Doctors*; Kaufman, *Homeopathy in America*. On the problems faced by regulars in the South and South Carolina, see Waring, *History of Medicine in South Carolina*, esp. 2:114–21, 143–44; Shryock, "Medical Practice in the Old South," in *Medicine in America: Historical Essays* (Baltimore: Johns Hopkins University Press, 1966), pp. 62–63; Keeney, "Unless Powerful Sick."

41. T. C. Pool to Peter Griffin, March 30, 1888, in CP, no. 5139.

42. Dr. F. M. E. Fant to Physician of the Lunatic Asylum, in CP, no. 3723; Shryock, "Medical Practice," p. 64.

43. *The Cottage Physician* (Springfield, Mass., 1895), title page. At least one edition of Buchan was published in South Carolina. See William Buchan, *Domestic Medicine* (Charleston 1807); Anonymous, *The Medical Vade-Mecum* (Charleston, 1800); J. Hume Simons, *The Planter's Guide and Family Book of Medicine* (Charleston, 1848); Alfred M. Folger, *The Family Physician* (Spartanburg, S.C., 1845); Simon Abbott, *The Southern Botany Physician* (Charleston, 1844); John Gunn, *Gunn's Domestic Medicine* (Knoxville, 1830; reprint, with an introduction by Charles E. Rosenberg, Knoxville: University of Tennessee Press, 1986); James

Ewell, *The Medical Companion, or Family Physician*, 8th ed. (Philadelphia, 1834); Joseph Laurie and Robert J. McClatchey, *The Homeopathic Domestic Medicine* (New York, 1872). On the literature and practice of domestic medicine in the nineteenth century, see Keeney, "Unless Powerful Sick," pp. 276-94; Risse et al., *Medicine Without Doctors*. On the use of the manuals for home care of the insane, see Samuel B. Thielman, "Community Management of Mental Disorders in Antebellum America," *Journal of the History of Medicine* 44 (1989): 352-59.

44. Abbott, *Southern Botany Physician*, pp. 281-83, 236-39; Buchan, *Domestic Medicine*, pp. 276-79, 290-91; Ewell, *Medical Companion*, pp. 480-90; *Cottage Physician*, pp. 190-91.

45. Simons, *Planter's Guide*, pp. 100-101; Ewell, *Medical Companion*, pp. 120, 125; Buchan, *Domestic Medicine*, p. 290.

46. Ewell, *Medical Companion*, pp. 484-85; Folger, *Family Physician*, pp. 136, 138-39.

47. Folger, *Family Physician*, pp. 258-59.

48. *Cottage Physician*, pp. 190-91, 206-7.

49. *Charleston Mercury*, January 5, 1837, advertisement for *Southern Botanic Journal*; Daniel Drake, "Diseases of the Negro Population," *Southern Medical and Surgical Journal* 1, n.s. (1845): 341-43; Thomas B. Affleck, "On the Hygiene of Cotton Plantations and the Management of Negro Slaves," *Southern Medical Reports* 2 (1850): 429-36. See also Keeney, "Unless Powerful Sick," pp. 280-81.

50. Cartwright, "Diseases and Peculiarities of the Negro Race," *De Bow's Review* 11 (1851): 331-35.

51. Waring, *History of Medicine in South Carolina* 2:114-16; Joseph F. Kett, *Formation of the American Medical Profession* (New Haven, Conn.: Yale University Press, 1968), pp. 17-19; Barnwell County, Sessions Journal, November 4, 1817, SCL.

52. *Southern Botanic Journal* 2 (1839): 27-28. On the Thomsonians, see Alex Berman, "The Thomsonian Movement and Its Relation to American Pharmacy and Medicine," *Bulletin of the History of Medicine* 25 (1951): 405-8; John Duffy, *The Healers: A History of American Medicine* (Urbana: University of Illinois Press, 1979), pp. 110-12; Ronald L. Numbers, "Do It Yourself the Sectarian Way," in *Sickness and Health in America: Readings in the History of Medicine and Public Health*, ed. Judith Walzer Leavitt and Ronald L. Numbers (Madison: University of Wisconsin Press, 1978), pp. 87-89.

53. *Southern Botanic Journal* 2 (1839): 27-28, 396-97; Dain, *Concepts of Insanity*, p. 161.

54. *Charleston Mercury*, May 25, 1836; Waring, *History of Medicine in South Carolina* 2:95, 100, 115; Kett, *Formation of the American Medical Profession*, pp. 22-23, 111-12; William G. Rothstein, *American Physicians in the Nineteenth Century: From Sects to Science* (Baltimore: Johns Hopkins University Press, 1972), pp. 145-47

55. Folger, *Family Physician*, pp. 244-46.

56. Kaufman, *Homeopathy in America*, pp. 23–33; Numbers, "Do It Yourself," pp. 89–91; Duffy, *Healers*, pp. 112–19; Dain, *Concepts of Insanity*, pp. 161–64. An example of a homeopathic domestic manual is Laurie and McClatchey, *Homeopathic Domestic Medicine*.

57. Bleser, *Hammonds of Redcliffe*, pp. 101–2; Faust, *Design for Mastery*, pp. 77–81.

58. E. Don Herd Jr., *The South Carolina Upcountry, 1540–1980* (Greenwood, S.C.: Attic Press, 1980), p. 243; Kaufman, *Homeopathy in America*, pp. 15–16; Waring, *Medicine in South Carolina* 2:114–16; Shryock, "Medical Practice in the Old South," pp. 62–63.

59. John Hawkins, "Magical Medical Practice in South Carolina," *Popular Science Monthly* (1907): 165–68, 172, copy in SCL.

60. George P. Rawick, ed., *The American Slave: A Composite Autobiography*, vols. 2 and 3, *South Carolina Narratives* (Westport, Conn.: Greenwood Publishing, 1972), vol. 2, pt. 1, pp. 12, 24, 39, 125, 171, 193, 271–72, 241–42, 307, 346, pt. 2, pp. 2, 38, 146, 175–76, vol. 3, pt. 3, pp. 87, 106–7, 128, 160, 246, 254, pt. 4, pp. 6, 53, 90, 103, 156, 221, 263; Kiple and King, *Black Diaspora*, p. 170.

61. Rawick, *American Slave*, vol. 2, pt. 1, p. 346, pt. 2, pp. 175–76, 345, vol. 3, pt. 3, pp. 106–7, 246, 254, pt. 4, pp. 6, 53, 90, 103; Genovese, *Roll Jordan Roll: The World the Slaves Made* (New York: Pantheon Books, 1974), pp. 221–30; Charles Joyner, *Down By the Riverside: A South Carolina Slave Community* (Chicago: University of Illinois Press, 1984), pp. 144–50; Elliott J. Gorn, "Black Magic: Folk Beliefs of the Slave Community," in Numbers and Savitt, *Science and Medicine in the Old South*, pp. 295–326; Margaret Washington Creel, *"A Peculiar People": Slave Religion and Community Culture Among the Gullahs* (New York: New York University Press, 1988), pp. 56–58. Root medicine remains viable in the South Carolina low country in the late twentieth century. See J. E. McTeer, *High Sheriff of the Low Country* (Beaufort, S.C.: Beaufort Book, 1970); Wilber H. Watson, ed., *Black Folk Medicine* (New Brunswick, N.J.: Transaction Books, 1985).

62. CH, 25, no. 12340.

63. In the case histories of the South Carolina State Hospital between 1877 and 1913, I found thirty-seven cases of patients who claimed to be the victims of conjure, spells, hoodoo, voodoo, witchcraft, and so forth. Of these, twelve were white, twenty-four black, and one could not be identified by race. See CH, 3–31.

64. CH, 8, no. 4240.

65. *Charleston Mercury*, January 3, 1840; *Charleston Courier*, October 2, 1870; *Columbia State*, December 6, 1895.

66. *Charleston Courier*, May 30–June 1, 1824, January 3, 1850, January 31, 1860; *Charleston Mercury*, January 2, 3, 12, 1839, January 3, 1840; *Charleston City Directory*, 1852, p. 217; *Columbia State*, December 4–7, 1895. For the history of proprietary medicines, see James Harvey Young, *The Toadstool Millionaires: A Social History of Patent Medicines in America Before Federal Regulation* (Princeton, N.J.:

Princeton University Press, 1961) and "Patent Medicines and the Self-Help Syndrome," in Risse et al., *Medicine Without Doctors*, pp. 95–116.

67. *Charleston Courier*, January 31, 1860. On patent medicines in the South, see James Harvey Young, "Patent Medicines: An Element of Southern Distinctiveness," in *Disease and Distinctiveness in the American South*, ed. Todd L. Savitt and James Harvey Young (Knoxville: University of Tennessee Press, 1988), pp. 154–93.

68. *Charleston Courier*, January 3, 11, 1839. On Brandreth, see Young, *Toadstool Millionaires*, pp. 75–89.

69. *Charleston Mercury*, June 14, 1850.

70. *Clinton Gazette*, March 21, 1912, clipping in Babcock Papers, SCL.

71. Elizabeth W. Etheridge, *The Butterfly Caste: A Social History of Pellagra in the South* (Westport, Conn.: Greenwood Publishers, 1972), p. 38; Roe, *A Plague of Corn*, pp. 95–97; Kenneth F. Kiple and Virginia H. Kiple, "Black Tongue and Black Men: Pellagra and Slavery in the Antebellum South," *Journal of Southern History* 43 (1977): 420.

72. *Charleston Courier*, January 3, 1839.

73. Keeney, "Unless Powerful Sick," pp. 287–88; Louis Manigault, Prescription Book, 1852, Charleston South Carolina, Medicine given to slaves at Gowrie Plantation, Manuscript Dept, Perkins Library, Duke University.

74. Mitchell King Diary, March 17, 1855, King Papers, SHC; CP, nos. 6952, 6993, 7099, 4953, 5088, 5098, 5171, 11981; CH, 9, no. 4705, 17, no. 8697, 19, nos. 9715, 9732, 20, no. 10118, 21, nos. 10883, 10969, 22, no. 10930.

75. Folger, *Family Physician*, pp. 244–46.

76. John S. Haller Jr., *American Medicine in Transition: 1840–1910* (Urbana: University of Illinois Press, 1981), p. 89; Rothstein, *American Physicians*, p. 183; Ben Tillman to James W. Babcock, October 13, 1903, April 5, 1908, Babcock Papers, SCL.

77. CP, nos. 6983, 5626; PTR, 1, Edward Caldwell.

78. Duffy, *Healers*, p. 122; Dain, *Concepts of Insanity*, p. 160.

CHAPTER TEN

1. *AR*, 1876–77, in *RR*, 1877–78, p. 463. Ensor's assessment of the problems endured by the South Carolina Lunatic Asylum was shared by other asylum superintendents. See *American Journal of Insanity* 32 (1875–76): 556, 34 (1877): 183, 34 (1878): 566–67.

2. William Roark, *Masters Without Slaves* (New York: Norton, 1978), pp. 40–52, 77–78, 88–89.

3. *AR*, 1861, pp. 6–8; MBR, June 7, 1862.

4. *AR*, 1842, pp. 16–17, 1856, p. 10, 1860, in *RR*, pp. 256, 261, 1861, pp. 7–8,

1862, pp. 3–4; MBR, November 6, 1856, November 18, 1858, November 1, 1862; Report of the Committee on the Lunatic Asylum, 1859, GAP.

5. *AR*, 1863, pp. 3–8; MBR, January 9, 1864.

6. In 1863, after the legislature raised the fee for pauper patients to $212, the actual cost of their care, according to the asylum's report, was $428. *AR*, 1863, pp. 3–8, 1864, pp. 3–4, 10; MBR, July 19, 1862, August 1, 14, September 5, 1863.

7. J. H. Easterby, ed., *The South Carolina Rice Plantation as Revealed in the Papers of R. W. F. Allston* (Chicago: University of Chicago Press, 1945), p. 201 n. 2; *AR*, 1861, in *RR*, p. 135, 1863, in *RR*, pp. 125–26, 1865, p. 8.

8. MBR, 1860–65, esp. June 1862, January 31, 1863.

9. MBR, July 14, 1864; *AR*, 1853–65, patient statistics.

10. A. R. Childs, ed., *The Private Journals of Henry William Ravenel, 1859– 1887* (Columbia: University of South Carolina Press, 1947), p. 150.

11. Gilbert E. Sabre, *Nineteen Months a Prisoner of War* (New York, 1865), pp. 165–67; see also A. O. Abbot, *Prison Life in the South, 1864–1865* (New York, 1865), pp. 152–53.

12. MBR, December 2, 1864, February 4, 1865; M. B. Lucas, *Sherman and the Burning of Columbia* (College Station: Texas A&M Press, 1976), pp. 56–57; *War of the Rebellion: A Compilation of the Official Records of the Union and Confederate Armies* (Washington, D.C.: Government Printing Office, 1899), ser. 2, 7: 1062–63, 1179–80, 1184, 1196–97.

13. Mary Leverette to Caroline, March 18, 1865, SCL.

14. C. Vann Woodward, ed., *Mary Chesnut's Civil War* (New Haven, Conn.: Yale University Press, 1981), p. 676.

15. On the controversy over the burning of Columbia, see Lucas, *Sherman*.

16. Mrs. Campbell Bryce, *The Personal Experiences of Mrs. Campbell Bryce during the Burning of Columbia, South Carolina* (Philadelphia, 1899), pp. 34–36.

17. *Our Women in the War* (Charleston, 1885), p. 118; Lucas, *Sherman*, p. 156.

18. *Our Women in the War*, p. 118; Bryce, *Personal Experiences*, pp. 36–37; Mary Leverette estimated the number of refugees at five hundred. Mary Leverette to Caroline, March 18, 1865, SCL; *AR*, 1865, pp. 6, 8.

19. Bryce, *Personal Experiences*, pp. 36–37; *Our Women in the War*, p. 118; Lucas, *Sherman*, p. 156, *AR*, 1865, pp. 6, 8.

20. MBR, April 10, 11, May 6, 22, November 4, 1865; *AR*, 1865, pp. 6, 8–10; *Columbia Daily Phoenix*, July 14, 1865; Bryce, *Personal Experiences*, pp. 50–51.

21. John Hope Franklin, *Reconstruction: After the Civil War* (Chicago: University of Chicago Press, 1961), pp. 30–35, 42–44; Michael Perman, *Reunion Without Compromise: The South and Reconstruction, 1865–1868* (London: Cambridge University Press, 1973).

22. *AR*, 1866–69; MBR, May 5, June 2, July 7, Oct. 6, 1866; SCSH, Admission Book, October 9, 1865, February 8, 27, April 13, 1866; PTR, 3, Thomas Crimmager.

23. Bureau of Freedmen and Abandoned Lands, Correspondence of W. J. Harkesheimer and Thomas Stark, 1867, SCL; Marlboro County, Commissioners of the Poor, Minutes, August 22, 1866, SCDAH; *AR*, 1871, p. 18.

24. Franklin, *Reconstruction*, pp. 2–6; Roark, *Masters Without Slaves*, pp. 77–78, 132–53, 170–80; E. M. Lander, *A History of South Carolina, 1865–1960* (Chapel Hill: University of North Carolina Press, 1960), pp. 3–5.

25. *AR*, 1860, in *RR*, p. 256, 1868, p. 6.

26. *AR*, 1866, p. 5, 1870, pp. 43–45.

27. *AR*, 1866, pp. 5–9; MBR, February 2, March 2, 1867; *RR*, 1868, pp. 114–16; *Anderson Intelligencer*, December 8, 1870.

28. South Carolina, *The Statutes at Large of South Carolina* (Columbia, S.C., 1836), 14:24.

29. *Charleston Daily News*, January 13, 1869. The composition of the regents changed during Reconstruction, but the board retained its black majority until 1876. See *AR*, 1870–75 for lists of regents. Thomas Holt, *Black over White* (Urbana: University of Illinois Press, 1977) contains information on black officeholders during Reconstruction in South Carolina.

30. *House Journal*, 1869, pp. 27–28; *Columbia Daily Phoenix*, November 25, 1869; Dorothy C. Wilson, *Stranger and Traveler: The Story of Dorothea Dix, American Reformer* (Boston: Little, Brown, 1975), pp. 313–15; John S. Reynolds, *Reconstruction in South Carolina* (Columbia, S.C.: State, 1905), pp. 123–25; *Charleston Daily News*, November 26, 1868.

31. *Columbia Daily Phoenix*, January 18, 1870; S. Sumter to John Waties, March 29, 1868, Waties-Parker Family Papers, SCL; Reynolds, *Reconstruction in South Carolina*, pp. 223–25.

32. MBR, February 24, May 10, June 4, 1870. The black assistant physician, Dr. J. D. Harris, was removed by the regents in 1871. I have been unable to discover anything about his previous or subsequent career.

33. Reynolds, *Reconstruction in South Carolina*, pp. 123–24.

34. S. Sumter to John Waties, March 29, 1868, Waties-Parker Family Papers, SCL.

35. The traditional view of Reconstruction derives from the work of William Dunning and his students early in this century. See, for example, William Dunning, *Reconstruction, Political and Economic, 1865–1877* (New York: Harper Brothers, 1907); Walter L. Fleming, *The Sequel to Appomattox* (New Haven, Conn.: Yale University Press, 1919); Claude G. Bowers, *The Tragic Era* (Cambridge, Mass.: Houghton Mifflin, 1929). For the traditional view of Reconstruction in South Carolina, see Reynolds, *Reconstruction in South Carolina*; David Duncan Wallace, *South Carolina: A Short History, 1520–1948* (Chapel Hill: University of North Carolina Press, 1951), chaps. 54–56. For a recent discussion of Reconstruction and its historiography, see Eric Foner, *Reconstruction, America's Unfinished Revolution, 1863–1877* (New York: Harper and Row, 1988).

36. Francis Tiffany, *The Life of Dorothea Lynde Dix* (Boston: Houghton Mifflin, 1890), p. 352. See also Wilson, *Stranger and Traveler*, pp. 313-15.

37. *A Biographical Directory of Contemporary American Physicians and Surgeons*, s.v. "J. F. Ensor" (Philadelphia, 1880); *Journal of the South Carolina Medical Association* 3 (1907): 152-53; David Duncan Wallace, *The History of South Carolina*, 4 vols. (New York: American Historical Society, 1934), 3:280-81.

38. For examples of the revisionist view of Reconstruction in South Carolina, see Joel Williamson, *After Slavery: The Negro in South Carolina During Reconstruction* (Chapel Hill: University of North Carolina Press, 1965); Peggy Lamson, *The Glorious Failure: Robert Brown Elliott and the Reconstruction in South Carolina* (New York: Norton, 1973); Thomas Holt, *Black over White* (Urbana: University of Illinois Press, 1977).

39. *AR*, 1870, pp. 3-11; MBR, August 20, 1870. Patient statistics are from *AR*, 1860, 1865, 1870, 1876-77.

40. *AR*, 1870, pp. 3-5, appendix 2.

41. *AR*, 1870, p. 12.

42. *AR*, 1870, appendix 1-3.

43. *AR*, 1871, pp. 5, 30-32.

44. *AR*, 1871, p. 19.

45. *AR*, 1871, pp. 37-38.

46. Senate Journal, 1871-72, p. 43; Wallace, *South Carolina: A Short History*, p. 584.

47. *AR*, 1871, pp. 37-39. For similar charges from some of the regents, see *AR*, 1872, pp. 7-8.

48. *AR*, 1874-75, pp. 20-21.

49. *Columbia Daily Phoenix*, May 8, September 8, 1872; *AR*, 1872, pp. 27-37; *Charleston Daily News*, September 19, 1872.

50. MBR, November 11, 1875, May 26, 1876.

51. MBR, May 6, 1871, April 4, May 4, 7, June 4, August 6, September 6, October 1, 1874, February 4, 1875; *AR*, 1870, appendix 2, 1872, pp. 7-8, 1874-75, pp. 20-21.

52. Ensor to the Board of Regents, December 1877, in Governor Hampton's Correspondence, SCDAH.

53. *AR*, 1873-74, pp. 48-49.

54. Alfred B. Williams, *Hampton and His Red Shirts* (Charleston: Walker, Evans, and Cogswell, 1935), pp. 55, 426-27.

55. *Charleston Daily News*, December 5, 1872.

56. *Columbia Daily Phoenix*, April 19, May 2, August 11, December 7, 1872; *Charleston Daily News*, September 19, 1872.

57. MBR, May 3, 1873.

58. *Charleston News and Courier*, May 7, 1873.

59. *AR*, 1873-74, pp. 49-50.

60. *Charleston News and Courier*, May 28, 1873.

61. *Aiken Tribune*, quoted in *Charleston News and Courier*, May 28, 1873.

62. *Charleston News and Courier*, May 15, 1873, reprinted from *Columbia Daily Phoenix*, May 6, 1873. Ensor generally received good press. See, for example, *Abbeville Press and Banner*, January 29, 1873, clipping in file on Ensor in WHL; *Anderson Intelligencer*, February 9, 1871; *Charleston News and Courier*, May 2, 1876.

63. See *Charleston News and Courier*, September 21, 1872.

64. Williamson, *After Slavery*, pp. 390–91, 397–403.

65. MBR, April 1, 1875.

66. MBR, January 6, May 6, 1876; *AR*, 1874–75, pp. 20–21; *Columbia Daily Phoenix*, January 25, 1873; *Charleston News and Courier*, May 7, 1873; Ensor to the Board of Regents, December 1877, in Governor Hampton's Correspondence, SCDAH.

67. Holt, *Black over White*, p. 181; Williamson, *After Slavery*, pp. 402–5.

68. Walter Allen, *Governor Chamberlain's Administration* (New York, 1888), pp. 51–52.

69. MBR, February 4, 1875; *AR*, 1874–75, pp. 5, 20–21, 1875–76, pp. 20–21; MBR, April 1, 1875.

70. Holt, *Black over White*, pp. 181–83; Allen, *Governor Chamberlain's Administration*, pp. 175–76, 245–46.

71. *American Journal of Insanity* 33 (1876): 179.

72. Robert J. Moore, "Governor Chamberlain and the End of Reconstruction in South Carolina," *Proceedings of the South Carolina Historical Association* (1977): 20–21; Williamson, *After Slavery*, pp. 406–12.

73. *AR*, 1876–77, p. 463.

74. Williams, *Hampton and His Red Shirts*, p. 427.

75. *AR*, 1876–77, in *RR*, p. 463; MBR, July 5, October 6, 1877.

76. William Gillette, *Retreat from Reconstruction* (Baton Rouge: Louisiana State University Press, 1979), pp. x–xi, 346; Avery Craven, *Reconstruction: The Ending of the Civil War* (New York: Holt, Rinehart and Winston, 1969), pp. 302–7; Kenneth M. Stampp, *The Era of Reconstruction, 1865–1877* (New York: Alfred Knopf, 1970), pp. 204–11.

77. MBR, July 5, November 13, December 6, 1877.

78. *Report of the Commission Appointed to Examine into the Condition of the Penal and Charitable Institutions of the State*, *RR*, 1877–78, p. 814.

79. Williams, *Hampton and His Red Shirts*, p. 427; Henry Thompson, *Ousting the Carpetbagger from South Carolina* (Columbia, S.C.: R. L. Bryan, 1926), p. 67; Reynolds, *Reconstruction in South Carolina*, p. 125; see also Wallace, *History of South Carolina* 3:280–81.

80. *Anderson Intelligencer*, February 9, 1871; Thompson, *Ousting the Carpetbagger*, p. 66; Reynolds, *Reconstruction in South Carolina*, p. 125.

81. *AR*, 1871, p. 18, 1872, pp. 24–25, 1876–77, in *RR*, pp. 460–61; MBR, Febru-

ary 24, May 10, June 4, 1870, January 14, 1871; John W. Parker to Dorothea Dix, October 20, 1870, Dix Papers, Houghton Library, Harvard University.

82. Williamson, *After Slavery*, pp. 414-15; Martin Abbott, "The Freedmen's Bureau and Its Carolina Critics," *Proceedings of the South Carolina Historical Association*, 1962, p. 23.

83. Ensor to Board of Regents, December 1877, Governor Hampton Correspondence, SCDAH.

84. MBR, February 4, 1875, May 6, 1876; *AR*, 1875-76, p. 11.

85. MBR, July 5, 1877; *AR*, 1876-77, in *RR*, 1877-78, p. 460.

86. Williams, *Hampton and His Red Shirts*, p. 427; see also note 15.

87. *AR*, 1870-1877, statistics on movement of population.

88. *AR*, 1872, p. 25, 1874, p. 40; CH, 3, nos. 2772, 2805, 2815, 2816, 2825, 2831; Thielman, "Madness and Medicine: Trends," pp. 25-46.

89. *AR*, 1872, p. 25, 1871, pp. 20, 22, 1873, in *RR*, pp. 475, 499.

90. On the decline of therapeutic optimism among American alienists see Gerald Grob, *Mental Institutions in America: Social Policy to 1875* (New York: Free Press, 1973), chaps. 7-8; David Rothman, *The Discovery of the Asylum: Social Order and Disorder in the New Republic* (Boston: Little, Brown, 1971), chap. 11.

91. For the years 1873-77, Ensor estimated that more than 90 percent of his patients were incurable. See *AR*, 1873, Exhibit 16, 1874, Exhibit 16, 1874-75, Exhibit 18, 1876-77, Exhibit 20.

92. *Charleston News and Courier*, May 7, 1873.

CHAPTER ELEVEN

1. By 1880 the asylum accounted for almost one-third of state appropriations. *House Journal*, 1881, p. 29.

2. David Carlton, *Mill and Town in South Carolina* (Baton Rouge: Louisiana State University Press, 1982), pp. 6-8, 15-25; William J. Cooper Jr., *The Conservative Regime in South Carolina* (Baltimore: Johns Hopkins University Press, 1968), pp. 16, 133-42; E. M. Lander, *A History of South Carolina, 1865-1960* (Chapel Hill: University of North Carolina Press, 1960), pp. 106-7; Peter Coclanis, *The Shadow of a Dream: Economic Life and Death in the South Carolina Low Country, 1670-1920* (New York: Oxford University Press, 1989), pp. 128-32, 154-55.

3. Cooper, *Conservative Regime*, pp. 133-42; *AR*, 1883-84, pp. 25-26, 1885-86, p. 14; MBR, January 14, 1886.

4. *Charleston News and Courier*, December 3, 1877.

5. MBR, November 7, 1878.

6. *Cyclopedia of Eminent and Representative Men of the Carolinas of the Nineteenth Century*, s.v. "Peter Griffin," 1:336.

7. *Charleston News and Courier*, November 20, 1877.

8. Cooper, *Conservative Regime*, pp. 20, 39-40.

9. On the Farmer's Movement and the career of Tillman, see Francis Butler Simkins, *Pitchfork Ben Tillman* (Baton Rouge: Louisiana State University Press, 1944); Diane Neal, "Benjamin Ryan Tillman: The South Carolina Years, 1847–1894" (Ph.D. diss., Kent State University, 1976).

10. *House Journal*, 1890, pp. 139–40; MBR, December 11, 1890, January 8, 1891; *Statutes-at-Large of South Carolina* (1891) 20:1117.

11. Julius J. Fleming to Benjamin Tillman, December 13, 1890, Governor Tillman Papers, SCDAH; Simkins, *Tillman*, p. 188.

12. *Charleston News and Courier*, April 23, 1891; L. G. Corbett to Benjamin Tillman, April 24, 1891, Governor Tillman Papers, SCDAH. Tillman offered to provide the entire text of the committee report to any newspaper that agreed to publish it in full, but none took up the offer. The testimony was not printed with the *Reports and Resolutions*, and no manuscript of it appears to have survived. The regents and Griffin agreed to the decision to publish only a part of the testimony in synopsis form, according to the *News and Courier*, April 21, 1891. See also *House Journal*, 1891, pp. 35–36 for Tillman's own summary of the investigation.

13. *Columbia Daily Register*, April 2, 1891; *Charleston News and Courier*, April 2, 1891. The report did not name anyone but referred to the officers "immediately in charge."

14. T. J. Strait to Tillman, March 1891, Governor Tillman Papers, SCDAH.

15. *Columbia Daily Register*, March 17, 1891. Ironically, on the same day the paper reported the suicide of a patient, the first in thirteen years.

16. *Charleston News and Courier*, April 21, 1891; *House Journal*, 1891, pp. 34–35.

17. MBR, April 20–28, 1891, *Columbia Daily Register*, April 22, 30, May 2, 1891, *Charleston News and Courier*, April 23, 1891.

18. *Columbia Daily Register*, May 19–22, 1891; *Charleston News and Courier*, May 20, 22, 1891; *Sumter Watchman and Southron*, May 27, 1891; MBR, May 14–20, 1891; Griffin to Tillman, May 20, 1891, Governor Tillman Papers, SCDAH.

19. *Charleston News and Courier*, May 20, 1891.

20. Tillman to Jones and others, March 10, 1892, in Governor Tillman Papers, SCDAH, quoted in Simkins, *Pitchfork Ben Tillman*, p. 182; *Statutes of South Carolina* (1891) 20:1117.

21. W. F. Babcock to James W. Babcock, May 22, 1891, Babcock Papers, SCL.

22. *Columbia Daily Register*, April 4, 1891; *Charleston News and Courier*, April 3, May 22, 1891; *Columbia State*, May 21, 1891. See also *Sumter Watchman and Southron*, April 8, 1891.

23. *Columbia Daily Register*, May 19, 1891.

24. *Columbia Daily Register*, April 2, 1891; MBR, April 9, 1891. Bunch was married to Tillman's niece.

25. William A. Harrison to Tillman, January 5, 1891, S. F. Blakeley to Tillman, January 5, 1891, Dr. T. B. Hinnant to Tillman, December 19, 1890, W. J. Bramlett to Tillman, December 15, 1890, Governor Tillman Papers, SCDAH.

26. S. F. Blakeley to Tillman, January 19, 1891, Governor Tillman Papers, SCDAH.

27. J. M. Beasley to Tillman, May 3, 1891, Governor Tillman Papers, SCDAH; Simkins, *Pitchfork Ben Tillman*, pp. 182–83; Neal, "Benjamin Ryan Tillman," pp. 160, 223–25.

28. Tillman to J. G. Withers, June 8, 1891, Thomas N. Berry to James W. Babcock, June 3, 1891, W. F. Babcock to James W. Babcock, May 24, 1891, Babcock Papers, SCL.

29. J. M. Beasley to Tillman, May 3, 27, 1891, Governor Tillman Papers, SCDAH.

30. *Charleston News and Courier*, May 22, 1891; J. M. Thompson to Tillman, April 8, 1891, Governor Tillman Papers, SCDAH; *Columbia Daily Register*, May 20, 1891; W. F. Babcock to James W. Babcock, May 22, 1891, Babcock Papers, SCL.

31. J. H. Taylor, *James Woods Babcock: An Appreciation* (Columbia, 1926), pp. 1–4; William S. Hall, "Psychiatrist, Humanitarian, and Scholar, James Woods Babcock, M.D.," *Journal of the South Carolina Medical Association* (1970) 66: 366–71; "James Woods Babcock," *Dictionary of American Biography*; "Obituary of James Woods Babcock," *American Journal of Psychiatry* 1 (1921–22): 709–10; *National Cyclopedia of American Biography*, s.v. "James Woods Babcock," 22:222.

32. *Testimony Taken Before the Legislative Committee to Investigate the State Hospital for the Insane at Columbia* (Columbia, S.C.: Gonzales and Bryan, 1910), p. 362; J. S. Withers to Tillman, June 5, 1891, Governor Tillman Papers, SCDAH. Withers was secretary of the Chester County Farmers Alliance.

33. Tillman to J. S. Withers, June 8, 1891, Governor Tillman Papers, SCDAH.

34. James W. Babcock to W. F. Babcock, May 25, 1891, Babcock Papers, SCL; Thomas N. Berry to Tillman, June 6, 1891, J. S. Withers to Tillman, June 5, 1891, Governor Tillman Papers, SCDAH.

35. Edward Cowles to Tillman, June 20, 1891, Governor Tillman Papers, SCDAH.

36. W. F. Babcock to James W. Babcock, May 24, 1891, Babcock Papers, SCL.

37. *Sumter Watchman and Southron*, July 8, 1891; "Obituary of James Woods Babcock," p. 710; Hall, "Psychiatrist, Humanitarian, and Scholar," pp. 366–71; Babcock Papers, SCL.

38. Dr. Herbert B. Howard to James W. Babcock, May 14, 1896, Babcock Papers, SCL. Howard was superintendent, Insane Department of the Massachusetts State Almshouse at Tewkesbury, where he and Babcock had met as interns.

39. T. O. Powell to P. L. Murphy, April 17, 1897, P. L. Murphy Papers, no. 535, SHC; Taylor, *James Woods Babcock*, p. 4.

40. MBR, September 10, 1891.

41. James W. Babcock to Katherine Guion, September 25, October 8, 25, 1891, Babcock Papers, SCL.

42. James W. Babcock to Katherine Guion, December 22, 1891, Babcock Papers, SCL.

43. James W. Babcock to Katherine Guion, December 22, 1891, June 29, 1892, C. Irving Fisher to James W. Babcock, May 1, 1892, Babcock Papers, SCL.

44. Corbett wrote Babcock expressing regret that the newspapers had implied that politics was behind his resignation. L. G. Corbett to James W. Babcock, October 15, 1892, Babcock Papers, SCL; James W. Babcock to Dr. Macy, October 22, 1892, Letters, 1892-93, SCSH; MBR, October 12, 1911; A. R. Woodson to Governor Martin Ansel, October 10, 1908, Ansel to James W. Babcock, October 12, 1908, Governor Ansel Papers, SCDAH.

45. James W. Babcock to P. L. Murphy, May 21, 24, 1897, P. L. Murphy Papers, SHC; Samuel Mather to James W. Babcock, March 29, May 21, 1897, James W. Babcock to Mather, May 24, 1897, C. Irving Fisher to James W. Babcock, April 8, 1897, Herbert B. Howard to James W. Babcock, April 7, 1897, Babcock Papers, SCL; MBR, June 11, 1897.

46. MBR, February 11, 1897, March 11, April 8, October 14, 1897.

47. Tillman to James W. Babcock, April 16, 1897, Babcock Papers, SCL.

48. James W. Babcock to P. L. Murphy, May 21, 1897, P. L. Murphy Papers, SHC.

49. AR, 1897, pp. 8, 17-18; MBR, June 11, 1897.

50. *Report and Proceedings of the Special Legislative Committee on the State Hospital, 1914* (Columbia, S.C.: Gonzales and Bryan, 1914), pp. 22-23, 131, 134-35, 189.

51. *Testimony, Legislative Committee*, p. 251.

52. *Testimony, Legislative Committee*, p. 251; MBR, March 11, 1897, April 13, 1899, May 8, 1907; Gov. Duncan C. Heyward to James W. Babcock, February 16, 1903, Resolution of Regents to James W. Babcock, April 12, 1906, Babcock Papers, SCL; James W. Babcock, "The Prevention of Tuberculosis in Hospitals for the Insane," reprint from *American Journal of Insanity* (October 1894): 9-13; MBR, September 13, 1906, January 1, 9, 1908, January 14, 1909, October 13, 1910; AR, 1899, pp. 17-19, 1902, pp. 11-12, 1907, pp. 12-14; James W. Babcock to B. R. Tillman, April 12, 1897, Babcock Papers, SCL.

CHAPTER TWELVE

1. Gerald Grob, *Mental Institutions in America: Social Policy to 1875* (New York: Free Press, 1973), pp. 205, 219-20, 291, and *Mental Illness and American Society, 1875-1940* (Princeton, N.J.: Princeton University Press, 1983), pp. 14-15, 195-98.

2. AR, 1890-91, p. 83; see also *Columbia State*, December 2, 1895; Newspaper clipping dated June 21, 1900, Babcock Papers, SCL.

3. MBR, February 7, 1878, December 4, 1879; AR, 1880-81, p. 18, 1882-83,

p. 24, 1883–84, pp. 25–26, 1885–86, p. 14, 1887–88, pp. 14–15, 1895–96, p. 13; 1898, pp. 7–8, 17, 1899, pp. 8–10, 1900, pp. 9–10, 17–19, 1903, p. 12, pp. 6–7, 16–17, 1905, pp. 16–19, 1906, pp. 15–16.

4. *AR*, 1880–81, p. 20, 1887–88, p. 16; *Testimony, Taken Before the Legislative Committee to Investigate the State Hospital for the Insane of Columbia* (Columbia, S.C.: Gonzales and Bryan, 1910), pp. 183–84, 398–99, 404–5.

5. See *ARs*, 1877–1914.

6. *AR*, 1882–83, pp. 22–25, 1887–88, pp. 15, 57–59, 1900, p. 9, 1906, pp. 15–16; *House Journal*, 1904, p. 24. Grob, *Mental Illness and American Society*, pp. 25–26.

7. *AR*, 1883–84, pp. 25–26, 1882–83, p. 22, 1885–86, p. 14, 1887–88, pp. 15–16.

8. MBR, January 14, 1886.

9. *Testimony, Legislative Committee*, pp. 398–99.

10. MBR, August 11, 1892.

11. MBR, August 11, 1892, September 13, 1893.

12. *Testimony, Legislative Committee*, p. 398; MBR, January 12, 1905, February 13, 1908; *AR*, 1900, pp. 18–19.

13. *House Journal*, 1890, p. 140; *AR*, 1881, p. 14. Efforts to reverse the trend and get patients' families to pay for at least part of the costs of asylum care had little success. By 1891 the number of beneficiaries had grown to 685, with 33 patients paying in full and 20 in part. *AR*, 1891, p. 19.

14. *AR*, 1877–78, in *RR*, p. 589; William J. Cooper Jr., *The Conservative Regime in South Carolina* (Baltimore: Johns Hopkins University Press, 1968), pp. 133–42; E. M. Lander, *A History of South Carolina, 1865–1960* (Chapel Hill: University of North Carolina Press, 1960), pp. 106–7; Peter Coclanis, *The Shadow of a Dream: Economic Life and Death in the South Carolina Low Country, 1670–1920* (New York: Oxford University Press, 1989), pp. 128–32, 154–55.

15. *AR*, 1871, p. 18, 1902, p. 34.

16. *AR*, 1890–91, p. 9; *Acts and Joint Resolutions of the General Assembly of South Carolina*, 1870–71 (Columbia, S.C., 1871), pp. 672–73.

17. *AR*, 1880–81, p. 14; MBR, April 1, 1875, July 13, 1876.

18. Senate Journal, 1881, pp. 23–24; *House Journal*, 1882, pp. 26–27; *AR*, 1880–81, p. 19.

19. *House Journal*, 1890, p. 141.

20. CP, nos. 4461, 7736; see also no. 4488.

21. *House Journal*, 1890, p. 141, 1881, p. 29, 1883, p. 19, 1892, p. 11; *AR*, 1880–81, p. 19, 1890–91, p. 11.

22. James W. Babcock to Mr. John F. Ficken, November 4, 1892, Letters, 1892–93, SCSH.

23. *AR*, 1891–92, pp. 10–11; *Statutes-at-Large of South Carolina* (1881) 17:927, 1882, 18:201–2.

24. *AR*, 1881–82, p. 11; 1882–83, p. 14. The problem of delayed transfer to

the asylum was dealt with to some extent by an act of 1896, which provided for emergency commitment in cases of violent and dangerous insanity. See *Statutes-at-Large of South Carolina* (1896) 22:180.

25. *Statutes-at-Large of South Carolina* (1894) 21: 837.

26. *AR*, 1894, p. 13, 1900, p. 21, 1904, p. 72.

27. AR, 1875-76, p. 11.

, 28. *AR*, 1878-79, p. 10, 1879-80, p. 10, 1881-82, p. 12, 1882-83, p. 13, 1893-94, pp. 7-8, 1894-95, p. 14.

29. *AR*, 1902, p. 12, 1894-95, p. 14, 1898, p. 5, 1899, pp. 16-17; MBR, February 11, October 14, 1909.

30. Grob, *Mental Institutions in America*, pp. 307-8, *Mental Illness and American Society*, pp. 24, 179-88, 195-96, and Gerald Grob, "Rediscovering Asylums: The Unhistorical History of the Mental Hospital," in *The Therapeutic Revolution: Essays in the Social History of American Medicine*, ed. Morris Vogel and Charles E. Rosenberg (Philadelphia: University of Pennsylvania Press, 1979), pp. 145-48; Ellen Dwyer, *Homes for the Mad: Life Inside Two Nineteenth-Century Asylums* (New Brunswick, N.J.: Rutgers University Press, 1987), pp. 186-187.

31. *AR*, 1880-81, p. 19; *AR*, 1869, in *RR*, p. 259, 1873-74, p. 38, 1874-75, p. 12; 1876-77, in *RR*, pp. 455-56, 1880-81, p. 19, 1883-84, pp. 15, 21-22, 1891-92, p. 6, 1894-95, pp. 9-10, 1897, p. 11.

32. *AR*, 1897, p. 11, 1899, p. 16, 1897, pp. 5-6, 1898, p. 6, 1900, p. 8; 1911, p. 12; MBR, September 14, 1911, June 11, 1912.

33. Grob, "Rediscovering Asylums," pp. 145-48.

34. *AR*, 1900, p. 8, 1891-92, pp. 6, 16, 1883-84, p. 21; House Journal, 1905, p. 38.

35. Grob, *Mental Institutions in America*, Chap. 8, and *Mental Illness and American Society*, pp. 24-25, 72-107; Dwyer, *Homes for the Mad*, pp. 2, 43-50; Peter McCandless, "'Build! Build!': The Controversy over the Care of the Insane in England, 1855-1870," *Bulletin of the History of Medicine* 53 (1979): 553-74; William L. Parry-Jones, "The Model of the Geel Lunatic Colony and Its Influence on the Nineteenth-Century Asylum System in Britain," in *Madhouses, Mad-Doctors, and Madmen*, ed. Andrew Scull (Philadelphia: University of Pennsylvania Press, 1981), pp. 201-17.

36. Peter L. Tyor and Leland V. Bell, *Caring for the Retarded in America: A History* (Westport, Conn.: Greenwood Press, 1984, pp. 18-19, 45; Albert Deutsch, *The Mentally Ill in America: A History of Their Care and Treatment from Colonial Times* (Garden City, N.Y.: Doubleday, Doran, 1937), pp. 338-85; Mark E. Lender and James K. Martin, *Drinking in America: A History* (New York: Free Press, 1982), p. 120.

37. *AR*, 1869, in *RR*, p. 259, 1876-77, in *RR*, pp. 456-57, 1879-80, pp. 11-12, 1882-83, pp. 16-17, 1887-88, pp. 13-14, 1888-89, p. 8.

38. *House Journal*, 1903, p. 51; *AR*, 1891-92, p. 12; 1898, p. 12, 1899, p. 19,

1902, p. 8, 1903, pp. 9–11, 1904, p. 16, 1905, pp. 14–15, 1906, p. 5, 1907, pp. 6, 14–15, 1908, pp. 3, 7.

39. *AR*, 1870, pp. 3–4; 1871, p. 27; *House Journal*, 1872, pp. 318–19; *RR*, 1871, p. 921, 1874, p. 870.

40. MBR, March 3, April 4, July 2, September 6, 1874, September 2, 1875, *AR*, 1874–75, pp. 12–13.

41. MBR, November 21, 1878, January 4, 1879, *AR*, 1878–79, pp. 10–11.

42. *AR*, 1878–79, pp. 10–11, 1879–80, p. 10; MBR, February 6, October 2, November 6, 1879, January 2, February 27, June 10, 1880.

43. *AR*, 1880–81, p. 17, 1881–82, p. 12, 1882–83, pp. 12–13, 1883–84, p. 20, 1884–85, p. 23; Samuel Sloan to Thomas Kirkbride, May 25, 1883, Kirkbride Correspondence; D. P. Robbins, *Descriptive Sketch of Columbia, S.C* (Columbia, 1888), p. 25.

44. *AR*, 1884–85, pp. 23–24.

45. *AR*, 1891–92, p. 12, 1877–78, in *RR*, p. 590, 1878–79, p. 12, 1879–80, pp. 9–19, 1880–81, pp. 9, 18, 1882–83, pp. 13, 17, 1885–86, pp. 11–12, 1887–88, pp. 8, 12, 1888–89, p. 6, 1890–91, p. 11, 1891–92, p. 12, 1892–93, pp. 11–15, 1897, p. 15, 1898, p. 6.

46. *Report of the Legislative Committee to Investigate the State Hospital for the Insane* (Columbia, S.C.: Gonzales and Bryan, 1910), p. 7; I. A. Newby, *Black Carolinians* (Columbia: University of South Carolina Press, 1973), chap. 2; Lander, *History of South Carolina*, pp. 106–7.

47. *AR*, 1880–81, p. 18, 1887–88, pp. 12–13, 1892–93, pp. 6, 11–15, 1902, p. 12, 1904, p. 68, 1908, p. 24; *Charleston News and Courier*, February 11, 12, 18, 20, 1910.

48. *AR*, 1887–88, pp. 12–13, 1888–89, pp. 7–8, 1892–93, pp. 14–15; *Columbia Register*, December 24, 1887; House Journal, 1887, p. 25; *Statutes-at-Large of South Carolina* (1889) 20:317–18.

49. *Report and Proceedings of the Special Legislative Committee to Investigate the State Hospital for the Insane and State Park* (Columbia, S.C.: Gonzales and Bryan, 1914), pp. 69–70, 59–60.

50. *AR*, 1887–88, pp. 12–13, 1888–89, pp. 7–8, 1892–93, pp. 14–15; *House Journal*, November 22, 1887, p. 25; *Statutes-at-Large of South Carolina* 20:317–18; *Statutes-at-Large of South Carolina* (1909–10) 26: no. 597.

51. *AR*, 1893–94, p. 12, 1894–95, p. 16, 1895–96, pp. 5, 12, 1897, pp. 15–17, 1898, p. 15; Notes on Page Ellington, Babcock Papers, SCL; MBR, February 8, 1912; *Testimony, Legislative Committee*, pp. 393–95.

52. MBR, May 2, 1857; *AR*, 1860, p. 12; Parker to J. L. McColl, July 25, 1863, in Marlboro County, Commissioners of the Poor, Minutes, 1857–1868, SCDAH.

53. Quoted in *Columbia Daily Phoenix*, May 4, 1872; *AR*, 1971, pp. 26–27; *Statutes-at-Large of South Carolina* (1872) 15:56, 67; SCSH, Admissions and Discharges, 1860–74; York County, Board of Commissioners, Minutes, November 29, 1872, SCL.

54. *AR*, 1883–84, p. 14, 1884–85, p. 8; MBR, April 8, 1885; *Statutes-at-Large of South Carolina* 18:827–828; *House Journal*, 1891, p. 36.

55. *AR*, 1884–85, p. 9; MBR, March 10, September 8, 1898; *Charleston News and Courier*, July 16, 1891.

56. *House Journal*, 1875, pp. 466–67; MBR, April 4, 1874, Feb. 4, 1875.

57. *AR*, 1874–75, p. 13.

58. *AR*, 1899, p. 20. According to a report by Governor Tillman in 1891, seven counties (out of thirty-five) did not have poorhouses. But one of the counties he listed as not having a poorhouse, Charleston, had an almshouse for each race. *House Journal*, 1891, p. 37.

59. *AR*, 1878–79, p. 10, 1879–80, pp. 10–12.

60. *AR*, 1890–91, pp. 6–8, 1894–95, p. 14, 1899, p. 20, 1900, p. 16, 1902, p. 13, 1905, p. 15; MBR, August 14, 1902. The State Board of Health took the same view in its report of 1888. The removal of harmless patients to the counties, the board argued, had allowed the asylum to save some money, but by inflicting "suffering upon the epileptics, idiots, and non-violent insane, etc., who are now, many of them, forced into poorhouses, jails, etc., not adapted for the reception or the support of such incurables." South Carolina State Board of Health, *The State Board of Health and the State Hospital for the Insane, 1880–1908* (Columbia, S.C.: Gonzales and Bryan, 1909–10), p. 9.

61. *AR*, 1883–84, p. 21.

62. MBR, May 12, 1892, September 13, 1893, September 13, 1894, January 10, 1895.

63. *AR*, 1883–84, p. 15.

64. E. H. Heins to James W. Babcock, December 26, 1910, in CP, no. 14882.

65. CP, no. 5032; *AR*, 1884–85, p. 9. Some local authorities were quite accommodating in removing patients when requested. See for example, Greenville County, Board of Commissioners, Minutes, February 4, 1885, SCL; MBR, April 8, 1885; *Charleston News and Courier*, July 16, 1891.

66. CP, no. 7192.

67. *AR*, 1881–82, pp. 10–11, 1882–83, p. 38, 1883–84, p. 16, 1884–85, p. 10, 1891–92, p. 11; Dr. A. S. Dozier to James W. Babcock, December 15, 1891; in CP, no. 6249.

68. J. J. Gentry to James W. Babcock, January 15, 1896, in CP, no. 7453; MBR, March 11, 1897, September 10, 1908. See also SRR, August 2, 1917.

69. CP, no. 9992.

70. Dr. James C. Mullins to Griffin, November 17, 1881, in CP, no. 3023; CP, no. 4881; CH, 25, no. 12826; CP, no. 6187.

71. J. B. Broom to Charlie, November 1893, CH, 14, no. 6875.

72. Sarah Allan, Diary, 1900, typescript of original, WHL; *Testimony, Legislative Committee*, pp. 372–75.

73. *AR*, 1890–91, p. 9.

74. *AR*, 1883-84, pp. 21-22; "Dr. Griffin's Remarks on the State Lunatic Asylum," *Transactions of the South Carolina Medical Association* (1879): 33-35; *AR*, 1880-81, p. 20.

75. See, for example, CP, nos. 4138, 4140, 4141, 4158, 4166, 4172, 4201, 4204, 4206, 4207, 4220, 4221, 4350, 4351, 4378, 4379.

76. CP, no. 4196.

77. CH, 21, no. 11098, CH, 23, no. 11774.

78. CP, no. 4450.

79. MBR, March 4, 1880, March 8, 1873, April 1, 1875, January 6, 1876, July 5, 1877, November 7, 1878; *AR*, 1875-76, p. 10, 1877-78, in *RR*, p. 587.

80. *Statutes-at-Large of South Carolina* (1884) 18:827-828.

81. *Statutes-at-Large of South Carolina* (1884) 18:827-828, (1894) 21:835-836.

82. CP, no. 15383. See also CH, 17, no. 8402.

83. MBR, April 14, July 14, 1898, November 12, 1903, June 9, 1904; *AR*, 1899, p. 16, 1897, pp. 5-6, 1898, p. 6, 1900, p. 8.

84. CP, no. 3872, 4471. For similar examples, see CP, nos. 3150, 3230, 3231, 3257, 4317, 4472, 5713, 5724, 5741, 6996.

85. J. D. Edwards to Babcock, July 9, 1906, in CP, no. 12432.

86. *AR*, 1875-76, pp. 11-12.

87. *AR*, 1883-84, p. 21.

88. *Testimony, Legislative Committee*, pp. 372-74.

89. CP, no. 7742; See also CP, nos. 8045, 8402, 8716.

90. CH, 17, no. 8716; Babcock to J. H. McDaniel, February 11, 1910, in CP, 1910, no. 14543; CP, no. 14441; *AR*, 1911, p. 12; MBR, June 11, 1912; *State Board of Health and the State Hospital*, pp. 36-37; *House Journal*, 1904, pp. 24-25.

91. MBR, July 13, 1893, February 11, 1897.

92. *AR*, 1895-96, p. 8

93. *Testimony, Legislative Committee*, p. 15.

94. *House Journal*, 1903, p. 51.

CHAPTER THIRTEEN

1. Thomas W. Doar to Annie D. Doar, August 23, 1908, Middleton-Doar Papers, SCHS. See also J. Y. J. to the regents, Nov. 13, 1901, CP, no. 9958.

2. E. M. Heyward to Annie D. Doar, November 23, 1900, Middleton-Doar Papers.

3. "By-Laws," in *AR*, 1890-91, p. 82.

4. *AR*, 1892-93, pp. 9-10, 1895-96, p. 8.

5. *AR*, 1870-77, 1902-1913, statistics on movement of population.

6. *Report of the Legislative Committee to Investigate the State Hospital for the Insane* (Columbia, S.C.: Gonzales and Bryan, 1910), pp. 47-48. On the decline in recovery rates and the general retreat to custodialism in the later nineteenth century, see Grob, *Mental Institutions in America*, pp. 204-6, 263, 302-8, and *Mental*

Illness and American Society, pp. 14–15, 39; Rothman, *Discovery of the Asylum*, pp. 265–87.

7. "Reports of American Asylums," *American Journal of Insanity* 21 (1865): 558. Norman Dain, *Concepts of Insanity in the United States, 1789–1965* (New Brunswick, N.J.: Rutgers University Press, 1964), pp. 129–39, 205–6; Grob, *Mental Institutions in America*, pp. 202–4; Rothman, *Discovery of the Asylum*, pp. 265–87.

8. *AR*, 1877–78, in *RR*, p. 592, 1878–79, pp. 13–14, 1879–80, pp. 12–13, 1883–84, p. 27, 1885–86, p. 15, 1886–87, p. 9, 1887–88, pp. 16–17, 1893–94, p. 11; MBR, November 11, 1875, November 2, 1876, May 2, July 7, 1878, March 6, October 2, 1879; James Thompson, *Of Shattered Minds: Fifty years at the South Carolina State Hospital*, ed. Anita W. Roof (Columbia, S.C.: Department of Mental Health, 1988), pp. 14, 22, 52–53.

9. MBR, January 3, 1878; *Report of Legislative Committee on the State Hospital*, p. 23; *Report and Proceedings of the Special Legislative Committee on the State Hospital for the Insane, and State Park, 1914*, (Columbia, S.C.: Gonzales and Bryan, 1914), p. 363.

10. *Testimony Taken Before the Legislative Committee to Investigate the State Hospital for the Insane of Columbia*, 1909 (Columbia, S.C.: Gonzales and Bryan, 1910), pp. 88–89, 302–5; *AR*, 1892–93, p. 17.

11. Ibid., p. 414.

12. *Report of Legislative Committee on the State Hospital*, pp. 31–35, *Testimony, Legislative Committee*, p. 160.

13. *Testimony, Legislative Committee*, pp. 63, 132, 166–67; *AR*, 1880–81, p. 22, 1883–84, p. 27, 1884–85, p. 9, 1888–89, p. 10, 1892–93, p. 17, 1893–94, p. 11; Grob, *Mental Illness and American Society*, pp. 23–24, argues that economic considerations played a minor role in occupational programs at most late nineteenth-century state asylums. According to Ellen Dwyer, *Homes for the Mad: Life Inside Two Nineteenth-Century Asylums* (New Brunswick, N.J.: Rutgers University Press, 1987), pp. 131–36, work programs at New York's Willard Asylum for the Chronic Insane had a strong economic emphasis.

14. MBR, May 2, 1878, February 6, April 3, 1879, July 14, 1887; *AR*, 1892–93, pp. 17–18; Newspaper clipping, June 21, 1900, Babcock Papers, SCL.

15. *AR*, 1877–78, in *RR*, p. 592.

16. *Testimony, Legislative Committee*, p. 408; *AR*, 1877–78, in *RR*, p. 592, 1879–80, p. 13, 1886–87, p. 9., 1890–91, p. 13, 1891–92, p. 13; *Report of Legislative Committee on the State Hospital*, p. 34; Thompson, *Of Shattered Minds*, p. 25.

17. *Testimony, Legislative Committee*, p. 395.

18. Ibid., pp. 334, 163–164, 287, 300, 310, 316, 321, 385, 393–95; *AR*, 1895–96, p. 11; Thompson, *Of Shattered Minds*, p. 8.

19. *Report of Legislative Committee on the State Hospital*, pp. 31–35; MBR, August 1, 1908; *Testimony, Legislative Committee*, pp. 61–63, 72–73, 80, 88–90, 158–59, 259–61, 279–82, 302–3, 305, 414, 430; *Report and Proceedings of the Special*

Legislative Committee to Investigate the State Hospital for the Insane, and State Park, 1914, p. 509. By 1914, motion picture shows and automobile rides had been added to the list of amusements.

20. *Testimony, Legislative Committee*, p. 110.

21. Thomas W. Doar to Annie D. Doar, February 7, 11, 1908, April 2, July 22, 1908, Middleton-Doar Papers, SCHS; *Testimony, Legislative Committee*, pp. 319–20, 425.

22. *Testimony, Legislative Committee*, p. 386.

23. Allan was a graduate of Women's Medical College of New York and had spent a year in postgraduate study at Johns Hopkins Hospital. Sarah Allan Diary, WHL; *AR*, 1894–95, p. 24.

24. CH, vols. 3–31, 1875–1913, SCDAH; C. F. Williams to Dr. W. A. Stober, December 21, 1921, in CP, no. 13256.

25. Most of the information about therapies is drawn from CH, 3–30; see also Sarah Allan Diary, WHL; Thompson, *Of Shattered Minds*; *Report and Proceedings of the Special Legislative Committee*, 1914, pp. 124–26, 307–8, 500–501, 513; MBR, February 8, 1894. On syphilis therapy, see Allan M. Brandt, *No Magic Bullet: A Social History of Venereal Disease in the United States Since 1880* (New York: Oxford University Press, 1985), pp. 40–41.

26. *Report of Legislative Committee on the State Hospital*, pp. 35–39; MBR, September 8, November 10, December 8, 1910; *Testimony, Legislative Committee*, pp. 409–10, 437.

27. Dain, *Concepts of Insanity*, pp. 112–13, 204–6; Grob, *Mental Institutions in America*, chaps. 7–8; Rothman, *Discovery of the Asylum*, chap. 11.

28. Saunders was a graduate of the Medical College of South Carolina. *AR*, 1907, p. 16. The sources for Saunders's medical innovating and views about medical treatment for insanity are cited in the following note.

29. *Testimony, Legislative Committee*, pp. 158, 161, 278–79, 414–15, 439; *Report and Proceedings of the Special Legislative Committee*, 1914, pp. 26–27, 37–39, 301, 363, 499–501, 505–7, 513; Thompson, *Of Shattered Minds*, p. 62; Brandt, *No Magic Bullet*, pp. 40–42.

30. *Report and Proceedings of the Special Legislative Committee*, 1914, p. 500.

31. *Testimony, Legislative Committee*, pp. 58, 64, 79, 86.

32. CH, 20, no. 9713. See CH, 14–30, for many similar examples.

33. *Report of Legislative Committee on the State Hospital*, pp. 40–42, 64–65; *Testimony, Legislative Committee*, pp. 406–7; Sarah Allan Diary, WHL. The investigating committee of 1909 estimated the percentage of patients under restraint at the South Carolina State Hospital by counting the number they saw restrained during several visits. The effort to reduce the use of mechanical restraint in late-nineteenth- and early-twentieth-century American mental institutions is discussed in Grob, *Mental Illness in America*, pp. 17–19; Dwyer, *Homes for the Mad*, pp. 22–24, 74, 140–41; Nancy Tomes, "The Great Restraint Controversy: A Comparative Perspective on Anglo-American Psychiatry in the Nineteenth Century," in

The Anatomy of Madness, ed. W. F. Bynum, Roy Porter, and Michael Shepherd (London: Tavistock, 1985).

34. Thomas Doar to Annie D. Doar, August 2, 1908, Middleton-Doar Papers, SCHS.

35. *Report of Legislative Committee on the State Hospital*, pp. 42, 31-47, *Testimony, Legislative Committee*, pp. 406-7, 428, 242-43, 145, 185, 254, 264-66.

36. *Testimony, Legislative Committee*, pp. 406-7.

37. MBR, February 7, March 7, 1878.

38. MBR, January 9, 1884; see also April 14, 1887.

39. MBR, May 8, 1890.

40. W. F. Babcock to James W. Babcock, May 24, 1891, Babcock Papers, SCL; MBR, July 12, 1894.

41. *Report of Legislative Committee on the State Hospital*, pp. 24-30, 60-61; *Testimony, Legislative Committee*, pp. 351-52. According to statistics in the hospital's annual reports, the deaths of more than eleven hundred patients were ascribed to pellagra between 1907 and 1914. On pellagra, see Elizabeth W. Etheridge, *The Butterfly Caste: A Social History of Pellagra in the South* (Westport, Conn.: Greenwood Publishing, 1972).

42. *Testimony, Legislative Committee*, pp. 46-51, 69.

43. Ibid., pp. 104-8.

44. David R. Reid to Governor Richard I. Manning III, January 26, 1915, Governor Richard I. Manning III Papers, SCDAH.

45. Tom Doar to Annie D. Doar, February 14, 1908, November 6, 1909, Middleton-Doar Papers, SCHS.

46. MBR, March 4, 1880; see also ibid., October 6, 1877.

47. *Testimony, Legislative Committee*, pp. 143, 165-66, 209, 425, 434.

48. MBR, January 3, 1912, July 10, 1913, November 13, 1913, April 9, 1914; *Report and Proceedings of the Special Legislative Committee*, 1914, pp. 430-32, 521-22.

49. *AR*, 1891-1913 (1901 missing), statistical tables; *Report of Legislative Committee on the State Hospital*, pp. 48-50.

50. According to the figures taken by the investigating committee of 1909 from the census report, the mortality rate for all American state hospitals for 1904 was 9.61 percent of the total number of patients resident; the South Atlantic average was 11.17. At the South Carolina State Hospital, the mortality rate was 21.54. This was more than three times the rate of the state hospitals in North Carolina. *Report of Legislative Committee on the State Hospital*, pp. 47-50; U.S. Bureau of the Census, *Insane and Feeble-Minded in Hospitals and Institutions, 1904* (Washington, D.C.: Government Printing Office, 1906), table 37, pp. 196-98.

51. Edward H. Beardsley, *A History of Neglect: Health Care for Blacks and Mill Workers in the Twentieth-Century South* (Knoxville: University of Tennessee Press, 1987), pp. 11-41; I. A. Newby, *Black Carolinians* (Columbia: University of South Carolina Press, 1973), pp. 114-21, 211-17. According to Beardsley, the black death rate from tuberculosis in 1900 was three times the white rate.

52. *Report of Legislative Committee on the State Hospital*, p. 56; *AR*, 1907, p. 11, 1908–14, statistical tables.

53. *AR*, 1893–94, pp. 9–11, 1894–95, pp. 11–12, 1902, p. 12, *Testimony, Legislative Committee*, pp. 400–401.

54. *Report of Legislative Committee on the State Hospital*, pp. 50–53; *Testimony, Legislative Committee*, 1909, pp. 422–24, 432; *Columbia State*, February 18, 1910.

55. James W. Babcock, "The Prevention of Tuberculosis in Hospitals for the Insane," reprint from *American Journal of Insanity* 51 (1894–95): 14, 8–14; *AR*, 1893–94, p. 9, 1894–95, pp. 11–12, 1895–96, p. 8, 1900–1908; *Report of Legislative Committee on the State Hospital*, pp. 48–49.

56. *Report of Legislative Committee on the State Hospital*, pp. 48–50, 58; *AR*, 1898, p. 12, 1899, pp. 18–19, 23, 1900, p. 13, 1901, pp. 11–12, 1906, p. 9, 1907, pp. 12–14; 1908, pp. 3–4, 7–10; *Testimony, Legislative Committee*, pp. 21, 161, 411–12, 432–33, 438, 440; *AR*, 1898, p. 12, 1899, pp. 18–19, 1900, p. 13.

57. *AR*, 1877–78, 1891, 1909, 1911, statistical tables; James W. Babcock to P. L. Murphy, April 18, 1907, P. L. Murphy Papers, SHC; *Report and Proceedings of the Special Legislative Committee*, 1914, pp. 5–6, 272–73, 343, 498; MBR, May 18, 1909; Sarah Allan Diary, WHL; Grob, *Mental Illness and American Society*, p. 19; U.S. Bureau of the Census, *Patients in Hospitals for Mental Diseases in 1923* (Washington, D.C.: Government Printing Office, 1926), p. 240.

58. Sarah Allan Diary, WHL.

59. MBR, February 11, 1897.

60. *Testimony, Legislative Committee*, pp. 405, 147, 177, 190, 245, 267, 294, 300.

61. Samuel A. Weber to James W. Babcock, January 21, 1910, Babcock Papers, SCL; R. H. Crosby to Board of Regents, June 9, 1914, in CH, 26, pp. 406–7.

62. Thomas W. Doar to Annie D. Doar, January 7, 11, February 7, 14, September 28, 1908, March 27, 1909, Middleton-Doar Papers, SCHS.

63. *Testimony, Legislative Committee*, pp. 70, 90, 95, 126–27, 301, 304–6.

64. A. and D. Harris to James W. Babcock, May 28, 1895, in CP, no. 7307; Gov. Martin Ansel to James W. Babcock, October 4, 1907, October 28, 1908, J. A. Cope to Gov. Ansel, October 27, 1908, Governor Martin Ansel Papers, 1a, State Officers, 1908–1909, SCDAH; *Testimony, Legislative Committee*, p. 87; Thompson, *Of Shattered Minds*, p. 3.

65. *Report of Legislative Committee on the State Hospital*, pp. 21–23; *Testimony, Legislative Committee*, pp. 153–57, 161, 273–76; *Report and Proceedings of the Special Legislative Committee*, 1914, pp. 5–6, 295–96, 301, 307, 424–25, 499–500, 505–6, 516–18.

66. MBR, July 5, 1877, June 11, 1891, June 15, 1893; *AR*, 1876–77, p. 21; *Report of Legislative Committee on the State Hospital*, p. 24; *Testimony, Legislative Committee*, 1909, p. 423; J. H. Schreiner to Gov. Benjamin Tillman, Governor Tillman Papers, SCDAH; Sarah Allan Diary, January–May 1900, WHL; Grob, *Mental Illness and American Society*, p. 19.

67. U.S. Bureau of the Census, censuses for 1860, 1870, 1880, 1900, Population

Schedules for Richland Co., South Carolina. Less than 1 percent of the population of South Carolina (five thousand) was foreign born in 1900. By comparison, New York had nearly two million immigrants. See U.S. Bureau of the Census, *A Century of Population Growth* (Baltimore: Genealogical Publishing, 1967), chap. 13.

68. Sarah Allan Diary, January 24, 25, March 24, March 29, 1900, WHL; *AR*, 1890–91, pp. 85–86.

69. *Testimony, Legislative Committee*, 1909, pp. 148–50, 289, 382.

70. *Acts Concerning the Lunatic Asylum of South Carolina and By-Laws for Its Government, Revised and Passed by the Board of Regents* (Columbia, 1857), pp. 15–16; *AR*, 1890–91, pp. 82–92; MBR, October 1, November 19, 1874; July 13, 1876; *Testimony, Legislative Committee*, p. 253.

71. MBR, May 12, June 10, 1892, May 9, 1912.

72. MBR, July 5, 14, 1877, January 3, 1878, February 7, March 7, April 4, 1878; *Testimony, Legislative Committee*, pp. 149, 229, 422.

73. MBR, February 7, 1878; see also June 7, 1887, April 11, 1889.

74. MBR, December 4, 1879, March 4, 1880.

75. W. F. Babcock to James W. Babcock, May 24, 1891, Babcock Papers, SCL.

76. Sarah Allan Diary, March 16, February 15, 23, April 1900, WHL; *Testimony, Legislative Committee*, pp. 201–2.

77. MBR, February 5, 1873, June 4, October 1, 1874, March 1, July 14, 1877, January 4, 1879, September 10, 1884, October 8, 1892, June 15, 1893, August 10, 1893, January 11. 1894, July 13, 1911; *Testimony, Legislative Committee*, pp. 422–23.

78. *Testimony, Legislative Committee*, pp. 176–82, 223–27, 240–42, 257–59.

79. On the early training schools for nurses, see Rosenberg, *The Care of Strangers*, pp. 219–28; Susan M. Reverby, *Ordered to Care: The Dilemma of American Nursing, 1850–1945* (Cambridge: Cambridge University Press, 1987), pp. 39–71.

80. *AR*, 1890–91, p. 11; Charleston, *Yearbook*, 1881, pp. 126–29; Grob, *Mental Illness and American Society*, p. 20; Dwyer, *Homes for the Mad*, pp. 179–80.

81. *AR*, 1890–91, pp. 11–13, 1892–93, p. 15; Zella (Blakely) Robinson, Classroom Notebook, 1902–3, Manuscript Department, Perkins Library, Duke University.

82. James W. Babcock to Katherine Guion, September 25, October 8, 25, 1891, Babcock Papers, SCL; MBR, October 8, 1891, February 11, 1897.

83. *Testimony, Legislative Committee*, p. 426.

84. *AR*, 1910, p. 16. MBR, December 10, 1891, June 15, 1893, October 15, 1910; *AR*, 1890–91, p. 12, 1891–92, p. 12, 1892–93, p. 16, 1894–95, pp. 19–20, 1897, pp. 75–76, 1908, pp. 53–55, 1910, pp. 16, 53–56, 1911, p. 6; *Testimony, Legislative Committee*, pp. 151, 186, 228, 277–78; Thompson, *Of Shattered Minds*, pp. 23–24.

85. Sarah Allan Diary, February 18, 1900, WHL.

86. David R. Reid to Governor Richard I. Manning, January 26, 1915, Governor Richard I. Manning III Papers, SCDAH; *Testimony, Legislative Committee*, pp. 37–46, 53, 79–80, 100–105, 137–40, 175, 178, 216–17.

87. Thomas W. Doar to Annie D. Doar, February 7, 1908, Middleton-Doar Papers, SCHS; *Report of Legislative Committee on the State Hospital*, p. 61.

88. Thomas W. Doar to Annie D. Doar, April 2, 1908, Middleton-Doar Papers, SCHS.

89. *Testimony, Legislative Committee*, pp. 134-36, 228-29, 51-56, 83, 86, 98-99, 110-13, 128-32, 141-45, 148, 161-63, 176-80, 188, 203-8, 216, 282-85, 296-97, 304-5, 382-83, 423, 436; *Report of Legislative Committee on the State Hospital*, pp. 24-26; MBR, April 11, 1912; *Report and Proceedings of the Special Legislative Committee*, 1914, p. 355.

90. *Report and Proceedings of the Special Legislative Committee*, 1914, pp. 493, 501-2.

91. *Testimony, Legislative Committee*, p. 408.

92. *Report and Proceedings of the Special Legislative Committee*, 1910, p. 50.

CHAPTER FOURTEEN

1. On Progressivism in the South, see Dewey W. Grantham, *Southern Progressivism: The Reconciliation of Progress and Tradition* (Knoxville: University of Tennessee Press, 1983); C. Vann Woodward, *Origins of the New South, 1877–1913* (Baton Rouge: Louisiana State University Press, 1980); George B. Tindall, *The Emergence of the New South, 1913–1945* (Baton Rouge: Louisiana State University Press, 1967). For Progressivism in South Carolina, see David Carlton, *Mill and Town in South Carolina* (Baton Rouge: Louisiana State University Press, 1982), esp. chap. 5. On Progressivism in the United States, see Robert Wiebe, *The Search for Order, 1877–1920* (New York: Hill and Wang, 1967).

2. MBR, March 9, 1893, April 12, 1894, January 4, 1897, June 9, 1899, February 9, 1900; "Dream Notes" and other unpublished writings of Babcock in the Babcock Papers, SCL. These writings show that Babcock kept up with the psychiatric literature of his time, including the works of Maudsley, Mercier, Freud, and Jung.

3. Isaac M. Taylor to P. L. Murphy, January 27, 1900, P. L. Murphy Papers, no. 535, SHC. Taylor was then assistant physician at the North Carolina State Hospital at Morganton, under Superintendent P. L. Murphy; *Testimony, Legislative Committee on the State Hospital, 1909* (Columbia, S.C.: Gonzales and Bryan, 1910), p. 398.

4. MBR, March 11, 1897, April, 13, 1899.

5. MBR, July 9, September 10, December 10, January 14, 1908.

6. Copy of a letter from Hunter A. Gibbes to the General Assembly of South Carolina, January 11, 1909, Babcock Papers, SCL.

7. *Charleston News and Courier*, January 23, 1909.

8. *Statutes-at-Large of South Carolina* (1909-10) 26: no. 231; David D. Wallace, *The History of South Carolina*, 4 vols. (New York: American Historical Society,

1934), 4:3-4; *Charleston News and Courier*, April 26-29, May 6, 7, 19, 20, 1909; *Journal of the South Carolina Medical Association* 5 (1909): 205, 238-39; *Honea Path Chronicle*, undated clipping in Babcock Papers, SCL; *Carolina Spartan*, May 26, 1909, in Babcock Papers, SCL.

9. The committee sent an inquiry to every state hospital superintendent in the U.S. The other members of the committee besides Christensen were Senators P. L. Hardin and George H. Bates, and Representatives J. P. Carey, George W. Dick, Olin Sawyer, and W. C. Harrison. See *Report of Legislative Committee on the State Hospital*, 1910.

10. *Report of Legislative Committee on the State Hospital* (Columbia: University of South Carolina Press, 1973), pp. 10-21.

11. Ibid., pp. 21-53.

12. Ibid., pp. 54-55.

13. Ibid., pp. 74-75.

14. Ibid., pp. 76-83.

15. Ibid., pp. 84-85.

16. Ibid., pp. 85-86.

17. *Charleston News and Courier*, January 21, 1910.

18. For a thorough discussion of the nature and importance of southern concepts of honor, see Bertram Wyatt-Brown, *Southern Honor: Ethics and Behavior in the Old South* (New York: Oxford University Press, 1982).

19. *Charleston News and Courier*, February 14, 1910; MBR, July 8, 1909.

20. *Charleston News and Courier*, February 13, 14, 1910; *Columbia Record*, February 14, 1910. See also *Charleston News and Courier*, May 20, 1909, *Journal of the South Carolina Medical Association* 5 (1909): 205, 238-39.

21. *Report of Legislative Committee on the State Hospital*, p. 76; *Charleston News and Courier*, February 17, 1910; Typescript of Speech by Senator Rogers, February 15, 1910, in Babcock Papers, SCL.

22. *Charleston News and Courier*, February 18, 1910; *House Journal*, 1910, pp. 163, 232, 531.

23. *Charleston News and Courier*, January 31, February 4, 1910; MBR, July 8, 1909.

24. *Charleston News and Courier*, February 12, 16, 17, 1910.

25. *Columbia State*, February 18, 1910.

26. *Charleston News and Courier*, February 12, 16, 17, 1910.

27. Ibid., February 7, 16, 17, 1910. After the state house rejected the bond bill, the *News and Courier* expressed regret that "the General Assembly did not give the people an opportunity" to vote on it. February 18, 1910.

28. *Charleston News and Courier*, February 11, 12, 1910.

29. Ibid., February 11, 12, 16, 1910.

30. Ibid., February 11-12, 16-17, 1910.

31. Ibid., February 19-20, 22, 1910; *House Journal*, 1910, pp. 914-15, 933-34; *Statutes-at-Large of South Carolina* (1909-10) 26: no. 597. In 1911, the assem-

bly increased the amount the commission was authorized to borrow to $200,000. *Statutes-at-Large of South Carolina* (1911–12) 27: no. 279.

32. Per capita expenditure increased from $144 in 1910 to $176 in 1914. Arthur P. Herring, *Report to the Hon. Richard I. Manning, Governor of South Carolina, on the State Hospital for the Insane* (Columbia, S.C.: Gonzales and Bryan, 1915), p. 9.

33. Babcock accused Drs. Thompson and H. H. Griffin of undermining his position as superintendent during the investigation of 1909 and after. See *Report and Proceedings of the Special Legislative Committee to Investigate the State Hospital for the Insane, and State Park*, 1914, pp. 22–23, 94–95; For examples of the tension at the hospital, see Thompson, *Of Shattered Minds*, pp. 62–64, 67–68; MBR, September 14, 20, 1911.

34. See *Annual Reports of the State Hospital Commission to the General Assembly of South Carolina*, 1911–13 (Columbia, S.C.: Gonzales and Bryan, 1912–14).

35. Carlton, *Mill and Town*, pp. 214–27; Clarence N. Stone, "Bleasism and the 1912 Election in South Carolina," *North Carolina Historical Review* 40 (1963): 54–74; Ronald D. Burnside, "Racism in the Administrations of Governor Cole Blease," *Proceedings of the South Carolina Historical Association* (1964): 43–57.

36. MBR, March 14, October 3, 1912, April 3, 1913, January 6, 1914. As governor, Blease had the right to replace members of the board of regents with his nominees when their terms ended or they resigned or died.

37. Stone, "Bleasism," p. 72; *Charleston News and Courier*, January 23, 1914; Messages etc. re Asylum Investigation of State Hospital, 1914, in Governor Blease Papers, SCDAH; *Senate Journal*, 1913, p. 709, 1914, pp. 573–75; *Report and Proceedings of the Special Legislative Committee*, 1914, p. 58.

38. *Report and Proceedings of the Special Legislative Committee*, 1914, pp. 36, 142.

39. Ibid., esp. 247, 425, 510–11; *AR*, 1911, p. 14, 1912, p. 11; James H. Cassedy, *Medicine in America* (Baltimore: John Hopkins Press, 1991), pp. 84–85.

40. *Columbia State*, February 18, 1910; Thompson, *Of Shattered Minds*, p. 62; *Report and Proceedings of the Special Legislative Committee*, 1914; Allan M. Brandt, *No Magic Bullet: A Social History of Venereal Disease in the United States Since 1880* (New York: Oxford University Press, 1985), pp. 7–51.

41. *Report and Proceedings of the Special Legislative Committee*, 1914, pp. 37–39, 102–3; Charleston *News and Courier*, February 12, 1914.

42. *Report and Proceedings of the Special Legislative Committee*, 1914, pp. 29–31, 19, 23–28.

43. Ibid., pp. 136–37.

44. MBR, December 12, 13, 1913, January 6, 15, 1914; *Report and Proceedings of the Special Legislative Committee*, 1914, pp. 72–85, 96–148, esp. 106–7, 142–47.

45. Benjamin Tillman to James W. Babcock, January 8, 15, 16, 18, 1914, Tillman Papers, Special Collections, Clemson University Library. See also favorable replies from Senators P. L. Hardin and Huger Sinkler to Tillman, January 14, 1914, in same collection.

46. Senate Journal, 1914, pp. 186–95, 310; *Columbia State*, January 21, 23, 24, 1914; *Charleston News and Courier*, January 21, 23, 24, 28, February 4, 12, 1914; John G. Evans to Benjamin Tillman, January 22, 1914, Tillman to Hon. D. C. Heyward, January 22, 1914, Tillman to Col. August Kohn, January 23, 25, 27, 1914, Tillman to J. G. Evans, January 24, 1914, James W. Babcock to Tillman, January 25, 1914, Tillman to James W. Babcock, January 26, February 5, 1914, Tillman to Mr. H. C. Tillman, February 27, 1914, Tillman to Mrs. F. T. Simpson, March 3, 1914, Tillman Papers, Clemson University; Coleman Blease to Hon. Charles Smith, Lt. Gov., January 27, 1914, in Messages etc. re Investigation of State Hospital, 1914, Blease Papers, SCDAH; Tillman to James W. Babcock, January 23, 25, 1914, Sen. C. T. Wyche to Tillman, January 23, 1914, Babcock Papers, SCL.

47. Tillman to D. C. Heyward, January 22, 1914, Tillman to James W. Babcock, January 23, 25, February 5, 1914. See also previous note.

48. *Report and Proceedings of the Special Legislative Committee*, 1914, pp. 300–301, 52–55, 260–261, 304.

49. Ibid., pp. 57–59, 61–62, 86, 234, 316, 374.

50. Ibid., pp. 9–10, 507–31.

51. Ibid., pp. 1–13.

52. *Columbia State*, undated clipping in Babcock Papers, SCL; *Charleston News and Courier*, February 8, 10, 11, 15, 20, 26, 27, March 5, 6, 1914; *Orangeburg Times and Democrat*, February 25, 1914, quoted in *News and Courier*; *Columbia State*, March 5, 6, 1914; *Sumter Watchman and Southron*, July 4, 1914.

53. *Senate Journal*, 1914, pp. 970–71; MBR, March 12, 26, 1914; *Charleston News and Courier*, February 27, 1914.

54. MBR, March 12–13, 1914; *Charleston News and Courier*, March 14, 1914; SRR, December 4, 1925. On Waverley Sanitarium and Babcock's career after leaving the state hospital, see Babcock Papers, SCL; Waring, *Medicine in South Carolina*, 3: 74–75; J. K. Hall to Dr. W. W. Fennell, May 1, 1922, J. K. Hall Papers, SHC.

55. MBR, March 26, 1914; *Charleston News and Courier*, March 14, 1914; On Strait, see Wallace, *History of South Carolina* 4:397.

56. On Manning, see R. M. Burts, *Richard Irvine Manning* (Columbia: University of South Carolina Press, 1974). On the various activities of the Board of Charities and Corrections, see its *Quarterly Bulletin* and annual reports. In 1920, it became the Board of Public Welfare. For a history of the State Training School for the Feeble Minded, see Benjamin O. Whitten, *A History of Whitten Village* (Clinton, S.C.: Jacobs Press, 1967). For discussion of the eugenics movement in the United States and the campaign against feeble-mindedness, see Daniel Kevles, *In the Name of Eugenics: Genetics and the Uses of Human Heredity* (New York: Alfred A. Knopf, 1985); Mark H. Haller, *Eugenics: Hereditarian Attitudes in American Thought* (New Brunswick, N.J.: Rutgers University Press, 1963).

57. On the foundation of the National Committee on Mental Hygiene and its early years, see Gerald Grob, *Mental Illness and American Society, 1875–1940*

(Princeton, N.J.: Princeton University Press, 1983), pp. 153–66; Norman Dain, *Clifford W. Beers: Advocate for the Insane* (Pittsburgh: University of Pittsburgh Press, 1980).

58. Herring, *Report*, pp. 9–18. See also Burts, *Richard Irvine Manning*, pp. 86–87.

59. Correspondence Relating to State Hospital, 1915–1918, Governor Richard I. Manning III Papers, SCDAH; *AR*, 1915, pp. 4–7, 15–27, 1916, pp. 3–4, 8–16; Burts, *Richard Irvine Manning*, pp. 87–91, 114–15; *House Journal*, 1916, pp. 80–84. The Governor Richard I. Manning III Papers contain correspondence with a number of specialists on mental diseases, including Herring; Thomas W. Salmon, director of Special Studies for the NCMH; and William A. White, superintendent of the Government Hospital for the Insane in Washington, D.C. Manning consulted with them on the selection of a new superintendent and other issues related to the state hospital.

60. The average daily cost per capita increased from about forty-eight cents in 1914 to fifty-four cents in 1917, but this was a time of rising prices for supplies. Herring, *Report*, p. 9; *AR*, 1917, p. 6.

61. See, for example, *AR*, 1925, pp. 4, 17, 1926, pp. 6, 18–19; *Annual Report of the State Board of Public Welfare of South Carolina* (Columbia: Gonzales and Bryan, 1920–26), 1921, p. 53, 1922, p. 12, 1923, pp. 76–86.

62. Grantham, *Southern Progressivism*, xx; Burts, *Richard Irvine Manning*, p. 215; Carlton, *Mill and Town*, pp. 171–74.

63. *AR*, 1921, pp. 11, 19, 1922, pp. 8, 16, 1930, pp. 8–9; *Annual Report of the South Carolina Board of Public Welfare*, 1920, p. 61, 1923, pp. 71–73, 79–86.

EPILOGUE

1. *Senate Journal*, 1831, pp. 65–66.

2. Andrew T. Scull, *Museums of Madness: The Social Organization of Insanity in Nineteenth-Century England* (New York: St. Martin's Press, 1979), p. 262.

Index

Nott, Josiah, 89
Nowland, Lucretia, 28–29
Nowland, Thomas, 28–29

O'Neall, Hugh, 28, 32
O'Neall, John B., 41, 70

Panic of 1819, 45–46
Panic of 1873, 228
Paris Clinical School, 192
Parish of Prince Frederick, Winyah, 28, 32
Parker, John W., 65–67, 77, 80, 85–86, 99, 102, 106–11, 124–25, 129–31, 143, 172, 224, 236, 250, 257, 261; appointed medical superintendent of South Carolina Lunatic Asylum, 67; treatment of insanity, 92–94, 114–23; conflict with Daniel Trezevant, 131–35; appointed chief medical officer of South Carolina Lunatic Asylum, 135; and Dorothea Dix, 136–39; and Civil War, 213–19; and Reconstruction, 219–21; dismissed, 221
Parker, Niles G., 224
Pellagra, 206, 284
Pennsylvania Hospital, 22, 28, 32, 33, 39, 115, 120–21, 129, 136, 145, 159
Perry, Benjamin, 129
Petigru, James L., 1, 217
Pinckney, Eliza Lucas, 25–27
Pinckney, Henry L., 69, 176
Pinel, Philippe, 38–39, 93, 189, 192
Porcher, Francis P., 179
Powell, T. O., 245, 298
Pringle, Robert, 26, 32
Prioleau, J. F., 172
Progressivism, 297–317 passim

Ramsay, David, 23, 33, 39
Ray, Isaac, 86
Read, William, 148–49
Retreat, York, 38–39, 51, 87, 110

Richardson, Manley, 16, 35
Richland County poorhouse, 262
Robert, Georgia, 148, 186–88
Roper Hospital, 157, 176, 179, 196
Rush, Benjamin, 28, 33–34, 39, 188–89, 191–92

St. Philip's Parish, 19, 20–24, 31
Sargent, George F., 315
Saunders, Eleanora B., 277–78, 289, 308–13
Saxon, Mary, 28, 90–91
Scott, Robert K., 220, 224–25
Shand, Gadsden, 300
Shecut, J. L. E. W., 191
Simmons, Susan, 148–50
Simms, William Gilmore, 63, 71, 76, 153–54, 157
Simons, J. Hume, 199
Simons, Thomas Y., 70–72, 189–90
Sloan, Samuel, 258
Smith, James, 156
Social control, 7
Solitary confinement, 85, 104–6, 171, 278
South Carolina College, 47–48
South Carolina Lunatic Asylum, 5–11, 82–83, 318; politics, 9–10, 64, 78, 213–32 passim, 235–36, 239, 250, 302–17; and Reconstruction, 9–10, 213, 219–32 passim, 235–36; and Civil War, 9–10, 213–19; establishment of, 40–59 passim; statutes relating to, 46, 64, 69, 73–74, 76, 255, 261, 266–67; Asylum Commission of, 50–57; Board of Trustees of, 58; Board of Regents of, 58, 64–65, 108–12, 114, 117, 124, 129, 131, 134–35, 139, 215, 220, 231, 242, 256, 260, 290, 293, 299, 301, 304, 308, 311–12; admissions to, 63, 68–76, 82–83, 112–13; staffing of, 65–68; attendants at, 67, 107, 118–22, 288–96; financial

DATE DUE

#47-0108 Peel Off Pressure Sensitive